IN THE NATION'S
COMPELLING
INTEREST

Ensuring Diversity in the Health-Care Workforce

Committee on Institutional and Policy-Level Strategies for Increasing the Diversity of the U.S. Health Care Workforce

Board on Health Sciences Policy

Brian D. Smedley, Adrienne Stith Butler, Lonnie R. Bristow, *Editors*

INSTITUTE OF MEDICINE
OF THE NATIONAL ACADEMIES

THE NATIONAL ACADEMIES PRESS
Washington, D.C.
www.nap.edu

THE NATIONAL ACADEMIES PRESS 500 Fifth Street, NW Washington, DC 20001

NOTICE: The project that is the subject of this report was approved by the Governing Board of the National Research Council, whose members are drawn from the councils of the National Academy of Sciences, the National Academy of Engineering, and the Institute of Medicine. The members of the committee responsible for the report were chosen for their special competences and with regard for appropriate balance.

This study was supported by Contract No. P009518 between the National Academy of Sciences and the W.K. Kellogg Foundation. Any opinions, findings, conclusions, or recommendations expressed in this publication are those of the author(s) and do not necessarily reflect the view of the organizations or agencies that provided support for this project.

Library of Congress Cataloging-in-Publication Data

In the nation's compelling interest : ensuring diversity in the health care workforce / Committee on Institutional and Policy-Level Strategies for Increasing the Diversity of the U.S. Health Care Workforce, Board on Health Sciences Policy ; Brian D. Smedley, Adrienne Stith Butler, Lonnie R. Bristow, editors.
    p. ; cm.
    Includes bibliographical references and index.
    ISBN 0-309-09125-X (hardcover)
    1. Discrimination in medical education—United States—Prevention. 2. Medical colleges—United States—Admission. 3. Minorities in medicine—United States. 4. Minorities—Education (Higher)—United States. 5. Medical personnel—Recruiting—United States. 6. Affirmative action programs—United States.
    [DNLM: 1. Cultural Diversity—United States. 2. Health Manpower—United States. 3. Accreditation—standards—United States. 4. Education, Medical—economics—United States. 5. Minority Groups—education—United States. 6. Personnel Selection—standards—United States. 7. Public Policy—United States. W 76 I355 2004] I. Smedley, Brian D. II. Butler, Adrienne Stith. III. Bristow, Lonnie R. IV. Institute of Medicine (U.S.). Committee on Institutional and Policy-Level Strategies for Increasing the Diversity of the U.S. Health Care Workforce. V. Institute of Medicine (U.S.). Board on Health Sciences Policy.
    R745.I5 2004
    610'.71'173—dc22
                  2004005891

Additional copies of this report are available from the National Academies Press, 500 Fifth Street, NW, Lockbox 285, Washington, DC 20055; (800) 624-6242 or (202) 334-3313 (in the Washington metropolitan area); Internet, http://www. nap.edu.

For more information about the Institute of Medicine, visit the IOM home page at: www.iom.edu.

The serpent has been a symbol of long life, healing, and knowledge among almost all cultures and religions since the beginning of recorded history. The serpent adopted as a logotype by the Institute of Medicine is a relief carving from ancient Greece, now held by the Staatliche Museen in Berlin.

"Knowing is not enough; we must apply.
Willing is not enough; we must do."
—Goethe

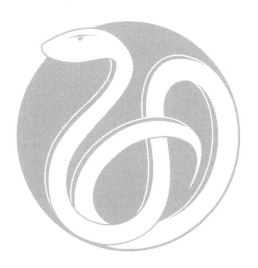

INSTITUTE OF MEDICINE
OF THE NATIONAL ACADEMIES

Adviser to the Nation to Improve Health

THE NATIONAL ACADEMIES
Advisers to the Nation on Science, Engineering, and Medicine

The **National Academy of Sciences** is a private, nonprofit, self-perpetuating society of distinguished scholars engaged in scientific and engineering research, dedicated to the furtherance of science and technology and to their use for the general welfare. Upon the authority of the charter granted to it by the Congress in 1863, the Academy has a mandate that requires it to advise the federal government on scientific and technical matters. Dr. Bruce M. Alberts is president of the National Academy of Sciences.

The **National Academy of Engineering** was established in 1964, under the charter of the National Academy of Sciences, as a parallel organization of outstanding engineers. It is autonomous in its administration and in the selection of its members, sharing with the National Academy of Sciences the responsibility for advising the federal government. The National Academy of Engineering also sponsors engineering programs aimed at meeting national needs, encourages education and research, and recognizes the superior achievements of engineers. Dr. Wm. A. Wulf is president of the National Academy of Engineering.

The **Institute of Medicine** was established in 1970 by the National Academy of Sciences to secure the services of eminent members of appropriate professions in the examination of policy matters pertaining to the health of the public. The Institute acts under the responsibility given to the National Academy of Sciences by its congressional charter to be an adviser to the federal government and, upon its own initiative, to identify issues of medical care, research, and education. Dr. Harvey V. Fineberg is president of the Institute of Medicine.

The **National Research Council** was organized by the National Academy of Sciences in 1916 to associate the broad community of science and technology with the Academy's purposes of furthering knowledge and advising the federal government. Functioning in accordance with general policies determined by the Academy, the Council has become the principal operating agency of both the National Academy of Sciences and the National Academy of Engineering in providing services to the government, the public, and the scientific and engineering communities. The Council is administered jointly by both Academies and the Institute of Medicine. Dr. Bruce M. Alberts and Dr. Wm. A. Wulf are chair and vice chair, respectively, of the National Research Council.

www.national-academies.org

HEALTH SCIENCES POLICY BOARD LIAISON

Sherman James, John P. Kirscht Collegiate Professor of Public Health and Chair, Department of Health Behavior and Education, University of Michigan, Ann Arbor, MI

IOM PROJECT STAFF

Brian D. Smedley, Study Director
Adrienne Stith Butler, Program Officer
Thelma L. Cox, Senior Project Assistant

IOM BOARD STAFF

Andrew M. Pope, Director, Board on Health Sciences Policy
Troy Prince, Administrative Assistant
Carlos Gabriel, Financial Associate

COPY EDITORS

James Ryan
Laura Penny

Reviewers

This report has been reviewed in draft form by individuals chosen for their diverse perspectives and technical expertise, in accordance with procedures approved by the NRC's Report Review Committee. The purpose of this independent review is to provide candid and critical comments that will assist the institution in making its published report as sound as possible and to ensure that the report meets institutional standards for objectivity, evidence, and responsiveness to the study charge. The review comments and draft manuscript remain confidential to protect the integrity of the deliberative process. We wish to thank the following individuals for their review of this report:

Marilyn Hughes Gaston, National Minority Health Month
Kevin Grumbach, University of California, San Francisco
George C. Hill, Vanderbilt University
Bob Montoya, Sacramento, CA
Thomas E. Perez, University of Maryland
Joan Y. Reede, Harvard University
Lynne D. Richardson, Mount Sinai Hospital
Susan C. Scrimshaw, University of Illinois
Jeanne C. Sinkford, American Dental Education Association
Richard M. Suinn, Colorado State University
Charles Terrell, Association of American Medical Colleges
William A. Vega, University of Medicine and Dentistry of New Jersey
Nancy Woods, University of Washington

Although the reviewers listed above have provided many constructive comments and suggestions, they were not asked to endorse the conclusions or recommendations nor did they see the final draft of the report before its release. The review of this report was overseen by **Elaine Larson**, Columbia University. Appointed by the National Research Council and Institute of Medicine, she was responsible for making certain that an independent examination of this report was carried out in accordance with institutional procedures and that all review comments were carefully considered. Responsibility for the final content of this report rests entirely with the authoring committee and the institution.

Acknowledgments

Several individuals and organizations made important contributions to the study committee's process and to this report. The committee wishes to thank these individuals but recognizes that attempts to identify all and acknowledge their contributions would require more space than is available in this brief section.

To begin, the committee would like to thank the sponsor of this report. Funds for the committee's work were provided by the W.K. Kellogg Foundation. The committee thanks Henrie Treadwell, Ph.D., and Bob DeVries, who served as the Project Officers on this grant.

The committee found the perspectives of many individuals and organizations to be valuable in understanding institutional and policy-level strategies for increasing the diversity of the health care workforce. Several individuals and organizations provided important information at open workshops of the committee. These include, in order of appearance, L. Natalie Carroll, M.D., President, National Medical Association; David Johnsen, D.D.S., President, American Dental Education Association; Hilda Richards, Ed.D., R.N., President, National Black Nurses Assocation, Inc.; Charles Terrell, Ed.D., Vice President, Division of Community Minority Programs, Association of American Medical Colleges; Barbara Blakeney, MS, APRN, BC, ANP, President, American Nurses Association; Phyllis Kopriva, Director, Women and Minority Services, and Kevin McKinney, M.D., Chair, Minority Affairs Consortium, American Medical Association; Geraldine Bednash, Ph.D., R.N., FAAN, Executive Director, American Association of Colleges of Nursing; Elena Rios, M.D., National Hispanic

Medical Association; Ben Muneta, M.D., President, Association of American Indian Physicians; Dean Whitla, Ph.D., Director, National Campus Diversity Project, Harvard Graduate School of Education; Ella Cleveland, Ph.D., Association of American Medical Colleges; Gabriel Garcia, M.D., Associate Dean of Medical School Admissions, Stanford University; Joshua Aronson, Ph.D., Assistant Professor, Department of Applied Psychology, New York University; Barbara Grumet, National League for Nursing Accrediting Commission; Charlotte Beason, Ed.D., R.N., C.N.A.A.A., Commission on Collegiate Nursing Education; Karen Hart, Commission on Dental Accreditation; David Stevens, M.D., Liaison Committee on Medical Education; Susan Zlotlow, Ph.D., American Psychological Association Committee on Accreditation; Kevin Barnett, Dr.PH., M.C.P., Public Health Institute; Paul Hattis, M.D., J.D., M.P.H., Tufts University; JudyAnn Bigby, M.D., Brigham and Women's Hospital and Harvard Medical School; Bradford Gray, Ph.D., New York Academy of Medicine; William Vega, Ph.D., UMDNJ-Robert Wood Johnson Medical School; Jeffery F. Milem, Ph.D., University of Maryland; Eric L. Dey, Ph.D., University of Michigan; Michael Rainey, Ph.D., Stony Brook University School of Medicine; Daryl G. Smith, Ph.D., Claremont Graduate University; William B. Harvey, Ed.D., American Council on Education; Beauregard Stubblefield-Tave, M.B.A., the Stubblefield-Tave Group; Karen Matherlee, Policy, Inc.; Henry Lopez, Jr., Bureau of Health Professions, Health Resources and Services Administration; and Howard Landesman, D.D.S., M.Ed., School of Dentistry, University of Colorado Health Science Center.

The committee also gratefully acknowledges the contributions of the many individuals who assisted the committee in its work, either by providing research support or by assisting in preparation of draft material. Dr. Paul Hattis of Tufts University served as an appointed consultant and assisted the committee in preparation of the chapter, "Community Benefit as a Tool for Institutional Reform." The committee would also like to thank the many other individuals who provided information pertinent to the committee's charge, including Linda E. Berlin, Dr.PH., R.N.C., Director of Research and Data Services, American Association of Colleges of Nursing; Melissa Connell, J.D., University of Colorado Health Sciences Center; Lin Jacobson, Ed.D., R.N., C.P.H.Q., Director of Research, National League for Nursing; Marlaine Smith, R.N., Ph.D., Professor & Associate Dean for Academic Affairs, and Pat Moritz, Ph.D., Dean, University of Colorado Health Sciences Center School of Nursing; Donna M. English, M.P.H., R.N., Deputy Director, Division of Nursing, Bureau of Health Professions, Health Resources and Services Administration; Ruth Beer Bletzinger, M.A., Director, Division of Community and Minority Programs, and Lois Colburn, Assistant Vice President, Division of Community and Minority Programs, Association of American Medical Colleges; Denis

Nissim-Sabat, Ph.D., Senior Policy Analyst, Public Policy Office, American Psychological Association (APA); Jessica Kohout, Ph.D., Director, Research Office, APA, and staff of the APA Research Office; and Kim Nickerson, Ph.D., Assistant Director, Minority Fellowship Program, APA.

Finally, the committee would also like to thank the authors whose papers contributed to the evidence base that the committee examined. These include Jeffery F. Milem, Ph.D., University of Maryland; Eric L. Dey, Ph.D., and Casey E. White, University of Michigan; Cathryn L. Nation, M.D., University of California; Gabriel Garcia, M.D., Stanford University; Neil Parker, M.D., University of California, Los Angeles; Karen Matherlee, Policy, Inc.; Norma E. Wagoner, Ph.D.; Leon Johnson, D.Ed., M.B.A.; and Harry S. Jonas, M.D.

Preface

For almost a decade, several state referenda and federal court decisions have limited the ability of many universities to consider race and ethnicity in admissions processes. With that background, in a real sense, this committee's assignment has been to examine the question of whether we, as a nation, are properly utilizing the pool of applicants to training in the health professions that we already have (or will have in the future). The need and desire of the American people for competent, compassionate health professionals who have the necessary communication skills for an increasingly diverse society already exists and will only rapidly increase. Are we getting all of the *qualified* students and faculty that we should from the available applicant pool? From its inception, the committee also recognized there is a need to answer the very important, but usually unspoken, question of how does the broader society benefit by having increased diversity among health care professionals, aside from the gratification of doing what is morally right?

Stated more narrowly and precisely, the IOM was asked for a study assessing the potential for institutional and policy-level strategies to increase under-represented minority participation in the health professions. In other words, do these two particular strata offer any unique potential to increase diversity?

Our exploration therefore required the committee to assess (a) whether our current institutional processes and policy-level factors are, at times unintentionally creating barriers to providing the nation with the culturally competent caregivers it needs, and (b) if so, how can they be improved? Can some of the assumptions we have made for a great many decades be fairly challenged, as to exactly what is "the best and the brightest?" Our committee believes they can be so challenged and, in fact, improved upon in light of the twenty-first century needs of America.

Much of that "unspoken question" about value to the broader society was addressed by the June 23, 2003, decision by the Supreme Court on the *Grutter v. Bollinger et al.* case, when the majority opinion found there is substantial evidence that the quality of the educational experience in a university that has achieved a "critical mass" of diversity is significantly greater than what is experienced without said diversity. It was necessary for our committee to carefully examine that evidence, and go beyond, to draw our own conclusions.

The Supreme Court further found that the need of the American society for such better-educated future leaders, who are also better accustomed to interacting with a diverse world community, as well as a more diverse American society, is indeed a "compelling governmental interest."

Logic would suggest the different problem-solving skills found amongst those of diverse ethnic and cultural backgrounds should lead to more creative thinking about clinical, research, patient satisfaction, and/or cost problems, which are the bottom lines for health care. Every student and every patient will be advantaged from the achievement of a critical mass of diversity in all health profession education, not just the minority students and minority patients.

The methodology employed by this committee involved researching the pertinent literature, inviting much valued input from all key interested parties in a series of six workshops, and, in particular, studying the existing models of success in this activity. We have tried to identify and spotlight those characteristics that seem to be essential to that success and to codify them in a series of recommendations. These recommendations should be seen as being generic, and applicable to each of the healing professions, not simply to only one or the other of Dentistry, Medicine, Nursing, and Psychology. We have also attempted to make due note when unique and innovative programs were encountered that merit continued interest because of their "thinking outside the box."

Identifying needed modifications, however, is not enough. One should not design a sailboat without identifying a realistic source of wind to make it move. Similarly, with the objective of increasing diversity, there must be such a credible source of wind to fill the sail. We believe that can best be done in any professional endeavor through the standards which are set by that profession. Accordingly, we invite the attention of the reader to the standard-setting process (and how it might be improved or stimulated to accept this task), of each of the components in health profession education.

Without coalescence around standards set by the professions themselves, little movement will occur.

Of significant importance, however, is the need to remember that, in the background remains the grim visage of the law. Justice O'Connor articulated the majority opinion in *Grutter v. Bollinger et al.* that, while the government's compelling interest currently justifies this continued exception to an unflinching application of the Equal Protection Amendment, it is not intended to be a permanent exception to that Amendment. She writes, "We see no reason to exempt race-conscious admissions programs from the requirement that all governmental use of race must have a logical end point. . . . We expect that 25 years from now, the use of racial preferences will no longer be necessary to further the interest approved today."

The lesson is not subtle. The challenge to American society is clear. In the view of the Court, 25 years (or one generation) from now, we as a nation should have reached a place where there is no longer a compelling need for an exception to the 14th Constitutional Amendment. This IOM committee's report offers important tools for that achievement, but keep in mind that *the clock is ticking.*

The committee benefited from excellent staff support, under the leadership of Study Director Brian D. Smedley, Ph.D., assisted by Adrienne Stith Butler, Ph.D., and Thelma L. Cox, all of whom rose to every challenge, including a tight time frame for the study. Our sponsor, the Kellogg Foundation, was clear in their stated objective and unflagging in their interest and support.

Our hope is that those who read this will find light for their paths and then take action accordingly. *Et facta est lux* ("light is made").

Lonnie R. Bristow, M.D.
Walnut Creek, CA
September 2003

Contents

Appendixes

Commissioned Papers

IN THE NATION'S
COMPELLING
INTEREST

Executive Summary

HEALTH CARE'S COMPELLING INTEREST:
ENSURING DIVERSITY IN THE HEALTH-CARE WORKFORCE

ABSTRACT

The United States is rapidly becoming a more diverse nation, as demonstrated by the fact that nonwhite racial and ethnic groups will constitute a majority of the American population later in this century. The representation of many of these groups (e.g., African Americans, Hispanics, and Native Americans) within health professions, however, is far below their representation in the general population. Increasing racial and ethnic diversity among health professionals is important because evidence indicates that diversity is associated with improved access to care for racial and ethnic minority patients, greater patient choice and satisfaction, and better educational experiences for health professions students, among many other benefits.

Many groups—including health professions educational institutions (HPEIs), private foundations, and state and federal government agencies—have worked to increase the preparation and motivation of underrepresented minority (URM) students to enter health professions careers. Less attention, however, has been focused on

1

strategies to reduce institutional- and policy-level barriers to URM participation in health professions training.

HPEIs can improve admissions policies and reduce barriers to URM admission by developing a clear statement of mission that recognizes the value of diversity in health professions education. Admissions policies should be based on a comprehensive review of each applicant, including an assessment of applicants' attributes that best support the mission of the institution (e.g., background, experience, multilingual abilities). Admissions models should balance quantitative data (i.e., prior grades and standardized test scores) with these qualitative characteristics.

The federal Health Resources and Services Administration (HRSA) is a major funder of health professions training that seeks to improve the quality and availability of diverse health professionals through an array of programs. These health professions programs should be evaluated to assess their effectiveness in increasing the numbers of URM students enrolling and graduating from HPEIs, and Congress should provide increased funding for programs shown to be effective in enhancing diversity. State and local entities should increase support for diversity efforts through programs such as loan forgiveness, tuition reimbursement, loan repayment, and other efforts. In addition, private entities should be encouraged to collaborate through business partnerships with HPEIs to support the goal of developing a more diverse health-care workforce.

The U.S. Department of Education should strongly encourage accreditation bodies to be more aggressive in formulating and enforcing standards that result in a critical mass of URMs throughout the health professions. In addition, health professions education accreditation bodies should develop explicit policies articulating the value and importance of diversity among health professionals, and monitor the progress of member institutions toward achieving these goals.

HPEIs should develop and regularly evaluate comprehensive strategies to improve the institutional climate for diversity. As part of this process, HPEIs should proactively and regularly engage and train students, house staff, and faculty regarding institutional diversity-related policies and expectations and the importance of diversity to the long-term institutional mission.

HPEI governing bodies should develop institutional objectives consistent with community benefit principles that support the goal of increasing health-care workforce diversity, including efforts to ease financial and nonfinancial obstacles to URM participation, *increase involvement of diverse local stakeholders in key decision-making processes, and undertake initiatives that are responsive to local, regional and societal imperatives. These objectives are best assessed and enforced via the accreditation process.*

EXECUTIVE SUMMARY

In a landmark decision that resolved over 5 years of litigation—and an even longer period of contentious national debate—the U.S. Supreme Court ruled in *Grutter v. Bollinger et al.* that the University of Michigan Law School's consideration of race and ethnicity as one of many factors in the admissions process was lawful, because the practice was "narrowly tailored" and did not violate the constitutional rights of nonminority applicants. Perhaps more importantly, the Court declared that the university's position that achieving a "critical mass" of racial and ethnic diversity in its law school was a compelling interest of the law school and the nation, a rationale that will have far-reaching implications, not just for URM students[1] but also for the nation as a whole.

Few professional fields will feel the impact of the decision in the *Grutter* case—and the potential influence of greater levels of racial and ethnic diversity—as profoundly as the health professions. Health professions disciplines are grappling with the impact of major demographic changes in the United States population, including a rapid increase in the proportions of Americans who are nonwhite, who speak primary languages other than English, and who hold a diverse range of cultural values and beliefs regarding health and health care. Efforts to increase the proportions of URMs in health professions fields, however, have met with limited success. To a great extent, efforts to diversify health professions fields have been hampered by gross inequalities in educational opportunity for students of different racial and ethnic groups. Primary and secondary education for URM students is, on average, far below the quality of education for non-URM

---

[1] For purposes of this report, the study committee defines "underrepresented minorities" as those racial and ethnic groups that are underrepresented in the heath professions relative to their numbers in the general population. This definition allows individual institutions to define which populations are underrepresented in its area of interest. The definition is consistent with the definition of "underrepresented minorities in medicine" recently adopted by the Association of American Medical Colleges (AAMC); previously, AAMC's definition was limited to historically disadvantaged groups (e.g., African Americans, some Hispanic/Latino groups, and Native Americans). The new definition takes into account the fact that many other groups, such as subpopulations of Asian Americans, Pacific Islanders, and Latinos, are also poorly represented among health professionals, and many in these communities face barriers to accessing appropriate health care.

students. The "supply" of URM students who are well-prepared for higher education and advanced study in health professions fields has therefore suffered.

Equally important, however, are efforts to reduce policy-level barriers to URM participation in health professions training, and to increase the institutional "demand" for URM students. For example, several events—including public referenda (i.e., the California Civil Rights Initiative [Proposition 209] and Initiative 200 in Washington state), judicial decisions (e.g., the Fifth District Court of Appeals finding in *Hopwood v. Texas*), and lawsuits challenging affirmative action policies in 1995, 1996, and 1997—forced many higher education institutions to abandon the use of race and ethnicity as factors in admissions decisions (in some cases temporarily, in light of the Supreme Court decision in *Grutter*), and to curtail race- and ethnicity-based financial aid.

Given these problems—an increasing need for URM health professionals, policy challenges to affirmative action, and little progress toward enhancing the numbers of URM students prepared to enter health professions careers—the W.K. Kellogg Foundation requested a study by the Institute of Medicine (IOM) to assess institutional and policy-level strategies for achieving greater diversity among health-care professionals. Specifically, the IOM was asked to:

- assess and describe potential benefits of greater racial and ethnic diversity among health professionals;
- assess institutional and policy-level strategies that may increase diversity within the health professions, including:
  o modifying HPEIs' admissions practices,
  o reducing financial barriers to health professions training among minority and lower-income students,
  o increasing the emphasis on diversity goals in HPEI program accreditation,
  o improving the HPEI campus "climate" for diversity, and
  o considering the application of community benefit principles to improve the accountability of nonprofit, tax exempt institutions (e.g., medical schools and teaching hospitals) to the diverse racial and ethnic communities they serve; and
- identify mechanisms to garner broad support among health professions leaders, community members, and other key stakeholders to implement these strategies.

This Executive Summary presents a shortened version of the study committee's full report, with summaries of the analysis, findings, and recommendations.[2] The reader is referred to the full report for a more detailed discussion of the committee's findings and recommendations.

Why Is Racial and Ethnic Diversity Important in Health Professions Fields?

A preponderance of scientific evidence supports the importance of increasing racial and ethnic diversity among health professionals. This evidence (some of which is summarized below) demonstrates that greater diversity among health professionals is associated with improved access to care for racial and ethnic minority patients, greater patient choice and satisfaction, better patient–provider communication, and better educational experiences for *all* students while in training.

Racial and Ethnic Diversity Among Health Professionals and Access to Health Care for Minority Patients

Racial and ethnic minority health care professionals are significantly more likely than their white peers to serve minority and medically underserved communities, thereby helping to improve problems of limited minority access to care. For example, URM physicians are more likely to treat patients of color (Komaromy et al., 1996), indigent patients, and patients that are sicker (Moy and Bartman, 1995; Cantor et al., 1996) than non-URM physicians. Racial and ethnic minority dentists (Solomon et al., 2001) and psychologists (Turner and Turner, 1996) are also more likely than their white peers to practice in racial and ethnic minority communities.

Diversity and Minority Patient Choice and Satisfaction

Minority patients who have a choice are more likely to select healthcare professionals of their own racial or ethnic background (Saha et al., 2000; LaVeist and Nuru-Jeter, 2002). Moreover, racial and ethnic minority patients are generally more satisfied with the care that they receive from minority professionals (Saha et al., 1999; LaVeist and Nuru-Jeter, 2002), and minority patients' ratings of the quality of their health care are generally higher in racially concordant than in racially discordant settings (Cooper-Patrick et al., 1999).

---

[2]Recommendations in this Executive Summary are presented in the order in which they appear and as they are designated in the full report. Enumeration is based on the chapter in which the recommendations are presented. Enumeration begins with recommendations presented in Chapter 2, which are designated as 2-1, 2-2, and so on.

Diversity and Quality of Training for Health Professionals

Diversity in health professions training settings may assist in efforts to improve the cross-cultural training and cultural competencies of *all* trainees. Interaction among students from diverse backgrounds in training settings may help students to challenge assumptions and broaden perspectives regarding racial, ethnic, and cultural differences (Cohen, 2003; Whitla et al., 2003). In addition, there is growing evidence, primarily from studies of college students' undergraduate experiences, that campus diversity experiences are associated with gains in *all* students' learning outcomes and community involvement (e.g., Gurin et al., 2002; Antonio et al., in press; Whitla et al., 2003).

Despite the importance of diversity in health professions, African Americans, American Indians and Alaska Natives, many Hispanic/Latino populations, and some Asian American (e.g., Hmong and other Southeast Asians) and Pacific Islander groups (e.g., Native Hawaiians) are grossly underrepresented among the nation's health professionals. A range of institutional and policy-level strategies to increase the presence of URMs in the health professions are discussed below.

Reconceptualizing Admissions Policies and Practices

Although admissions practices vary by institution and discipline, admission into many HPEIs remains a highly competitive process, in which many talented applicants compete for a limited number of slots. For a range of reasons, including efficiency in sorting through a large number of applicants, and to attain a reasonable expectation of how applicants can be expected to perform in HPEIs, many admissions committees rely heavily on quantitative information, such as applicants' prior grades and standardized test scores, in identifying those applicants that will receive serious consideration.

Standardized test scores are generally good predictors of subsequent academic performance but have been used—in some cases inappropriately—as a barometer of applicants' academic "merit," often to the detriment of URM students. Some higher education institutions, as well as many among the general public, cling to the belief that admissions tests measure a "compelling distillation of academic merit" (National Research Council, 1999). Yet standardized admissions tests do not measure the full range of abilities that are needed to succeed in higher education (Sternberg and Williams, 1997), nor were they designed to. In addition, test scores are malleable, and are not indicative of fine distinctions between individual applicants. Admissions tests, whether they measure aptitude or achievement, are therefore best viewed as imprecise estimates of how students might be expected to perform in specific educational contexts, and are best used to sort applicants into broad categories (National Research Council, 1999). URM students typically score lower than their white or Asian American peers on a range of standardized tests, including the SAT, GRE, and MCAT. This disparity occurs for a variety of reasons, but principally because of poorer educational opportunities afforded to African American, Latino, and American Indian/Alaska Native students. These students are more likely than non-URM students to attend schools that are racially and economically segregated, poorly funded, offer few (if any) advanced placement and college preparatory classes, have fewer credentialed teachers, and suffer from a climate of low expectations (American Sociological Association, 2003; Camara and Schmidt, 1999). Moreover, even among those URM students who are invested in high academic performance, social and psychological factors—such as the pressure to perform above levels suggested by stereotypes of low minority academic ability—may serve to suppress their test performance (Steele, 1997; Steele and Aronson, 1995).

When quantitative variables such as standardized test scores are weighted heavily in the admissions process, URM applicants, because of their generally poorer academic preparation and test performance, are less successful in gaining admission than non-URM applicants. Absent admissions practices that allow applicants' race or ethnicity to be considered along with other personal characteristics of applicants, URM student participation in health professions education is likely to decline sharply. States that have implemented "percent solution" admissions strategies (i.e., where a top percentage of high school graduates are guaranteed admission to the state university system) have found that URM admissions have generally not increased (Tienda et al., 2003; Horn and Flores, 2003; Marin and Lee, 2003). In addition, an analysis by the Association of American Medical Colleges of the likely impact of "race-neutral" admissions policies in medical schools reveals that 70 percent fewer URM students would gain admission under such conditions (Cohen, 2003).

These barriers to URM admission have led some HPEIs to reconceptualize their admissions policies and practices to place greater weight on applicants' qualitative attributes, such as leadership, commitment to service, community orientation, experience with diverse groups, and other factors. This shift of emphasis to professional and "humanistic" factors is also consistent with a growing recognition in health professions fields that these attributes must receive greater attention in the admissions process to maintain professional quality, to ensure that future health professionals are prepared to address societal needs, and to maintain the public's trust in the integrity and skill of health professionals (Edwards et al., 2001). Anecdotally, evidence suggests that this shift may also reduce barriers to admission of qualified URM applicants, thereby achieving the dual goals of improving both the quality and diversity of health professions students (Garcia et al., 2003; Maldonado, 2001). Several HPEIs have adopted admissions policies that:

• Encourage admissions procedures to closely follow the institutions' stated mission with regard to teaching, research, and service—particularly if the needs of medically underserved communities are a part of the institutional mission;
• Encourage a comprehensive review of applicants' files, to understand how students' personal, community, and professional backgrounds may influence students' prior academic performance and contribute to the learning environment;
• Require admissions committee members to receive training aimed at improving their ability to assess underrepresented applicants and sharpening interviewing skills;
• De-emphasize standardized test data in the admissions equation, after a diverse group of academically qualified candidates are identified; and
• Include representatives from groups affected by the institution's admissions decisions on admissions committees and increase incentives for faculty participation on admissions committees.

Recommendation 2-1: HPEIs[3] should develop, disseminate, and utilize a clear statement of mission that recognizes the value of diversity in enhancing its mission and that of the relevant health-care professions.

Recommendation 2-2: HPEIs should establish explicit policies regarding the value and importance the institution places on the teaching and provision of culturally competent care and the role of institutional diversity in achieving this goal.

Recommendation 2-3: Admissions should be based on a comprehensive review of each applicant, including an assessment of applicants' attributes that best support the mission of the institution (e.g., race/ethnicity, background, experience, multilingual abilities). Admissions models should balance quantitative data (i.e., prior grades and standardized test scores) with these qualitative characteristics.

Recommendation 2-4: Admissions committees should include voting representation from underrepresented groups. In addition, HPEIs

---

[3]Recommendations regarding admissions policies and practices are intended to apply to HPEIs, whether free-standing or affiliated with a university or embedded in another institution.

should provide special incentives to faculty for participation on admissions committees (e.g., by providing additional weight or consideration for service during promotion review) and provide training for committee members on the importance of diversity efforts and means to improve diversity within the committee purview.

Reducing Financial Barriers to URM Participation in Health Professions Education

The costs associated with health professions training pose a significant barrier for many URM students, whose economic resources are lower, on average, than non-URM students. In recent years, financial barriers to both undergraduate and graduate education have risen sharply due to shifts in policies and priorities at the federal, state, and institutional levels. Tuition and other educational costs have climbed steadily, while at the same time sources of grant aid have decreased (Advisory Committee on Student Financial Assistance, 2002). The trends toward increased tuition costs and decreased need-based aid have resulted in higher levels of unmet need for lower-income students. The impact of high unmet need can be considerable on low-income students, even those who are academically prepared for the challenges of higher education. Low-income students with high unmet need are significantly less likely to expect to finish college; plan to attend a 4-year college after graduating from high school; take entrance exams; and apply, enroll, and persist to degree completion than high-income students with low unmet need (Advisory Committee on Student Financial Assistance, 2002; College Board, 2003; U.S. Department of Education, 2003).

Student financial assistance for health professions education is provided by a number of federal, state, and private sources. At the federal level, the Health Resources and Services Administration (HRSA) is the primary funder for health professions programs that either target or in some way include URM students, practitioners, and/or faculty. HRSA is charged with administering Title VII and Title VIII of the Public Health Service Act. These titles authorize funding, through a variety of programs for students and institutions, in order to increase the quality of the education and training of the primary care provider workforce, with special attention to the geographic, racial, and ethnic diversity of the United States health-care workforce. Title VII applies to medicine and dentistry (and in many cases mental health), while Title VIII pertains to nursing. These programs have provided support for many URM health professions students, yet Congressional appropriations for these programs have fluctuated as a result of budget pressures.

Among private sources of funding for URM health professions students, several organizations have contributed significantly toward scholarships, loan repayment, and stipend programs, in addition to mentoring and other support programs to enhance URM representation in health professions. These include the National Medical Fellowships, The California Endowment, the California Wellness Foundation, the W.K. Kellogg Foundation, the Ford Foundation, and the Robert Wood Johnson Foundation.

The large variety and scope of public and private efforts for funding URMs in health profession education make it difficult to assess if and how well these programs work together and complement one another in their efforts. While there are many programs targeting URM students who are entering graduate education, many of these same programs, as well as a host of others, also engage in pipeline efforts. The result is "a discontinuity of interventions across regions and across stages of the educational pipeline, making it difficult to sustain gains from one educational stage to the next" (Grumbach et al., 2002). Coordination and communication among various programs will help allow programs to better plan their own efforts and determine additional needs.

Recommendation 3-1: HRSA's health professions programs should be evaluated to assess their effectiveness in increasing the numbers of URM students enrolling and graduating from HPEIs to ensure that they maximize URM participation.

Recommendation 3-2: Congress should increase funding for Public Health Service Act Titles VII and VIII programs shown to be effective in increasing diversity, and should develop other financial mechanisms to enhance the diversity of the health-care workforce.

Some public and private entities have developed innovative collaborations to provide student financial support and institutional diversity efforts in ways that may increase the number of URM students in health professions programs. For example, the University of Colorado Health Sciences School of Dentistry has partnered with the Orthodontic Education Company (OEC) to establish a new dental center that they hope will address the shortage of orthodontists, provide low-cost care to children in underserved areas, and attract individuals from these communities to dental careers. The OEC provides scholarships and stipends in exchange for service in OEC private or group practices following graduation. The University of Colorado will establish and administer the program, supported by an investment of almost $100 million by the OEC. In other efforts, New York State has initiated the Minority Participation in Medical Education Grant Program, which provides funds to institutions to enhance minority recruitment and retention, develop minority student mentoring programs, develop medical career pathways for minority students, and develop minority faculty role models. A second program initiated by the state, the Graduate Medical Education (GME) Reform Incentive Pool, seeks to increase the representation of minorities in graduate medical education, increase the number of residents in primary care, and promote practice in underserved areas, among other goals. The program provides funds to hospitals and groups of training institutions.

Recommendation 3-3: State and local entities, working where appropriate with HPEIs, should increase support for diversity efforts through programs such as loan forgiveness, tuition reimbursement, loan repayment, GME, and supportive affiliations with community-based providers.

Recommendation 3-4: Private entities should be encouraged to collaborate through business partnerships and other entrepreneurial relationships with HPEIs to support the common goal of developing a more diverse health-care workforce.

Accreditation as a Key to Increase Diversity in Health Professions

Accreditation is the process by which nongovernmental organizations set standards for and monitor the quality of educational programs provided by member institutions. Accreditation is a voluntary process of institutional self-regulation, often conducted within the broad framework of standards established by the U.S. Department of Education and the Council for Higher Education Accreditation (CHEA). By setting standards for educational programs and methods for institutional peer review, accrediting bodies advance academic quality, ensure accountability to the public, encourage institutional progress and improvement, and provide a mechanism for continual assessment of broad educational goals for higher education. As such, accreditation is an important vehicle for institutional change, and a potential means to enhance diversity in health professions.

The increasing diversity of the United States population requires that accreditation bodies be responsive to demographic changes and develop and enforce standards that ensure that health professionals are prepared to serve diverse segments of the population. As one accreditation official noted during a public workshop hosted by the study committee, "Our role is to serve the public." Given that almost all accreditation bodies view public service and accountability as central to their mission, establishing and monitoring goals related to diversity among health-care professions can be unambiguously viewed as an important aspect of this effort.

Accreditation bodies may take varying approaches in efforts to accomplish these goals. The standards and practices adopted by the American Psychological Association (APA), however, are instructive and offer several approaches for accreditation standards to address diversity concerns (APA Committee on Accreditation, 2002):

1. Develop a plan to achieve diversity, consistent with the institutional mission, and demonstrate efforts to reach diversity goals.

2. Develop standards that encourage the development and infusion of diversity-related curricula throughout the training program.

3. Regularly monitor and evaluate the efforts of accredited institutions in achieving their diversity goals.

4. Apply graduated sanctions and reinforcement from the accrediting body to "shape" appropriate diversity efforts.

5. Seek community representation on standard-setting bodies.

6. Seek diverse representation on peer review teams.

APA's accreditation standards have contributed to an increased level of attention and effort among psychology education and training institutions in addressing diversity concerns (Zlotlow, 2003). Some of these programs, for example, have developed new websites devoted to promoting and enhancing diversity-related institutional policies and curriculums, and accreditation standards have promoted greater sharing among training programs regarding strategies to improve minority recruitment and retention efforts (Zlotlow, 2003).

Recommendation 4-1: The U.S. Department of Education should strongly encourage accreditation bodies to be more aggressive in formulating and enforcing standards that result in a critical mass of URMs throughout the health professions.

Recommendations 4-2: Health professions education accreditation bodies should develop explicit policies articulating the value and importance of providing culturally competent health care and the role it sees for racial and ethnic diversity among health professionals in achieving this goal.

Recommendation 4-3: Health professions education accreditation bodies should develop standards and criteria that more effectively encourage health professions schools to recruit URM students and faculty, to develop cultural competence curricula, and to develop an institutional climate that encourages and sustains the development of a critical mass of diversity.

Recommendation 4-4: Accreditation standards should include criteria to assess the number and percentage of URM candidates, students admitted and graduated, time to degree, and number and level of URM faculty.

Recommendation 4-5: Accreditation-related advisory boards and accreditation bodies should include URMs and other individuals with expertise in diversity and cultural competence.

Recommendation 4-6: If diversity-related standards are not met, the institution should be required to declare formally what steps will be put in place to address the deficiencies. Repeated deficiencies should result in accreditation-related sanctions.

Transforming the Institutional Climate to Enhance Diversity

The institutional climate for diversity—defined as the perceptions, attitudes, and values that define the institution, particularly as seen from the perspectives of individuals of different racial or ethnic backgrounds—can exert a profound influence on diversity efforts. Diversity is most often viewed as the proportion and number of individuals from groups underrepresented among students, faculty, administrators, and staff (i.e., structural diversity). Diversity, however, can also be conceptualized as the *diversity of interactions* that take place on campus (e.g., the quality and quantity of interactions across diverse groups and the exchange of diverse ideas), as well as *campus diversity-related initiatives and pedagogy* (e.g., the range and quality of curricula and programming pertaining to diversity, such as cultural activities and cultural awareness workshops; Hurtado et al., 1999). Each of these elements of diversity must be carefully considered as institutions assess their diversity goals.

The institutional climate for diversity is influenced by several elements of the institutional context, including the degree of structural diversity, the historical legacy of inclusion or exclusion of students and faculty of color, the psychological climate (i.e., perceptions of the degree of racial tension and discrimination on campus), and the behavioral dimension (i.e., the quality and quantity of interactions across diverse groups and diversity-related pedagogy; Hurtado et al., 1999). Each of the dimensions of the institutional climate may influence diversity efforts, in both positive and negative ways. More importantly, the institutional climate is malleable and can be altered through interventions aimed at each element of the institutional context.

How Can Health Professions Education Institutions Enhance the Institutional Climate for Diversity?

Building on this research and theory, Hurtado et al. (1999) outline 12 strategies for helping institutions to achieve an improved climate for diversity and to maximize the benefits of diversity. The first four principles (i.e., affirm the value of diversity, systematically assess the climate, develop a plan of action, and institute on-going evaluation of the plan) are "core" to any institutional efforts for change, while the remaining eight offer guidance for the development of new programs and policies. Hurtado and colleagues stress that these principles represent a comprehensive, "holistic" approach to institutional change and require that institutions possess strong leadership, adequate resources to support change efforts, strong planning and evaluation, and a long-term commitment to diversity goals.

Recruitment, Hiring, and Retention of Underrepresented Minority Faculty

Enhancing the racial and ethnic diversity of health professions education faculty can provide support for URM students in the form of role models and mentors, lead to important pedagogical changes, and "bring new kinds of scholarship to an institution, educate students on issues of growing importance to society, and offer links to communities not often connected to our campuses" (Smith, 2000, p. 51). HPEIs can take several steps to improve their efforts to recruit minority faculty. To begin, institutions should carefully examine their mission statement and assess how faculty diversity assists the institution to meet its goals. Identifying and recruiting qualified URM faculty candidates can be improved by utilizing active search processes that go beyond simply posting positions and recruiting though networks that are familiar to the faculty. Search committees should be diverse, to help in assessing and evaluating candidates of different backgrounds, and should have a close working relationship with the university administration to ensure the success of the search process. Finally, post-hiring support is critical for many URM faculty members to address the challenges of earning tenure, balancing teaching and research, and other faculty concerns (Smith, 2000).

Minority Student Recruitment and Retention

Several HPEIs have implemented successful URM student recruitment and retention programs. Some elements of successful recruitment efforts include developing academic and educational partnerships with minority-serving institutions, addressing financial barriers, targeting outreach to URM students, and engaging pre-health advisors. As significantly, institutions should develop comprehensive strategies to retain URM students, by instituting a range of academic and social supports, including faculty and peer mentoring, tutoring and academic skills assessment, and teaching study skills. Institutions may increase opportunities for URM students to integrate themselves into the campus community (and take advantage of support programs) through both ethnic- and racial-group interest organizations, as well as general campus programs, such as orientation programs that clearly outline the institutions' expectations regarding diversity-related policies and goals, and sensitivity training programs that increase awareness and understanding of diversity in the campus context. A confidential ombudsman program may assist efforts to improve the campus climate for diversity by providing an informal mediation process to gather information about complaints, advise individuals about how to resolve disputes informally, mediate disputes, seek "win–win" resolution of problems, and advise individuals about more formal grievance procedures should informal efforts fail (Steinhardt and Connell, 2002).

Recommendation 5-1: HPEIs should develop and regularly evaluate comprehensive strategies to improve the institutional climate for diversity. These strategies should attend not only to the structural dimensions of diversity, but also to the range of other dimensions (e.g., psychological and behavioral) that affect the success of institutional diversity efforts.

Recommendation 5-2: HPEIs should proactively and regularly engage and train students, house staff, and faculty regarding institutional diversity-related policies and expectations, the principles that underlie these policies, and the importance of diversity to the long-term institutional mission. Faculty should be able to demonstrate specific progress toward achieving institutional diversity goals as part of the promotion and merit process.

Recommendation 5-3: HPEIs should establish an informal, confidential mediation process for students and faculty who experience barriers to institutional diversity goals (e.g., experiences of discrimination, harassment).

Recommendation 5-4: HPEIs should be encouraged to affiliate with community-based health-care facilities in order to attract and train a more diverse and culturally competent workforce and to increase access to health care.

Community Benefit Principles and Diversity

Community benefit is a legal term that applies to charitable activities that benefit the community as a whole. For over 100 years, federal tax law has recognized the significant role of charitable trusts (nonprofits that serve "religious, charitable, scientific, literary, or educational purposes) in furthering governmental and social goals, providing for income tax exemption for qualifying organizations. The framework of charitable trust has been adopted and maintained in every update of the tax code since the original ruling. Historically, this framework has expanded beyond early "relief of poverty" criteria for hospitals to qualify for tax exemption as 501(c)(3) nonprofit organizations, to more recent IRS rulings that removed the requirement to provide services for the poor, and identified the promotion of health (i.e., community benefit) as a charitable purpose.

Since then, some states have established formal guidelines for nonprofit hospitals and nursing homes. States such as New York have required the development and implementation of "community service plans" by nonprofit hospitals. Requirements include an annual review of the hospital mission statement, publication of hospital assets and liabilities, an assessment of community needs and hospital strategies to address them, and the solicitation of input from community stakeholders. The Utah State Tax Commission issued a set of formal guidelines for nonprofit hospitals and nursing homes that included a requirement for a minimum financial threshold of contributions that exceed the annual property tax liability of each facility. The legal requirements New York and Utah placed upon nonprofit health-care providers reflect two alternative approaches that have marked subsequent state actions in this arena: a general reporting requirement (NY) and the establishment of a minimum financial threshold (UT).

Between 1990 and 2001, a total of eleven states implemented some form of legal mechanism to increase the accountability of nonprofit healthcare providers. Eight of the eleven took the general reporting requirement approach; three took the minimum financial threshold approach. In addition, states are requiring such activities as:

- community assessments to identify local unmet needs,
- solicitation of community input in the development of community benefit plans, and
- review of organizational mission statements to reflect a commitment to address community health needs.

These efforts have yielded mixed results, primarily because of inconsistencies in the application of community benefit regulations and inadequate administrative resources for states to provide oversight regarding compliance. States with reporting requirements, for example, find that there are numerous examples of promising programs, but substantial variability in the quality and specificity of reporting make it impossible to conduct a reliable comparative analysis of performance. Many states lack uniform guidelines for reporting. In addition, many nonprofit hospitals lack the infrastructure and competencies to design, implement, and monitor community benefit activities.

A central question of this study is to what extent community benefit principles can assist policy efforts to enhance diversity in health professions. Though community benefit principles offer an attractive framework for holding health professional training programs and their institutional sponsors accountable for advancing goals tied to racial and ethnic diversity of their students and trainees, from a legal perspective, it is important that the principles be applied in the most effective venue. In that regard, while community benefit laws and associated public expectations have evolved out of a tax exemption context, the most practical application of concepts for increased institutional accountability are outside of the tax exemption arena, and are best applied in the accreditation world.

Community benefit principles provide insights for the public expectations of both nonprofit health-care providers and institutions that train these providers. Just as nonprofit hospitals are expected to play a role in addressing priority unmet needs in local communities, HPEIs can appropriately be expected to play a direct role in responding to priority unmet health needs at the local and/or societal level. Furthermore, for publicly sponsored colleges and universities, community benefit concepts might also link governmental subsidies for these public institutions of higher education to performance measures related to student and trainee diversity goals. Community benefit principles should therefore form a conceptual cornerstone by which health professions education accreditation organizations and state governments can set expectations for the advancement of societal goals tied to racial and ethnic diversity of the health-care workforce.

Recommendation 6-1: HPEI governing bodies should develop institutional objectives consistent with community benefit principles that support the goal of increasing health-care workforce diversity including, but not limited to efforts to ease financial and nonfinancial obstacles to URM participation, increase involvement of diverse local stakeholders in key decision-making processes, and undertake initiatives that are responsive to local, regional, and societal imperatives (see Recommendation 5-4).

Recommendation 6-2: Health professions accreditation institutions should explore the development of new standards that acknowledge and reinforce efforts by HPEIs to implement community benefit principles as they relate to increasing health-care workforce diversity.

Recommendation 6-3: HPEIs should develop a mechanism to inform the public of progress toward and outcomes of efforts to provide equal health care to minorities, reduce health disparities, and increase the diversity of the health-care workforce.

Recommendation 6-4: Private and public (e.g., federal, state, and local governments) entities should convene major community benefit stakeholders (e.g., community advocates, academic institutions, health-care providers), to inform them about community benefit standards and to build awareness that placing a priority on diversity and cultural competency programs is a societal expectation of all institutions that receive any form of public funding.

Mechanisms to Garner Support for Diversity Efforts

Several mechanisms offer promise to increase the general public and key stakeholders' understanding of the need for and benefits of greater diversity among health professionals. This kind of understanding is necessary in order to effectively develop and implement institutional and policy-level strategies to increase diversity among health professionals. Implementation of these strategies should begin with efforts to collect data and conduct additional research to assess diversity among health professionals and in health professions education and to further identify the benefits of diversity for health care service delivery. Educational initiatives should begin with health professionals, HPEIs, and the communities that they serve. Other stakeholders—including business and corporate leaders, community and grassroots groups, organized labor, policy makers, and elected representatives, among many others—should also be involved in diversity efforts, specifically by forming broad coalitions to advocate for policies to enhance diversity. Several innovative examples of such efforts are underway nationwide, and should be expanded.

Recommendation 7-1: Additional data collection and research are needed to more thoroughly characterize URM participation in the health professions and in health professions education and to further assess the benefits of diversity among health professionals, particularly with regard to the potential economic benefits of diversity.

Recommendation 7-2: Local and national efforts must be undertaken to increase broad stakeholders' understanding of and consensus regarding steps that should be taken to enhance diversity among health professionals.

Recommendation 7-3: Broad coalitions should advocate to vigorously encourage HPEIs, their accreditation bodies, and federal and state sources of health professions student financial aid to adopt policies to enhance diversity among health professionals.

BOX ES-1
Summary of Recommendations

IMPROVING ADMISSIONS POLICIES AND PRACTICES. HPEIs should:
• Develop, disseminate, and utilize a clear statement of mission that recognizes the value of diversity;
• Establish explicit policies regarding the value and importance of culturally competent care and the role of institutional diversity in achieving this goal;
• Base admissions decisions on a comprehensive review of each applicant, and balance the consideration of quantitative and qualitative data; and
• Include voting representation from underrepresented groups on admissions committees and provide special incentives to faculty for participation.

REDUCING FINANCIAL BARRIERS TO HEALTH PROFESSIONS TRAINING
• HRSA's health professions training programs should be evaluated to ensure that they maximize URM participation;
• Congress should increase funding for Public Health Service Act Titles VII and VIII programs shown to be effective in increasing diversity;
• Federal and state health agencies should increase support for diversity efforts through programs such as loan forgiveness, tuition reimbursement, loan repayment, GME, and supportive affiliations with community-based providers; and
• Public–private collaboration should be encouraged to support the common goal of developing a more diverse health-care workforce.

ENCOURAGING DIVERSITY EFFORTS THROUGH ACCREDITATION. Accreditation bodies should:
• Formulate and enforce diversity-related standards;
• Develop explicit policies articulating the value and importance of culturally competent health care and the role for racial and ethnic diversity in achieving this goal;
• Develop standards and criteria that encourage and support URM student and faculty participation;
• Include criteria and standards to assess the success of diversity efforts;
• Include URMs and other individuals with expertise in cultural competence and diversity on accreditation bodies and advisory groups; and
• Apply sanctions if diversity-related standards are not met.

IMPROVING THE INSTITUTIONAL CLIMATE FOR DIVERSITY. HPEIs should:
• Develop and regularly evaluate comprehensive strategies to improve the institutional climate for diversity;
• Proactively and regularly engage and train students, house staff, and faculty regarding institutional diversity-related policies and expectations and the importance of diversity;
• Establish an informal, confidential mediation process for students and faculty who experience barriers to institutional diversity goals; and
• Affiliate with community-based health-care facilities in order to attract and train a more diverse and culturally competent workforce and to increase access to health care.

Continued

BOX ES-1 Continued

APPLYING COMMUNITY BENEFIT PRINCIPLES TO DIVERSITY EFFORTS.
HPEIs and relevant public and private groups should:
- Develop institutional objectives consistent with community benefit principles that support the goal of increasing health-care workforce diversity, and reinforce these efforts through program accreditation;
- Explore the development of new standards that acknowledge and reinforce efforts to implement community benefit principles as they relate to increasing health-care workforce diversity;
- Develop a mechanism to inform the public of progress toward diversity efforts; and
- Convene major community benefit stakeholders to inform them about community benefit standards and their relationship to diversity.

MECHANISMS TO ENCOURAGE SUPPORT FOR DIVERSITY EFFORTS include:
- Additional research and data collection on diversity and its benefits;
- Efforts to increase broad stakeholders' understanding of and consensus regarding steps that should be taken to enhance diversity among health professionals; and
- The development of broad coalitions to encourage HPEIs, their accreditation bodies, and federal and state sources of health professions student financial aid to adopt policies to enhance diversity among health professionals.

REFERENCES

Advisory Committee on Student Financial Assistance. 2002. *Empty Promises. The Myth of College Access in America*. Washington, DC: U.S. Department of Education.
American Psychological Association (APA) Committee on Accreditation. 2002. *Guidelines and Principles for Accreditation of Programs in Professional Psychology*. Washington, DC: American Psychological Association.
American Sociological Association. 2003. *Brief of the American Sociological Association et al., as Amicus Curiae in Support of Respondents*. Merritt DJ, Lee BL, Attorneys for Amici Curiae. Washington, DC: American Sociological Association.
Antonio AL, Chang MJ, Hakuta K, Kenny DA, Levin SL, Milem JF. In press. Effects of racial diversity on complex thinking in college students. *Psychological Science*.
Camara WJ, Schmidt AE. 1999. *Group Differences in Standardized Testing and Social Stratification*. College Board Report No. 99-5. New York: College Board Publications. Pp. 1–18.
Cantor JC, Miles EL, Baker LC, Barker DC. 1996. Physician service to the underserved: Implications for affirmative action in medical education. *Inquiry* 33:167–181.
Cohen JJ. 2003. The consequences of premature abandonment of affirmative action in medical school admissions. *Journal of the American Medical Association* 289(9):1143–1149.
College Board. 2003. *Trends in College Pricing*. Washington, DC: College Board.
Cooper-Patrick L, Gallo JJ, Gonzales JJ, Vu HT, Powe NR, Nelson C, Ford DE. 1999. Race, gender, and partnership in the patient–physician relationship. *Journal of the American Medical Association* 282(6):583–589.

Edwards JC, Elam CL, Wagoner NE. 2001. An admission model for medical schools. *Academic Medicine* 76(12):1207–1212.

Garcia JA, Paterniti DA, Romano PS, Kravitz RL. 2003. Patient preferences for physician characteristics in university-based primary clinics. *Ethnicity & Disease* 13:259–267.

Grumbach K, Coffman J, Munoz C, Rosenoff E. 2002. *Strategies for Improving the Diversity of the Health Professions*. University of California, San Francisco: Center for California Health Workforce Studies.

Gurin P, Dey EL, Hurtado S, Gurin G. 2002. Diversity and higher education: Theory and impact on educational outcomes. *Harvard Education Review* 72(3):330–366.

Horn CL, Flores SM. 2003. *Percent Plans in College Admissions: A Comparison of Three States' Experiences*. Cambridge, MA: The Civil Rights Project, Harvard University.

Hurtado S, Milem J, Clayton-Peterson A, Allen W. 1999. *Enacting Diverse Environments: Improving the Climate for Racial/Ethnic Diversity in Higher Education*. ASHE-ERIC Higher Education Report Volume 26, No. 8. Washington, DC: George Washington University, Graduate School of Education and Human Development.

Komaromy M, Grumbach K, Drake M, Vranizan K, Lurie N, Keane D, Bindman AB. 1996. The role of black and Hispanic physicians in providing health care for underserved populations. *New England Journal of Medicine* 334(20):1305–1310.

LaVeist TA, Nuru-Jeter A. 2002. Is doctor–patient race concordance associated with greater satisfaction with care? *Journal of Health and Social Behavior* 43(3):296–306.

Maldonado F. 2001. Rethinking the admissions process: Evaluation techniques that promote inclusiveness in admissions decisions. In: Smedley BD, Stith AY, Colburn L, Evans CH, eds. *The Right Thing to Do, The Smart Thing to Do: Enhancing Diversity in Health Professions*. Washington, DC: National Academy Press.

Marin P, Lee EK. 2003. Appearance and reality in the sunshine state: The Talented 20 Program in Florida. Cambridge, MA: The Civil Rights Project, Harvard University.

Moy E, Bartman A. 1995. Physician race and care of minority and medically indigent patients. *Journal of the American Medical Association* 273(19):1515–1520.

National Research Council. 1999. *Myths and Tradeoffs: The Role of Tests in Undergraduate Admissions*. Beatty A, Greenwood MRC, Linn RL, eds. Washington, DC: National Academy Press.

Saha S, Komaromy M, Koepsell TD, Bindman AB. 1999. Patient–physician racial concordance and the perceived quality and use of health care. *Archives of Internal Medicine* 159:997–1004.

Saha S, Taggart S, Komaromy K, Bindman AB. 2000. Do patients choose physicians of their own race? *Health Affairs* 19(4):76–83.

Smith D. 2000. How to diversify the faculty. *Academe* 86(5):48–52.

Solomon ES, Williams CR, Sinkford JC. 2001. Practice location characteristics of black dentists in Texas. *Journal of Dental Education* 65(6):571–574.

Steele CM. 1997. A threat in the air. How stereotypes shape intellectual identity and performance. *American Psychologist* 52(6):613–629.

Steele CM, Aronson J. 1995. Stereotype threat and the intellectual test performance of African Americans. *Journal of Personality and Social Psychology* 69(5):797–811.

Steinhardt R, Connell M. 2002. Reporting of wrongdoing and resolving disputes: The value of ombudsmen and hotlines in the corporation. In: Banks TL, Banks FZ, eds. *Corporate Legal Compliance Handbook*. New York: Aspen Publishers.

Sternberg, RJ, Williams WM. 1997. Does the *Graduate Record Examination* predict meaningful success in the graduate training of psychologists? A case study. *American Psychologist* 52(6):630–641.

Tedesco L. 2001. The role of diversity in the training of health professionals. In: Smedley BD, Stith AY, Colburn L, Evans CH, eds. *The Right Thing to Do, The Smart Thing to Do: Enhancing Diversity in Health Professions*. Washington, DC: National Academy Press.

Tienda M, Leicht KT, Sullivan T, Maltese M, Lloyd K. 2003. *Closing the Gap?: Admissions & Enrollments at the Texas Public Flagship Before and After Affirmative Action*. [Online]. Available: http://www.texastop10.princeton.edu/publications/tienda012103. pdf [accessed January 15, 2004].

Turner CB, Turner BF. 1996. Who treats minorities? *Cultural Diversity in Mental Health* 2(3):175–182.

U.S. Bureau of the Census. 2003. Hispanic population reaches all-time high of 38.8 million, new Census Bureau estimates show. Press release. [Online]. Available: www.census.gov/ press-release/www/2003/cb03-100.html [accessed June 18, 2003].

U.S. Department of Education, National Center for Education Statistics. 2003. *How Families of Low- and Middle-Income Undergraduates Pay for College: Full-Time Dependent Students in 1999–2000*. NCES report # 2003-162. Washington, DC: U.S. Department of Education.

Whitla DK, Orfield G, Silen W, Teperow C, Howard C, Reede J. 2003. Educational benefits of diversity in medical school: A survey of students. *Academic Medicine* 78(5):460–466.

Zlotlow S. 2003. Presentation to the IOM Committee on Institutional and Policy-Level Strategies to Increase the Diversity of the U.S. Health Care Workforce. April 9, 2003, Washington, DC.

1

Introduction

INSTITUTIONAL AND POLICY-LEVEL STRATEGIES FOR INCREASING THE DIVERSITY OF THE U.S. HEALTH-CARE WORKFORCE

The United States is rapidly transforming into one of the most racially and ethnically diverse nations in the world. Groups commonly referred to as *minorities*—including Asian Americans, Pacific Islanders, African Americans, Hispanics, American Indians, and Alaska Natives—are the fastest-growing segments of the population and are emerging as the nation's majority. Since 2000, for example, Hispanics accounted for 3.5 million—or over one-half—of the population increase of 6.9 million individuals in the United States. The number of Asian Americans grew at a larger proportion (9 percent) than any other racial or ethnic group during this same time period. And in at least three states (California, Hawaii, and New Mexico) and the District of Columbia, these groups constitute a majority of the population (U.S. Bureau of the Census, 2003).

Despite the rapid growth of racial and ethnic minority groups in the United States, their representation among the nation's health professionals has grown only modestly at best over the past 25 years, producing a trend in which the proportion of minorities in the population outstrips their representation among health professionals by several fold.[1] Hispanics, for

---

[1]This is not meant to imply that racial and ethnic minority patients receive better health care when treated by providers who are of the same race or ethnicity, or that nonminority

23

example, comprise over 12 percent of the U.S population, but only 2 percent of the registered nurse population, 3.4 percent of psychologists, and 3.5 percent of physicians. Similarly, one in eight individuals in the United States is African American, yet less than one in twenty dentists or physicians is African American.

These stark figures, in part, have prompted many major health professions organizations and health professions educational institutions (HPEIs) to develop initiatives to increase the proportion of underrepresented minorities (URM)[2] in health professions fields. These efforts, however, have met with limited success. To a great extent, efforts to diversify health professions fields have been hampered by gross inequalities in educational opportunity for students of minority racial and ethnic groups. Primary and secondary education for URM students is, on average, far below the quality of education for non-URM students. Proportionately fewer URM students enter higher education than their white or Asian American peers, and an even smaller percentage of these go on to graduate (post-baccalaureate) study. The "supply" of URM students who are well-prepared for higher education and advanced study in health professions fields has therefore suffered.

Equally important, however, are efforts to reduce policy-level barriers to URM participation in health professions training, and to increase the institutional "demand" for URM students. For example, several events— including public referenda (i.e., Proposition 209 in California and Initiative 200 in Washington state), judicial decisions (e.g., the Fifth District Court of Appeals finding in *Hopwood v. Texas*), and lawsuits challenging affirmative action policies in 1995, 1996, and 1997—forced many higher education institutions to abandon the use of race and ethnicity as factors in admissions decisions (in some cases temporarily, in light of the June 2003 Supreme Court decision in *Grutter v. Bollinger*, in which white plaintiffs sued—unsuccessfully—in an effort to halt the University of Michigan's admissions policies that consider applicants' race and ethnicity as one of

---

providers are less capable than minorities of providing high-quality care to these populations. Rather—as will be discussed later in this chapter and throughout the report—greater racial and ethnic diversity in health professions may offer broad benefits to help improve health-care access for minorities and improve the cultural competency of *all* health-care providers and the health systems in which they work.

[2]URMs are defined as those racial and ethnic populations that are underrepresented in the heath professions relative to their numbers in the general population. This definition allows individual institutions to define which populations are underrepresented in its area of interest. See the subsection on "Which Racial and Ethnic Groups Are Examined?" later in this chapter for a fuller explanation of this definition.

many factors in the admissions process[3]), and to curtail race- and ethnicity-based financial aid.

Given these problems—an increasing need for minority health professionals, policy challenges to affirmative action, and little progress toward enhancing the numbers of URM students prepared to enter health professions careers—the W.K. Kellogg Foundation requested a study by the Institute of Medicine to assess institutional and policy-level strategies for achieving greater diversity among health-care professionals. Institutional and policy-level strategies are defined as specific policies or programs of health professions schools, associations, accreditation bodies, health-care organizations/systems, or state and federal governments, designed to increase access to health professions careers among underrepresented racial and ethnic minority groups, as a means of increasing the likelihood that "pipeline" efforts[4] to increase diversity will succeed. Specifically, the IOM was asked to:

• assess and describe potential benefits of greater racial and ethnic diversity among health professionals;
• assess institutional and policy-level strategies that may increase diversity within the health professions, including:
   o modifying graduate health professions training programs' admissions practices;
   o increasing the emphasis in health professions program accreditation on enhancing diversity in training programs and developing cross-cultural skills and competencies of health professions trainees;
   o improving the campus "climate" for diversity, including efforts to recruit and support URM students and faculty and facilitate learning within a context of diversity;
   o modifying the financing and funding of health professions training in order to reduce financial barriers to health professions training among minority and lower-income students; and

---

[3]In a landmark decision that resolved over five years of litigation—and an even longer period of contentious national debate—the U.S. Supreme Court ruled in *Grutter v. Bollinger et al.* that the University of Michigan Law School's consideration of race and ethnicity as one of many factors in the admissions process was lawful, because the practice was narrowly tailored and did not violate the constitutional rights of nonminority applicants. Perhaps more importantly, the Court declared that the university's position that achieving a "critical mass" of racial and ethnic diversity in its law school was a compelling interest of the law school and the nation—a rationale that will have far-reaching implications, not just for URM students, but also for the nation as a whole.

[4]"Pipeline" efforts refer to strategies that aim to increase the numbers of well-prepared URM students (in grades K-16) motivated to enter health professions fields.

> **BOX 1-1**
> **Fast Facts—Diversity and Health Care**
>
> • Nearly one in five Spanish-speaking U.S. residents delayed or refused needed medical care because of language barriers (Robert Wood Johnson Foundation, 2001).
> • Nearly 2 in 5 Latinos, 27 percent of Asian Americans, 23 percent of African Americans, and 16 percent of whites reported communication problems with their doctor (Collins et al., 1999).
> • Nearly half of Asian Americans and Pacific Islanders have problems with availability of mental health services because of limited English proficiency and lack of providers who have appropriate language skills (U.S. Surgeon General, 2001).
> • African Americans, Latinos, and Asian Americans with mental health needs are less likely than whites to receive treatment . If treated, they are likely to have sought help in primary care, as opposed to mental health specialty care, and African Americans are less likely than whites to receive evidence-based mental health care in accordance with professional treatment guidelines (U.S. Surgeon General, 2001).
> • Less than 13 percent of the 8.6 million patients seen in community health centers (CHCs), which primarily serve minority and low-income patients, received preventive and basic dental care in 1998 (Mertz and O'Neill, 2002).
> • About 45 percent of Californians who have low incomes or who have low English proficiency did not receive dental care in the past year (Kaiser Daily Health Policy Report, 2003).
> • An increase of more than 20,000 minority nurses is needed to increase the proportion of minority nurses by just 1 percent (National Advisory Council on Nurse Education and Practice, 2000).

o considering the application of community benefit principles to improve the accountability of nonprofit, tax exempt institutions (e.g., medical schools and teaching hospitals) to the diverse racial and ethnic communities they serve; and

• identify mechanisms to garner broad support among health professions leaders, community members, and other key stakeholders to implement these strategies.

WHY EXAMINE INSTITUTIONAL AND POLICY-LEVEL STRATEGIES FOR INCREASING DIVERSITY IN HEALTH PROFESSIONS?

Historically, the efforts of HPEIs and professional associations to increase the presence of URM students in health professions careers have focused on enhancing students' preparation to pursue these careers. Appropriately, many of these efforts have focused on improving URM students' math and science education, particularly at the primary and secondary school levels, "bridging" K-12 training with undergraduate pre-health curricula and graduate training, and other academic and social supports. These programs have achieved some notable successes in a range of health disciplines. The Robert Wood Johnson Foundation-supported Minority Medical Education Program, for example, a 6-week summer intensive medical school preparatory program, has assisted 63 percent of its graduates to gain admission into medical school (Cantor et al., 1998).

Institutional and policy-level strategies for increasing diversity in health professions, however, have been relatively understudied. This lack of emphasis may lead to a void of strategies should future policy changes erode efforts to increase diversity (e.g., despite the U.S. Supreme Court decision in the *Grutter* case reaffirming the use of race/ethnicity in admissions decisions, some opponents of this decision plan to establish ballot initiatives in several states and localities to prohibit higher education institutions from adopting or continuing "race-conscious" admissions policies). As will be discussed in a later chapter (see "Reconceptualizing Admissions Policies and Practices"), "race-neutral" admissions policies, as have been practiced by some states over the past few years, have profoundly changed the landscape for diversity and have adversely affected health professions' efforts to increase minority representation in training programs. Failure to address these changes may therefore undercut some of the significant gains achieved by pipeline enhancement programs.

This focus is not to diminish the importance of pipeline development efforts. Rather, these strategies should be viewed as complementary. Strategies at the institutional and policy level, in conjunction with pipeline efforts, may have reciprocal effects; for example, the successful development and implementation of institutional and policy-level strategies to increase diversity in health professions may increase the demand for expanded emphasis and investment in pipeline enhancement strategies.

WHICH RACIAL AND ETHNIC GROUPS AND HEALTH PROFESSIONS ARE EXAMINED?

For purposes of this report, the study committee defines URMs as those racial and ethnic groups that are underrepresented in the heath professions relative to their numbers in the general population. This definition allows individual institutions to define which populations are underrepresented in its area of interest. It is also consistent with the definition of underrepresented minorities recently adopted by the Association of American Medical Colleges (AAMC). Previously, AAMC's definition was limited to historically disadvantaged groups (i.e., African Americans, mainland Puerto

Ricans, and Native Americans, including American Indians, Alaska Natives, and Native Hawaiians). The new AAMC definition takes into account the fact that many other groups, such as subpopulations of Asian Americans, Pacific Islanders, and Latinos, are also poorly represented among health professionals, and many in these communities face barriers to accessing appropriate health care.

While the study committee defines URMs broadly, it should be noted that the racial and ethnic groups identified in AAMC's previous definition of URM groups (e.g., African Americans, some Hispanic/Latino groups, American Indians) are historically underrepresented and face long-standing barriers to greater inclusion among health professionals—including persistent discrimination, educational inequality, and few role models for students of these racial and ethnic groups. The persistent underrepresentation of these groups among health professionals suggests that a sustained emphasis on increasing access to health professions careers among historically underrepresented populations is critically important.

The study committee recognizes that a broad range of health professionals contribute invaluably to the health-care enterprise. These disciplines—including dental hygienists, pharmacists, allied health professionals, physician assistants, nutritionists, occupational therapists, and clinical social workers, among many others—are critically important to ensuring that America's health-care systems provide the best quality health care, health promotion, and disease prevention services. This study, however, will focus on medicine, nursing, dentistry, and professional psychology. This is not to suggest that diversity is unimportant or has already been achieved in other health professions. Rather, this study is limited in its scope because a comprehensive analysis of all health-related fields is not feasible given the time frame of the current study. Over 15 million Americans work in over two-dozen health-care and health-related occupations and an even greater array of specialties and subspecialties (Matherlee, this volume), making the task of assessing health workforce trends daunting. In addition, medicine, nursing, dentistry, and professional psychology are among the largest health professions, and the availability and concentration of diverse professionals in these fields will therefore have significant implications for health service delivery. Furthermore, more complete data are available from these fields to evaluate minority participation and diversity efforts. It is the study committee's expectation that strategies adopted to increase diversity in these fields may be applicable, in some cases, to other health professions.

WHY IS RACIAL AND ETHNIC DIVERSITY IMPORTANT IN HEALTH PROFESSIONS FIELDS?

The U.S. Supreme Court's review of the University of Michigan admissions lawsuits prompted an avalanche of amicus brief filings from both proponents and opponents of affirmative action and the use of race and ethnicity in university admissions processes. Many of these arguments have been summarized elsewhere, particularly by the plaintiffs' and defendants' respective legal counsel (see especially amicus brief filings at the University of Michigan Internet website http://www.umich.edu/~urel/admissions/legal). The weight of scientific evidence, however, supports the necessity of ensuring that health professionals reflect the diversity of the U.S. population. This evidence (summarized below) demonstrates that greater diversity among health professionals is associated with improved access to care for racial and ethnic minority patients, greater patient choice and satisfaction, and better patient–clinician communication. In higher education settings, greater diversity is associated with improved student learning and community participation. Indirectly, evidence suggests that greater diversity can improve the cultural competence[5] of health professionals and health systems, and that such improvements may be associated with better health-care outcomes. In addition, greater diversity among health professionals has the potential to improve the clinical research enterprise and to lead to new developments and improvements in health care and how care is delivered.

Racial and Ethnic Diversity Among Health Professionals and Access to Health Care for Minority Patients

Racial and ethnic minority health-care clinicians are significantly more likely than their white peers to serve minority and medically underserved communities, thereby helping to improve problems of limited minority access to care. Several studies document this trend across a range of health professions, although the bulk of this research has focused on the practice patterns of physicians.

Turner and Turner (1996), for example, studied the practice characteristics of psychological service providers, using a random sample of psychologists listing the National Register of Health Service Providers. Racial

---

[5]Cultural competence is defined as "a set of behaviors and attitudes and a culture within the business or operation of a system that respects and takes into account the person's cultural background, cultural beliefs, and their values and incorporates it into the way health care is delivered to that individual" (Betancourt et al., 2002, p.3).

and ethnic minority psychologists treated more than twice the proportion
of racial and ethnic minority patients than nonminority psychologists (24.0
percent vs. 11.7 percent, respectively), and those psychologists who utilized
cognitive/behavioral theoretical orientations saw a larger percentage of minority patients than psychologists who used psychoanalytic or other theoretical orientations. These findings are especially important in light of consistent findings that racial and ethnic minority patients underutilize mental
health services (U.S. Surgeon General, 2001).

Moy and Bartman (1995), in a nationwide survey of households, found
that minority patients were more than four times more likely than white
patients to receive health care from nonwhite physicians. Medically indigent patients were also between 1.4 and 2.6 times more likely to receive
care from minority physicians than were more affluent patients. In addition, minority physicians tended to see patients who were sicker than the
patients seen by their white peers. Minority physicians' patients were more
likely to report being in poor health, with more acute complaints, more
chronic conditions, and greater functional limitations. These findings held
true even after controlling for physician gender, specialization, workplace,
and geographic location.

Relative to nonminority communities, minority neighborhoods tend to
face shortages of physicians, yet physicians of color are disproportionately
more likely to serve in these communities. Komaromy et al. (1996), in a
survey of over 1,000 physicians in California, found that African American and Hispanic physicians were five and two times more likely, respectively, than their white peers to practice in communities with high proportions of African American and Hispanic residents. Over half of the patients
seen by African American and Hispanic physicians, on average, were members of these clinicians' racial or ethnic group. Hispanic and black physicians tended to practice in areas with fewer primary care physicians per
capita, but even after adjustment for the proportion of minority residents
in the communities studied, African American and Hispanic physicians
were more likely to care for African American and Hispanic patients,
respectively. Similarly, Cantor et al. (1996) found that minority and women
physicians, as well as those from lower socioeconomic backgrounds, were
disproportionately more likely to serve minority, low-income, and Medicaid populations, even after adjustment for physician specialty, practice
setting, and practice location.

Racial and ethnic minority dentists are also more likely than their white
peers to practice in racial and ethnic minority communities. Solomon, Williams, and Sinkford (2001), in a study of African American and white
dentists in Texas, found that a larger percentage of African American dentists practiced in communities with a high residential African American
population than white dentists. African American dentists were also found

to be more likely to practice in communities characterized by lower levels of education and income than white dentists. Similarly, Mertz and Grumbach (2001), in an assessment of the availability of dental services in California, found that approximately one in five California communities—disproportionately minority, low-income, and rural—have a shortage of dentists and that minority dentists were more likely to practice in minority communities.

Diversity and Minority Patient Choice and Satisfaction

Minority patients who have a choice are more likely to select clinicians of their own racial or ethnic background. Lopez, Lopez, and Fong (1991), for example, in a study of Mexican-American college students, found that these students expressed a clear preference for ethnically similar mental health counselors or psychotherapists. These findings held among both men and women and among those who had and had not sought counseling. Similarly, Bichsel and Mallinckrodt (2001) surveyed a sample of American Indian women living in the Warm Spring (Oregon) Reservation regarding preferences for mental health counseling and found that respondents expressed preferences for female, ethnically similar counselors who understand and are sensitive to the respondents' culture.

Saha et al. (2000) investigated whether minority patients tend to see physicians of their own race because of convenience (e.g., location) or as a matter of choice. Using data from a national survey of heath-care consumers, the authors found that African American and Hispanic patients who had a choice of clinician were more likely to choose a physician of their own race or ethnicity. Among Hispanic patients, over 40 percent responded that the physician's ability to speak the patient's language was a significant consideration in choosing a physician. These associations remained even after controlling for the physician's office location (e.g., location in a predominantly minority neighborhood).

In light of these findings, it is not surprising that racial and ethnic minority patients are generally more satisfied with the care that they receive from minority physicians. Saha et al. (1999), for example, found that African American patients who receive care from physicians of the same race were more likely than African Americans with nonminority clinicians to rate their physicians as excellent in providing health care, in treating them with respect, in explaining their medical problems, in listening to their concerns, and in being accessible. In addition, the investigators found that although Hispanic patients who received care from Hispanic physicians did not rate their doctors as significantly better than Hispanic patients with non-Hispanic health-care clinicians, patients with an ethnically concordant provider were more likely to be satisfied with their overall health care.

Similarly, Cooper-Patrick and her colleagues (1999) found that minority patients' ratings of the quality of their health care were generally higher in racially and ethnically concordant than racially and ethnically discordant settings. Using a measure of physicians' participatory decision-making style, Cooper-Patrick surveyed over 1,800 adults who were seen in 1 of 32 primary care settings by physicians who were either African American (25 percent of the physician sample), white (56 percent), Asian American, (15 percent), or Latino (3 percent). Overall, African American patients rated their visits as significantly less participatory than whites, after adjusting for patient age, gender, education, marital status, health status, and length of the patient–physician relationship. Patients in race- and ethnic-concordant relationships, however, rated their visits as significantly more participatory than patients in race- and ethnic-discordant relationships. In addition, Cooper and Roter have found, through independent ratings of videotaped clinical encounters, that physician visits by African American patients were longer, were characterized by less physician dominance of the discussion, and were more patient-centered when the physician was African American than when the physician was white (Cooper and Roter, 2003).

Similarly, LaVeist and Nuru-Jeter (2002) examined predictors of racial concordance between patient and clinician and the effect of race concordance on satisfaction among a sample of white, African American, and Hispanic patients. Among all racial and ethnic groups, patients who reported having at least some choice in selecting a physician were more likely to have a race- or ethnic-concordant physician. Having a race-concordant physician was also associated with higher income for African Americans and not speaking English as a primary language among Hispanics. After adjusting for patients' age, sex, marital status, income, health insurance status, and whether the respondent reported having a choice in physician, African American patients in race-concordant relationships were found to report higher satisfaction than those African Americans in race-discordant relationships. Furthermore, Hispanic patients in ethnic-concordant relationships reported greater satisfaction than patients from other racial and ethnic groups in similarly concordant relationships.

Diversity and Quality of Health Care for Minority Populations

Racial and ethnic minorities tend to receive a lower quality of health care than nonminorities. Much of this disparity may be explained by the overrepresentation of some minority groups among the uninsured, given that uninsured and underinsured individuals face greater difficulties in accessing care and are less likely to receive needed services. Yet a large body of research demonstrates that even when insured at the same levels as whites, minority patients receive fewer clinical services and receive a lower quality of care (Institute of Medicine, 2003a). This disparity is apparent across a range of disease areas (e.g., diabetes, cancer, HIV/AIDS) and clinical services, and in a range of clinical settings (e.g., teaching and non-teaching hospitals, public and private clinics). At least some of these disparities may result from aspects of the clinical encounter and attitudes, both conscious and unconscious, of health-care clinicians (Institute of Medicine, 2003a), raising the question of whether greater diversity among health-care professionals may help to mitigate health-care disparities.

While no direct link has been established as yet between diversity among health-care clinicians and health outcomes for patients, research indicates that health-care processes and outcomes are influenced by cultural and linguistic barriers that minority clinicians are sometimes able to address. Perez-Stable, Napoles-Springer, and Miramontes (1997), for example, assessed the effects of ethnicity and language concordance between patients and their physicians on health outcomes, use of health services, and clinical outcomes among a sample of Spanish-speaking and non-Spanish-speaking Hispanic and non-Hispanic patients with hypertension or diabetes. Of the 74 Spanish-speaking Latinos, 60 percent were treated by clinicians who spoke Spanish, while 40 percent were treated by non-Spanish-speaking clinicians. After controlling for patient age, gender, education, number of medical problems, and number of prescribed medications, the authors found that having a language-concordant physician was associated with better patient self-reported physical functioning, psychological well-being, health perceptions, and lower pain.

In addition, as noted above, some research indicates that minority physicians display better process-of-care behaviors with minority patients than nonminority clinicians (Cooper-Patrick et al., 1999). Hispanic patients display better satisfaction and adherence to treatment plans when their physician not only speaks Spanish, but also shares the same cultural background (Perez-Stable et al., 1997). These "intermediate" outcomes may affect patients' health care outcomes, in that patient satisfaction is associated with greater patient compliance with treatment regimens, participation in treatment decisions, and use of preventive care services (Betancourt et al., 2002).

Diversity and Quality of Training for All Health Professionals

Racial and ethnic minority patients, when given a choice, tend to choose health-care clinicians from similar backgrounds, as noted above. But because the proportion of racial and ethnic minority health-care clinicians is low relative to the proportion of racial and ethnic minorities in the general population (see below), it is clear that all health-care professionals must develop the skills and competencies to serve diverse patient populations. Diversity in health professions training settings may therefore assist in efforts to improve the cross-cultural training and cultural competencies of *all* trainees. Students from diverse background interacting with each other in training settings may help to challenge assumptions and broaden students' perspectives regarding racial, ethnic, and cultural differences (Whitla et al., 2003; Cohen, 2003). Whitla and colleagues (2003), for example, in a survey of medical school graduates' attitudes regarding diversity in medical education, found that students reported experiencing greater levels of diversity in medical school than in their prior educational experiences, as the percentage of students reporting contact with other groups increased from 50 percent prior to college to 85 percent in medical school. Overwhelmingly, these students viewed diversity among their medical student peers as a positive; 86 percent thought that classroom diversity enhanced discussion and was more likely to foster serious discussions of alternate viewpoints. Over three-quarters of the students surveyed found that diversity helped them to rethink their viewpoints when racial and ethnic conflicts occurred, and the same percentage felt that diversity provided them with a greater understanding of medical conditions and treatments. The pattern of responses did not differ by respondents' racial or ethnic group (Whitla et al., 2003).

In addition, diversity among students in training settings may enrich classroom discussions and spur changes in curriculums to address students' cross-cultural education needs. There is growing evidence—primarily from studies of college students' undergraduate experiences—that student diversity is associated with greater gains in students' learning and community involvement (e.g., Gurin et al., 2002; Antonio et al., in press). Gurin and colleagues, for example, utilized data from longitudinal surveys of undergraduate students to assess whether students' diversity experiences as undergraduates were related to their "learning outcomes" (defined as the use of active thinking, intellectual engagement and motivation, and academic skills) and "democracy outcomes" (i.e., citizenship engagement, belief in the compatibility of group differences and democracy, the ability to take the perspective of others, and cultural awareness and engagement). The investigators found that diversity experiences were significantly related to learning outcomes after graduation, even after adjusting for students' academic and socioeconomic background (i.e., gender, SAT scores, high school grades, parents' educational level, racial composition of high school and neighborhood growing up), institutional characteristics, and initial (pretest) scores on learning outcome measures. Informal interactions across racial and ethnic lines were especially significant for all racial/ethnic groups in predicting intellectual engagement and academic skills. Similarly, diversity experiences were found to significantly predict students' democracy outcomes, even after adjustment for students' prior academic and socioeconomic background and pre-college racial exposure, as well as measures of democracy orientation upon initial assessment. For all racial groups, informal interactions across racial and ethnic lines were associated with higher levels of citizenship engagement and awareness and appreciation of racial and cultural diversity (Gurin et al., 2002).

These studies suggest that students' classroom experiences and personal growth are enhanced by the presence of a diverse campus community. These benefits are explored in greater detail in Chapter 5, "Transforming the Institutional Climate for Diversity."

Diversity and Research on Racial and Ethnic Minority Health Disparities

Diversity among health professionals may improve scientific understanding of the causes and consequences of racial and ethnic health disparities and may help to eliminate these gaps. Minority scientists and researchers bring a wide range of cultural perspectives and experiences to research teams, which increases the likelihood that sociocultural issues influencing health outcomes will be addressed in research design and study questions (Institute of Medicine, 1999). In turn, a greater examination of health status and health risks among some racial and ethnic minorities will likely yield information that may prove helpful to improve health outcomes among *all* racial and ethnic groups. For example, public health scholars and epidemiologists have noted that some racial and ethnic minorities experience better health status than the majority population, despite relatively less advantaged environmental and socioeconomic circumstances (e.g., the "epidemiologic paradox" of better health status among new immigrant Latino populations, relative to second- and third-generation Latinos living in the United States), suggesting that these groups possess culturally determined coping styles, social supports, or health attitudes and behaviors that may reduce risks for poor health (Institute of Medicine, 1999).

Minority investigators may also prove valuable in efforts to increase the enrollment of minority patients in clinical trials. Minority participation in clinical research as human subjects is typically lower than among non-minority populations, even though some minorities experience higher rates of chronic and infectious diseases than whites. Low participation rates among minorities may be traced to a variety of historic and cultural factors (e.g., the legacy of abuse and mistreatment of minorities at the hands of the scientific and medical establishment, as exemplified in the infamous Tuskegee syphilis experiment). Yet more minorities are needed to participate in clinical research to better understand how to improve the health of these populations and close the health gap. As a result of their generally broader cross-cultural experiences, minority investigators are often able to address minority patient mistrust and improve communication between the scientific and lay communities (Institute of Medicine, 1999).

Equally important, minority scientists and researchers, because of their personal experiences and interests, are more likely to study health needs of minority and underserved populations. As Jordan Cohen has noted,

> Our country's research agenda is influenced significantly by those who choose careers in investigation. It is also true that individual investigators tend to research problems that they see and feel. Since what people see as problems depends greatly on their particular cultural and ethnic filters, it follows that finding solutions to some of our country's most recalcitrant heath problems, even being able to conceptualize what the real problems actually are, will require a research workforce that is much more diverse racially and ethnically than we now have (Cohen, 2003, p. 1144).

The nation's premiere health research institution, the National Institutes of Health, has recognized the need for greater racial/ethnic diversity among health researchers and offers a number of grant programs to enhance the career development of minority health researchers.

Diversity and Health Policy and Health Research Leadership

Racial and ethnic diversity in health professions is also critical to enhance the representation of minority groups among the leadership in the health policy and health research enterprises. Racial and ethnic minority health professionals are often able to bring diverse and underrepresented perspectives to both health policy and health systems leadership, which may lead to organizational and programmatic changes that can improve the accessibility and cultural competence of health systems. Diversity in health systems leadership should not, however, be assumed to (in and of itself) lead to more culturally competent health systems; such diversity merely increases the likelihood that broader systems change will include and be guided by diverse perspectives.

Similarly, URM representation among health research policy leadership is important to broaden and improve the nation's health research agenda. Minority researchers often bring a sensitivity to and understanding of minority health concerns that can significantly influence the design and interpretation of minority health research. This sensitivity can also significantly influence decisions regarding resource allocation and research priorities, particularly with regard to the priorities of the nation's leading health research agency, the National Institutes of Health (NIH). Many NIH scientific advisory boards and councils lack significant racial and ethnic diversity

(Institute of Medicine, 1999), which NIH has attempted to address by identifying URM health researchers, policy analysts, and others who might be willing to serve in advisory capacities. Analogously, women's health research has grown exponentially and has benefited from the increased presence of women among health researchers and policy makers. As a result, scientific knowledge of women's health (and subsequent break-throughs in the understanding and treatment of women's health concerns) has improved dramatically over the past several decades. As above, this is not to suggest that women and minority scientists and clinicians should be expected to work exclusively in women's and minority health domains; rather, it suggests that gender and racial/ethnic diversity in the health re-search enterprise can lead to important development and expansion of these fields.

Diversity and Quality of Care for All Americans

While few empirical data bear directly upon the question, indirect evidence suggests that diversity among health professionals may bring fresh approaches to health care and new problem-solving skills that can enrich and improve health care for *all* Americans. Anecdotal evidence suggests that the skills and resources of many diverse groups can help to address the nation's health-care needs. Scientists and clinicians of color have contributed to many medical breakthroughs (e.g., Dr. Daniel Hale Williams, the African American physician credited with performing the first successful surgical repair of a heart wound; Dr. Charles R. Drew, the African American physician responsible for organizing the concept of the Blood Bank; Organ and Kosiba, 1987). As the U.S. Surgeon General's report on mental health, culture, and diversity notes, "Diversity has enriched our Nation by bringing global ideas, perspectives, and productive contributions to all areas of contemporary life" (U.S. Surgeon General, 2001).

TRENDS IN MINORITY PARTICIPATION IN NURSING, MEDICINE, DENTISTRY, AND PROFESSIONAL PSYCHOLOGY— WHERE ARE THE GAPS?

While the need for and benefits of a racially and ethnically diverse workforce are clear, nursing, medicine, dentistry, and psychology have yet to reflect the diversity of the nation among their clinicians, faculty, and students. Given the changing demographic composition of the United States and current trends in minority underrepresentation in the health-care workforce, the health professions appear to be in sharp contrast with broader population changes in the country. This section will review, where the data exist, a demographic profile of clinicians, faculty, and health professions students.[6] In this section, "URM" groups are defined as African Americans, American Indians and Alaska Natives, and Latinos, because most data collection efforts until recently used this definition. This is consistent with definitions used by AAMC prior to announcing its new, broader definition of URM in June 2003.

Nurses

The Nursing Workforce

In recent years, the nursing profession has seen modest growth in the number of underrepresented racial and ethnic minorities entering its ranks. Findings from the National Sample Survey of Registered Nurses (HRSA, 2002) indicate that the percentage of minority nurses increased from 7 percent in 1980 to 12 percent in 2000. These data must be interpreted with caution, however, because of a change in questionnaire construction in 2000 to reflect revisions in the Office of Management and Budget's (OMB) designated racial and ethnic categories. While the percentage of minority nurses increased, this percentage is still far below the minority representation in the population, which is approximately 30 percent (see Figure 1-1).

Rates of growth in the registered nurse (RN) workforce vary among racial and ethnic groups. Between 1977 and 1997, the percentage of African Americans among the nursing workforce increased from 2.6 to 4.2 percent, a 62 percent increase, while the representation of Hispanic RNs increased by 1.4 percent to 1.6 percent during the same period (a 17 percent increase; Buerhaus and Auerbach, 1999). During this same period, all "other ethnic groups"—including Asian Americans, Pacific Islanders, American Indians and Alaska Natives—increased among the RN workforce by over one-third (Buerhaus and Auerbach, 1999).

Despite these modest gains in URM representation among nurses, the nursing profession faces a critical shortage of nurses that threatens to impair the quality of care in many health-care settings (Kimball and O'Neil, 2002). In 2000, the estimated shortage of full-time equivalent RNs was

---

[6]Data on minority underrepresentation in health professions are inconsistent across health disciplines. In general, more published information is available regarding minority underrepresentation in medicine than in other health profession disciplines, a disparity that should be corrected in future research. This report therefore provides more information regarding URM participation in medicine than in other fields but attempts to cite, where available, comparable data on the racial and ethnic underrepresentation for all four health professions studied here.

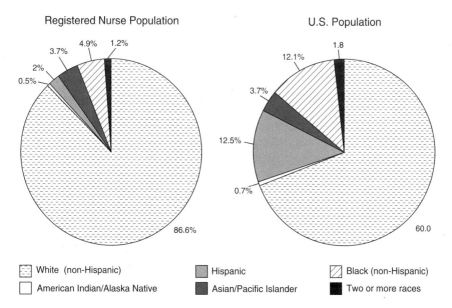

FIGURE 1-1 Distribution of registered nurses by racial/ethnic background: March 2000.
SOURCE: HRSA, 2002.

110,000, or 6 percent of the workforce. An initial slow rate of growth of this shortage is anticipated, reaching 12 percent of the workforce by 2010. At that point, the shortage will grow at an accelerated rate, reaching 20 percent by 2015. If trends continue and the problem remains unaddressed, the shortage will grow to 29 percent by 2020. Not unexpectedly—given their underrepresentation in the current nursing workforce—the shortage of minority nurses will be particularly difficult to address; an increase of more than 20,000 minority nurses is needed to increase the proportion of minority nurses by just 1 percent (National Advisory Council on Nurse Education and Practice, 2000).

The increased demand for nurses will be caused by increases in the population, growth of the elderly population, and medical advances that increase the need for nurses. The supply of potential nurses is affected by a decrease in the number of nursing graduates, decrease in relative earnings for nurses, aging of the workforce, and new and alternative job opportunities for nurses (HRSA, 2002). The shortage of nurses may have implications for patient safety in terms of hospital deaths and injuries and increased costs (through replacing nurses lost through turnover and caring for patients with poor outcomes (Institute of Medicine, 2003b).

URM *Participation in Nursing Education*

Among recent nursing graduates (those whose degrees were awarded in 2002), white nurses constituted the largest percentage of graduates in baccalaureate, associate, diploma, and RN programs, earning between 60–70 percent of diploma, associate, basic B.S.N., and all basic RN degrees (National League for Nursing, 2003) (Figure 1-2). Among minorities, African American and those nurses who classified their ethnicity as "other" received the largest percentage of degrees. More African American nurses received nursing diplomas than nursing degrees (B.S.N. and above). Less than 10 percent of degrees were awarded to Hispanic, Asian, and American Indian nurses.

Figure 1-3 presents enrollment trends for students in baccalaureate nursing programs (national annual data on other degree nursing programs were not available for all the years studied). URM enrollment has steadily increased between 1991 and 1999, increasing 48 percent from 11,661 to 17,303 baccalaureate nursing students.

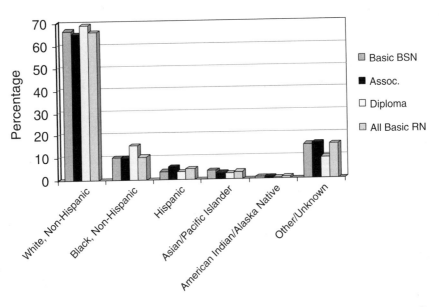

FIGURE 1-2 Estimated minority nursing graduations: baccalaureate, associate, diploma programs, 2001–2002 (preliminary and unpublished data).
SOURCE: National League for Nursing (2003). Figure included, with permission, from the National League for Nursing, New York, NY. Copyright 2004 by NLN.

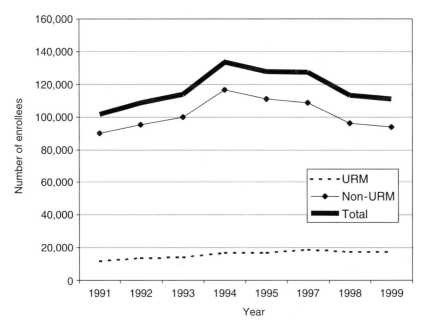

FIGURE 1-3 Enrollment in U.S. baccalaureate nursing programs.
SOURCE: Grumbach et al., 2001.

Both URM and non-URM enrollment in baccalaureate programs began to decline in the mid-1990s, although non-URM enrollment declined more sharply.

Nursing Faculty

Nursing faculty, like the broader population of nurses, does not reflect the nation's diversity (Figure 1-4). Data indicate geographic variations in faculty diversity, as the largest percentage of African American nursing faculty are represented among faculty in the south (nearly 10 percent). In addition, there are slightly more American Indian nursing faculty in the Midwest region of the country, while the representation of Asian American nursing faculty is only slightly larger in the West than in the rest of the nation (National League for Nursing, 2002). While minorities are starkly underrepresented among nursing faculty, opportunities to increase the presence of racial and ethnic minority nursing faculty may increase in the near future, as their will be a significant need to replace the current nursing faculty, whose average age is 51.2 years (American Association of Colleges of Nursing, 2003).

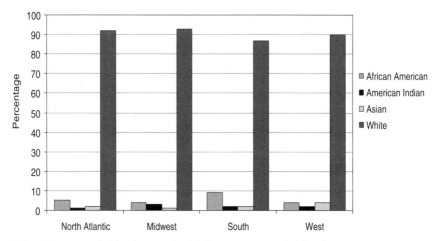

FIGURE 1-4 Racial background of full-time nursing faculty by region, 2002.
SOURCE: National League for Nursing (2003). Reproduced, with permission, from
the National League for Nursing, New York, NY. Copyright 2004 by NLN.

Physicians

URM Representation in the Physician Workforce

African Americans, Latinos, and American Indians, and Alaska Natives
are underrepresented among United States physicians (Figure 1-5), as these
groups constitute less than 8 percent of the physician population. Of these,
Hispanics/Latinos are the largest URM group, constituting approximately
3.5 percent of the physician population, followed by African Americans,
who represent approximately 2.6 percent of physicians. The majority of
United States physicians are white, a percentage that has slowly declined
over the past several decades.

URM Representation Among Medical School Faculty

URM representation among medical school faculty increased between
1980 and 2001, as the percentage of URM faculty increased while the
percentage of white faculty declined slightly (Figure 1-6; AAMC, 2002).
Whites, however, remain disproportionately the largest racial or ethnic
group among medical school faculty, composing just less than four of five
medical school faculties in 2001. The number of full-time clinical and non-
clinical URM faculty increased from 1,140 to 4,060 between 1981 and
2001, although they represent only 4.2 percent of current medical school

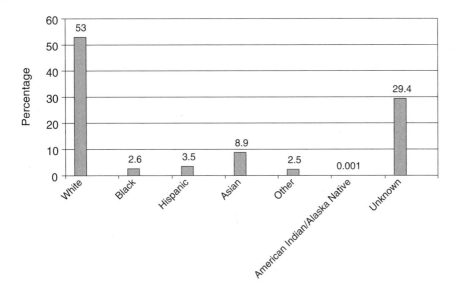

FIGURE 1-5 Total physicians by race/ethnicity, 2000.
SOURCE: AMA, *Physician Characteristics and Distribution in the US 2002–2003.*

faculties. Approximately 20 percent of these URM faculty members are located at Howard University School of Medicine, Meharry Medical College, Morehouse School of Medicine, and three Puerto Rican medical schools (Universidad Central del Caribe School of Medicine, Ponce School of Medicine, and the University of Puerto Rico School of Medicine).

In recent years, significant progress has been made in increasing the presence of URM faculty at many nonminority medical schools, while at other institutions their presence remains rare. Overall, the percentage of URM faculty has more than tripled in the past 20 years. In 1981, the majority of medical schools (82 of 111) had between one and nine URM faculty members and none had more than 39. In 2001, 22 (out of 112) schools had more than 40 URM faculty members, yet 27 had between one and nine URM faculty. There are still few schools that have a "critical mass" of URM faculty (AAMC, 2002).

URM Participation in Medical Education

Among medical students and recent graduates of medical schools, URM student enrollment and graduation rates generally show steady increases through the early and mid-1990s, followed by declines. URM students

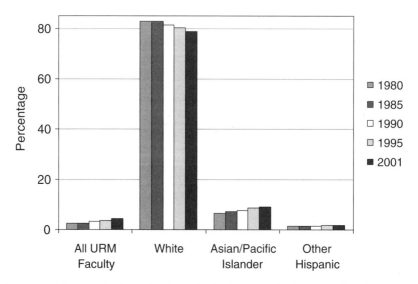

FIGURE 1-6 Distribution of U.S. medical school faculty by race/ethnicity, 1980 to 2001.
SOURCE: AAMC Faculty Roster System, December 2001. Reprinted, with permission, from the Association of American Medical Colleges, 2004. Copyright 2004 by AAMC.

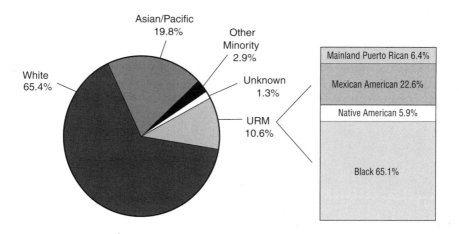

FIGURE 1-7 U.S. medical school graduates, 2001.
SOURCE: AAMC Student Record System, April 2002. Reprinted, with permission, from the Association of American Medical Colleges, 2004. Copyright 2004 by AAMC.

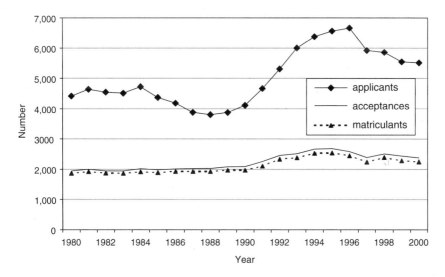

FIGURE 1-8 Allopathic medical school URM application, acceptance, and matriculation trends.
SOURCE: Grumbach et al., 2001.

constituted approximately 10 percent of medical graduates in 2001 (Figure 1-7; AAMC, 2002). The majority of these URM students (65 percent) were African American, with smaller percentages of Mexican American students (22.6 percent), mainland Puerto Ricans (6.4 percent), and Native Americans (5.9 percent). Trends from 1980 to 2001 revealed an increase in the number of URM graduates until 1998, with a gradual decline since that year. Trends in URM medical school applicants indicate an increase from the late 1980s to the mid-1990s (Figure 1-8). Since 1996–1997, there has been a steady decline. There were 6,663 URM applicants in 1996. By 2000, the number of applicants decreased to 5,511, which represents a 17 percent decrease. The decline in applicants corresponds to a decline in the number of acceptances and matriculants during the same period of time.

Dentists

URM Participation in the Dental Workforce

As in nursing and medicine, racial and ethnic minorities in dentistry are underrepresented compared to their proportions in the general population. Approximately 13 percent of dentists are nonwhite (Mertz and O'Neil, 2002), and African Americans, American Indians, and Hispanics constitute only 6.8 percent of the dental workforce (see Figure 1-9).

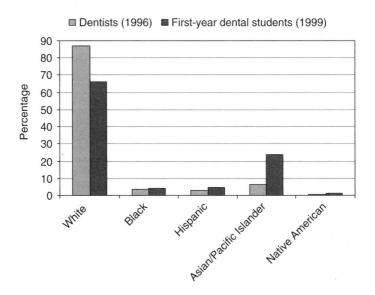

FIGURE 1-9 Variations in racial/ethnic representation in dentistry, 1996–1999. SOURCE: Valachovic et al., 2001. Reprinted, with permission, from the American Dental Education Association, 2004. Copyright 2004 by ADEA.

URM Participation in Dental Education

Among first-year dental students in 1999, 34 percent were nonwhite. Of this percentage, however, less than one-third (10.2 percent of the total student enrollment) were from URM groups. As in medicine, the number of URM matriculants in dentistry has declined in recent years. Matriculants dropped by 23 percent: from 525 in 1989 to 404 in 1999 (Figure 1-10). Other figures indicate a slight increase in the percent of URM graduates since 1999 (Figure 1-11).

URM Participation Among Dental School Faculty

Trends in the percentage of minority full-time faculty indicate that the number of URM faculty remained low and relatively stable during the 1990s (Figure 1-12). Between 1990 and 1998, the percentage of Native American faculty increased very slightly, from 0.3 percent to 0.6 percent. The percentage of African American faculty hovered around 5 percent during these 8 years and the percentage of Hispanic faculty remained stable at approximately 3 percent.

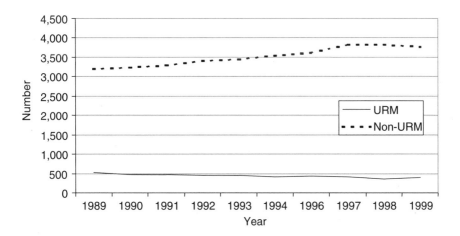

FIGURE 1-10 Dental school matriculants.
SOURCE: Grumbach et al., 2001.

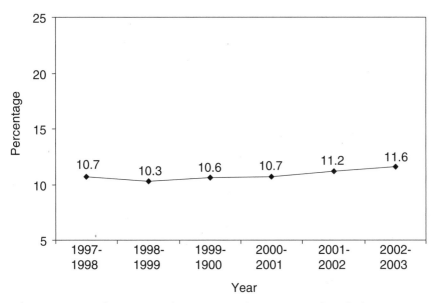

FIGURE 1-11 Underrepresented minority graduates in U.S. dental education programs: Black, Hispanic, Native American.
SOURCE: Total Minority Enrollment in U.S. Dental Education Programs, 1997–2003. American Dental Association Survey Center, Surveys of Predoctoral Dental Education. Reprinted, with permission, from American Dental Association, 2004. Copyright 2004 by ADA.

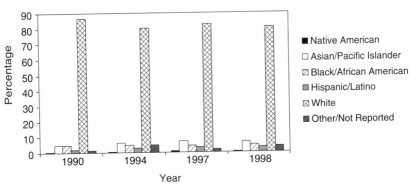

FIGURE 1-12 Minority full-time faculty in U.S. dental schools.
SOURCE: Haden et al., 2000. Reprinted, with permission, from the American
Dental Education Association, 2004. Copyright 2004 by ADEA.

Psychologists

URM Participation in the Psychology Workforce

Minority representation in the field of psychology is disproportionately low (Figure 1-13; Rapopor et al., 2000). Among all psychologists, 3.4 percent are African American, 3.4 percent are Hispanic, and 2.2 are Asian/Pacific Islander. The percentage of American Indian/Alaska Native psychologists is less than 1 percent.

URM Participation among Psychology Faculty

URMs are similarly underrepresented among faculty in departments of psychology (Figure 1-14). Among full professors, 94.1 percent are white, 1.7 percent are Asian, 2 percent are Hispanic, 1.9 percent are African American, and 0.3 percent are American Indian. Among all tenured professors, 2.5 percent are African American, 2.3 percent Hispanic, and 0.3 percent American Indian. However, URM faculty have slightly higher representation among tenure track professors (5.1 percent black, 4.6 percent Hispanic, and 0.9 percent American Indian).

URM Participation in Psychology Graduate Education

The percentage of URM graduate students in departments of psychology is greater than percentage of URM faculty. During the 2002–2003 academic year, 7 percent of first-year students in programs that offered a Ph.D. were African American, 6 percent were Hispanic, 1 percent were

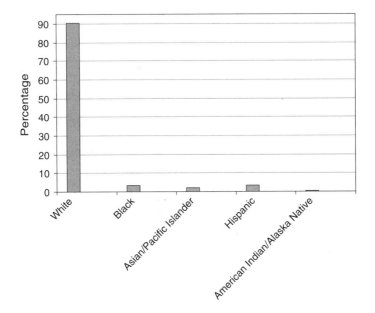

FIGURE 1-13 Employed doctoral psychologists (percent), 2001.
SOURCE: National Science Foundation/Division of Science Resources Statistics, 2001 Survey of Doctorate Recipients.

Native American, and 1 percent classified themselves as multiracial (Figure 1-15). Among 2000 graduates from clinical psychology programs, the largest subfield of practitioners, 5 percent were African American, 7 percent were Hispanic, and less than 1 percent were Native American.

SUMMARY

African Americans, American Indians and Alaska Natives, and many Hispanic/Latino populations are grossly underrepresented among the nation's physicians, nurses, dentists, and psychologists. These populations also experience generally poorer health status and face greater difficulties in accessing health care. Consequently, many health professions leaders have called for an expansion of efforts to increase diversity among health-care professionals as one means of assisting in the effort to increase access to health care for all populations and to close the health gap between minorities and nonminorities.

Recent policy developments, however, have had and may continue to have a significant negative impact on the ability of health professions train-

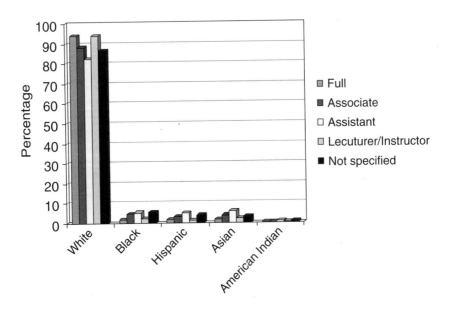

FIGURE 1-14 Academic rank of faculty in departments of psychology by race/ethnicity, 2002–2003.
SOURCE: Faculty Salary Survey, 2002–2003. Academic Rank and Tenure Status of Faculty in Graduate Departments of Psychology by Race/Ethnicity, 2002–2003. Reprinted, with permission, from the American Psychological Association, 2004. Copyright 2004 by APA.

ing programs and higher education institutions to admit URM students into the health professions training pipeline. The U.S. Supreme Court decision in the *Grutter v. Bollinger* lawsuit reaffirmed that higher education institutions may consider applicants' race or ethnicity as one of many factors in admissions decisions. But as a result of public referenda, judicial decisions, and lawsuits challenging affirmative action policies in 1995, 1996, and 1997, many higher education institutions abandoned (in some cases, temporarily) the use of race and ethnicity as factors in admissions decisions. To add to this challenge, significant financial disparities persist between minority and nonminority students, leaving many URM students with fewer financial resources to pursue careers in health professions. It is therefore important to assess whether opportunities exist at the level of higher education institutions, health professions leadership and accrediting bodies, and state and federal policy to reduce barriers to minority participation in health professions.

This chapter has presented a review of evidence regarding the impor-

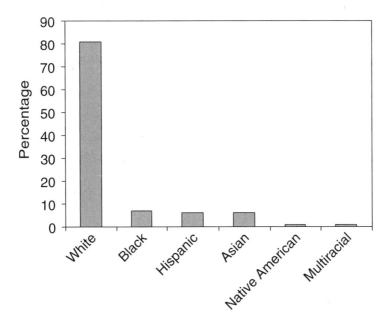

FIGURE 1-15 Race/ethnicity of newly enrolled students in doctoral departments of psychology, 2002–2003.
SOURCE: Graduate Study in Psychology, 2004. Compiled by APA Research Office. Reprinted, with permission, from the American Psychological Association, 2004. Copyright 2004 by APA.

tance of diversity in health professions. This evidence demonstrates that greater diversity among health professionals is associated with improved access to care for racial and ethnic minority patients, greater patient choice and satisfaction, and better patient–clinician communication. Indirectly, this evidence suggests that greater diversity can improve the cultural competence of health professionals and health systems and that such improvements may be associated with better health-care outcomes. In addition, greater diversity among health professionals has the potential to improve the clinical research enterprise and to lead to new developments and improvements in health care and how care is delivered.

Subsequent chapters of this report will explore the potential value of specific institutional and policy-level strategies to increase diversity in the health professions. These strategies include efforts to reconceptualize admissions procedures for health professions education programs, to improve public and private financing of health professions education, to place greater emphasis on faculty and student diversity in program accreditation standards, and to improve the campus climate for diversity. Finally, the study committee considers the potential application of community benefit principles to improve the accountability of nonprofit, tax-exempt institutions to the diverse racial and ethnic communities they serve.

REFERENCES

American Association of Colleges of Nursing. 2003. *AACN's Nursing Faculty Shortage Fact Sheet.* [Online]. Available: http://www.aacn.nche.edu/Media/Backgrounders/facultyshortage.htm [accessed January 16, 2004].
American Medical Association (AMA). 2003. *Physician Characteristics and Distribution in the US, 2002-2003.* Chicago: American Medical Association.
Anderson LM, Scrimshaw SC, Fullilove MT, Fielding JE, Normand J. 2002. Culturally competent healthcare systems: A systematic review. *American Journal of Preventive Medicine* 24(3 Suppl):68–79.
Antonio AL, Chang MJ, Hakuta K, Kenny DA, Levin SL, Milem JF. In press. Effects of racial diversity on complex thinking in college students. *Psychological Science.*
Association of American Medical Colleges (AAMC). 2002. *Minority Students in Medical Education: Facts and Figures XII.* Washington, DC: Association of American Medical Colleges.
Betancourt JR, Green AR, Carrillo JE. 2002. *Cultural Competence in Health Care: Emerging Frameworks and Practical Approaches.* New York: The Commonwealth Fund.
Bichsel RJ, Mallinckrodt B. 2001. Cultural commitment and the counseling preferences and counselor perceptions of Native American women. *The Counseling Psychologist* 29(6): 858–881.
Buerhaus PI, Auerbach D. 1999. Slow growth in the United States of the number of minorities in RN workforce. *Journal of Nursing Scholarship* 31(2):179–183.
Cantor JC, Bergeisen L, Baker L. 1998. Effect of intensive educational program for minority college students and recent graduates on the probability of acceptance into medical school. *Journal of the American Medical Association* 280:772–776.
Cantor JC, Miles EL, Baker LC, Barker DC. 1996. Physician service to the underserved: Implications for affirmative action in medical education. *Inquiry* 33:167–181.
Cohen JJ. 2003. The consequences of premature abandonment of affirmative action in medical school admissions. *Journal of the American Medical Association* 289(9):1143–1149.
Collins KS, Hall A, Neuhaus C. 1999. *U.S. Minority Health: A Chartbook.* New York: The Commonwealth Fund.
Cooper L, Roter D. 2003. Patient–provider communication: The effect of race and ethnicity on process and outcomes of health care. In: Smedley BD, Stith AY, Nelson AR, eds. *Unequal Treatment: Confronting Racial and Ethnic Disparities in Health Care.* Washington, DC: The National Academies Press.
Cooper-Patrick L, Gallo JJ, Gonzales JJ, Vu HT, Powe NR, Nelson C, Ford DE. 1999. Race, gender, and partnership in the patient–physician relationship. *Journal of the American Medical Association* 282(6):583–589.
Grumbach K, Coffman J, Rosenoff E, Muñoz C. 2001. Trends in underrepresented minority participation in health professions schools. In: Smedley BD, Stith AY, Colburn L, Evans CH, eds. *The Right Thing to Do, The Smart Thing to Do: Enhancing Diversity in the Health Professions.* Washington, DC: National Academy Press.
Gurin P, Dey EL, Hurtado S, Gurin G. 2002. Diversity and higher education: Theory and impact on educational outcomes. *Harvard Education Review* 72(3):330–366.

Haden NK, Beemsterboer PL, Weaver RG, Valachovic RW. 2002. Dental school faculty shortages increase: An update on future dental school faculty. *Journal of Dental Education* 64(9):666–682.

Health Resources and Services Administration (HRSA). 2002. *Projected Supply, Demand, and Shortages of Registered Nurses: 2000–2020.* [Online]. Available: http://bhpr.hrsa. gov/healthworkforce/rnproject/default.htm [accessed December 2, 2003].

Institute of Medicine (IOM). 1999. *The Unequal Burden of Cancer: An Assessment of NIH Programs and Research for Minorities and the Medically Underserved.* Haynes AM, Smedley BD, eds. Washington, DC: National Academy Press.

Institute of Medicine (IOM). 2001. *Crossing the Quality Chasm: A New Health System for the 21st Century.* Washington, DC: National Academy Press.

Institute of Medicine (IOM). 2003a. *Unequal Treatment: Confronting Racial and Ethnic Disparities in Healthcare.* Smedley BD, Stith AY, Nelson AR, eds. Washington, DC: The National Academies Press.

Institute of Medicine (IOM). 2003b. *Keeping Patients Safe: Transforming the Work Environment of Nurses.* Page A, ed. Washington, DC: The National Academies Press.

Kaiser Daily Health Policy Report. 2003. California seniors who are Latino or have limited English language skills more likely to report being in fair or poor health, study says. [Online]. Available: www.kaisernetwork.org/daily_reports [accessed October 31, 2003].

Kimball B, O'Neil E. 2002. *Health Care's Human Crisis: The American Nursing Shortage.* Princeton, NJ: The Robert Wood Johnson Foundation. [Online]. Available: http://www.rwjf.org/news/special/nursing_report.pdf [accessed January 16, 2004].

Komaromy M, Grumbach K, Drake M, Vranizan K, Lurie N, Keane D, Bindman AB. 1996. The role of black and Hispanic physicians in providing health care for underserved populations. *New England Journal of Medicine* 334(20):1305–1310.

LaVeist TA, Nuru-Jeter A. 2002. Is doctor–patient race concordance associated with greater satisfaction with care? *Journal of Health and Social Behavior* 43(3):296–306.

Lopez SR, Lopez AA, Fong KT. 1991. Mexican Americans' initial preferences for counselors: The role of ethnic factors. *Journal of Counseling Psychology* 38(4):487–496.

Matherlee K. This volume. The role of public financing in improving diversity in the health professions. In Smedley BD, Stith-Butler A, Bristow LR, eds. *In the Nation's Compelling Interest: Ensuring Diversity in the Health-Care Workforce.* Washington, DC: The National Academies Press.

Mertz E, O'Neil E. 2002. The growing challenge of providing oral health care services to all Americans. *Health Affairs* 21(5):65–77.

Mertz EA, Grumbach K. 2001. Identifying communities with low dentist supply in California. *Journal of Public Health Dentistry* 61(3):172–177.

Moy E, Bartman A. 1995. Physician race and care of minority and medically indigent patients. *Journal of the American Medical Association* 273(19):1515–1520.

National Advisory Council on Nurse Education and Practice. 2000. *A National Agenda for Nursing Workforce Racial/Ethnic Diversity.* Report to the Secretary of Health and Human Services and Congress. Washington, DC: U.S. Department of Health and Human Services.

National League for Nursing 2003. *Nurse Educators 2002: Report of the Faculty Census Survey of RN and Graduate Programs.* New York: National League for Nursing.

Nettles MT, Millet CM. 2001. Toward diverse student representation and higher achievement in higher levels of the educational meritocracy. In: Smedley SB, Stith AY, Colburn L, Evans CH, eds. *The Right Thing to Do, The Smart Thing to Do: Enhancing Diversity in Health Professions.* Washington, DC: National Academy Press.

Organ CH, Kosiba MM. 1987. *A Century of Black Surgeons—The U.S.A. Experience.* Volume I. Norman, OK: Transcript Press.

Perez-Stable EJ, Napoles-Springer A, Miramontes JM. 1998. The effects of ethnicity and language on medical outcomes of patients with hypertension or diabetes. *Medical Care* 35(12):1212–1219.

Rapoport AI, Kohout J, Wicherski M. 2000. *Psychology doctorate recipients: How much financial debt at graduation?* Issue Brief: Division of Science Resources Studies, National Science Foundation. [Online]. Available: http://www.nsf.gov/sbe/srs/issuebrf/sib00321/ htm [accessed August 18, 2003].

Robert Wood Johnson Foundation. 2001. New survey shows language barriers causing many Spanish-speaking Latinos to skip care. [Online]. Available: www.rwjf.org/news [accessed January 26, 2003].

Saha S, Taggart S, Komaromy K, Bindman AB. 2000. Do patients choose physicians of their own race? *Health Affairs* 19(4):76–83.

Saha S, Komaromy, M, Koepsell TD, Bindman AB. 1999. Patient–physician racial concordance and the perceived quality and use of health care. *Archives of Internal Medicine* 159:997–1004.

Sinkford JC, Harrison S, Valachovic W. 2001. Underrepresented minority enrollment in U.S. dental schools—The challenge. *Journal of Dental Education* 65(6):564–570.

Solomon ES, Williams CR, Sinkford JC. 2001. Practice location characteristics of black dentists in Texas. *Journal of Dental Education* 65(6):571–574.

Turner CB, Turner BF. 1996. Who treats minorities? Cultural diversity in mental health. *Cultural Diversity in Mental Health* 2(3):175–182.

U.S. Bureau of the Census. 2003. Hispanic population reaches all-time high of 38.8 million, new Census Bureau estimates show. [Online]. Available: www.census.gov/press-release/ www/2003/cb03-100.html [accessed September 24, 2003].

U.S. Surgeon General. 2001. *Mental Health: Culture, Race, and Ethnicity. A Supplement to Mental Health: A Report of the Surgeon General.* Washington, DC: U.S. Department of Health and Human Services.

Valachovic RW, Weaver RG, Sinkford JC, Haden K. 2001. Trends in dentistry and dental education. *Journal of Dental Education* 65(6):539–561.

Whitla DK, Orfield G, Silen W, Teperow C, Howard C, Reede J. 2003. Educational benefits of diversity in medical school: A survey of students. *Academic Medicine* 78(5):460–466.

2

Reconceptualizing Admissions Policies and Practices

Health professions training programs' admissions policies and practices vary widely from discipline to discipline and from institution to institution. These variations are reflected in differences in entrance requirements, discipline-specific criteria, and institutional mission. Almost all, however, rely upon a combination of quantitative information (e.g., high school and/or collegiate grade point average, particularly in science courses, and standardized admissions test data) and qualitative information (e.g., applicants' personal characteristics, background, and motivation to enter health professions fields) to arrive at admissions decisions.

This chapter will explore commonly used admissions policies and practices and their impact upon racial and ethnic diversity in graduate health professions training programs, with particular attention to the role of high-stakes, standardized, norm-referenced tests (e.g., the MCAT, DAT, GRE) in the admissions process. In addition, the chapter reviews data regarding minority applicants' standardized test performance and explores how these tests are used in typical admissions processes. The benefits and limits of the use of these tests are also discussed. Alternative admissions models are then reviewed, and their implications for underrepresented minitory (URM) applicant success in the admissions process are explored. Throughout this discussion, the committee attempts to reconcile two objectives that have often been viewed as competing concerns, but which, as outlined in the introductory chapter, can be seen as complementary. How can health professions training programs reconceptualize admissions policies and practices to reduce barriers to URM participation in health professions, while at the same time adopting admission practices that more accurately reflect the desired skills and attributes needed by future health professionals? In other words, how can diversity and quality goals coexist in admissions practices?

The chapter will begin with a brief description of the history, intent, and purposes of standardized tests used in higher education admissions. Though the discussion in this chapter is intended to provide general recommendations applicable to admissions policies for all health professions, it must be noted that admissions policies and practices vary considerably among the health profession disciplines studied here. Nursing education, for example, operates in a very different context for admissions decisions, with varying levels of "selectivity" depending on the type of degree program. Admission to many masters degree and doctoral level nursing programs is highly competitive, but admission to registered nurse (RN) education at the college or vocational institutional level is far less competitive than the post-graduate, doctoral educational settings of nursing, medicine, dentistry, and psychology. Many community college nursing education applicants are accepted if they meet minimum criteria for completing required courses, and in many states, community colleges are oversubscribed, and eligible applicants are put on a waiting list or go through a lottery process to matriculate. Even for baccalaureate-level nursing programs, the process is less competitive than for the doctoral health professions programs in other fields. Most of the baccalaureate nursing programs, for example, are at state colleges and not at "elite" universities.

STANDARDIZED TESTS AND HIGHER EDUCATION ADMISSIONS

A Brief Background on Standardized Tests

Historically, standardized admissions tests emerged from the early work of psychometric psychologists who attempted to quantify human intelligence through a variety of testing and assessment tools. In the late nineteenth and early twentieth centuries, these efforts were driven in large part by Darwinian theories of individual variation and natural selection (McGaghie, 2002) but were often accompanied by explicitly racist and eugenicist ideology regarding the racial superiority of European descendants and inferiority of non-Europeans. Many of the leading test developers, such as Alfred Binet, E.L. Thorndike, and others, saw the broad use of intelligence tests as not only an efficient means of distinguishing between individuals of differing intellectual ability, but also as a scientific means of verifying the intellectual superiority of Caucasians and inferiority of non-Caucasian racial groups, in accordance with laws of natural selection (Gould, 1996).

Early efforts to develop achievement tests that could be administered in large groups led to their widespread use, particularly by the Army, which during World War I sought a means to identify promising officer candidates. The Army's Alpha and Beta tests served as early precursors of school-based intelligence and aptitude tests, which became broadly used in schools following the war. An early developer of the Army's tests, Carl Brigham, was commissioned by the College Board to develop a test that could be administered to high school students, and in 1926 Brigham experimentally administered the first Scholastic Aptitude Test (SAT) to 10,000 students. This test, modeled on the Army Alpha test, was soon adopted by several Ivy League colleges, which sought an efficient means to screen applicants and "expand opportunities throughout the country for students who did not come from the upper class" (Calvin, 2000, p. 24). By the beginning of World War II, the SAT became widely used by selective colleges and universities as part of the admissions process (National Research Council, 1999).

Following World War II, the demand for standardized admissions tests increased sharply as the number of applicants—fueled in part by expanded opportunities to attend college as a result of the GI Bill—rose (Wightman, 2003). Standardized tests scores were viewed as an efficient mechanism with which college admissions committees could assess the talent and skills of a growing applicant population (increasingly composed of individuals who were not part of the existing educated class) with which admissions officials were largely unfamiliar. Tests were therefore viewed by many, including college administrators, applicants, and the general public, as an opportunity to "open the doors of educational opportunity to a broad range of students . . . particularly . . . to the elite schools in the northeast" (Wightman, 2003, p. 2).

Health professions training programs also experienced needs for standardized tests to assist admissions decisions, given greater public demand for access to medical education and the wide range of academic preparation of applicants. In 1930 the first version of the Medical College Admissions Test (MCAT) (then called the Scholastic Aptitude Test for Medical School) was developed and implemented (Wightman, 2003). Its potential value in admissions was clear: given high rates of attrition among freshman medical students (chiefly for academic reasons), medical schools sought a means to predict success in medical education and avoid wasting student slots. With greater use of subsequent versions of the MCAT, national medical student attrition rates declined from 20 percent in 1925 to 7 percent in 1946 (McGaghie, 2002).

Admissions tests have evolved considerably since their early versions (the MCAT has undergone five substantive revisions; McGaghie, 2002), and in some cases reflect different purposes. The SAT, for example, was originally developed to assess general verbal and mathematical reasoning as a means of predicting applicants' aptitude to do college-level work. The

American College Test (ACT), which evolved primarily in the Midwestern United States, offered colleges a tool to assess students' explicit content knowledge and their ability to apply this knowledge in college. The ACT was therefore not only an admissions tool, but also offered a means of assisting students in course placement and academic planning (National Research Council, 1999). More recently, the SAT II (Scholastic Achievement Test) has been developed to assess content knowledge in academic subjects.

The Benefits of Standardized Tests

Standardized admissions tests remain beneficial in assisting admissions decisions for at least three reasons. First, the educational experiences of applicants vary considerably, as the U.S. educational system emphasizes local control of educational standards, funding, and curricula. In addition, applicants often have different educational experiences and opportunities. Standardized tests offer an efficient means of comparison among students who have diverse educational backgrounds.

Second, standardized test data are often useful for higher education institutions that must sort through a large number of applications, often with limited resources and time constraints. Standardized tests can be administered at low costs to students and the institutions that use test data and therefore offer efficiencies for admissions officials. Finally, standardized tests offer an opportunity for students to demonstrate their academic abilities, particularly in instances where students' classroom performance is not indicative of their abilities, and help students to realistically assess their chances of gaining admission to the institution of their choice (National Research Council, 1999).

In this context, standardized admissions tests offer an efficient way to compare diverse applicants. Their appropriate use can be summarized as follows: tests are designed to *sort applicant pools into broad categories,* "those who are quite likely to succeed academically at a particular institution, those who are quite unlikely to do so, and those in the middle" (National Research Council, 1999, p. 24).

Common Misinterpretations and Misuses of Standardized Tests

Unfortunately, in some instances standardized tests have been employed beyond their original intents and current usefulness, and they are commonly misinterpreted, both by the general public as well as university officials, in ways that are inconsistent with their design and stated purpose. Two such misuses, as identified by the NRC (National Research Council, 1999), include:

The belief that admissions tests measure a "compelling distillation of academic merit." Admissions tests do not measure the full range of abilities that are needed to succeed in higher education—nor were they designed to. Important attributes such as persistence, maturity, intellectual curiosity, creativity, the ability to work with others, and motivation are all associated with high academic achievement but are not measured by admissions tests. Instead, these attributes must be assessed by other means, such as applicants' essays, letters of recommendation, and record of extracurricular and community activities. Admissions tests therefore provide only part of the information a university admissions officer might need to fully assess the likelihood of a student succeeding in higher education, or whether the student fits within the institution's mission.

The belief that admissions tests provide a precise measure of student performance. As noted above, standardized admissions tests are best used to sort applicants into broad categories. In some instances, however, academic institutions and the general public have viewed test data as an indication of fine distinctions between individual applicants. This perception is not only untrue, but it also leads to contentious debate regarding the fairness of using test data to sort applicants whose test performance varies only minimally. Admissions tests, whether they measure aptitude or achievement, are imprecise estimates of how students might be expected to perform in specific educational contexts. Student performance on admissions tests often varies, and therefore test scores are best viewed as a point within a range of possible scores. Individual variation in test performance can occur without special preparation (e.g., intensive test preparation courses), and marked variation can occur following such preparation. "Given that a score is a point in a range on a measure of a limited domain," the NRC notes, "the claim that a higher score should guarantee one student preference over other another is not justifiable. Thus, schools that rely too heavily on scores to distinguish among applicants are extremely vulnerable to the charge of unfairness" (National Research Council, 1999, p. 24).

An additional misconception regarding standardized tests is brought about by the use of test data in popular publications to "rank" the quality of academic institutions. Several popular publications, including the *U.S. News and World Report*, publicize "rankings" of U.S. colleges and universities, using average admission test scores of entering classes as part of the criteria to assess institutional "selectivity." The use of average admissions test scores in this fashion not only provides a misleading indicator of selectivity, it also results in pressure on some institutions to weigh test data more heavily in admissions, as a means of raising the average test scores of entering students. As noted above, almost all institutions (particularly selective private institutions) weigh test scores in concert with other information, such as prior grades, essays, and letters of recommendation. Other factors, such as whether the applicant's parents are alumni of the institution, are also given weight at many institutions. Test scores alone therefore provide little information about the "selectivity" of an institution. The pressure on institutions to weigh test data more heavily is perhaps a natural result of having average test scores published and compared with other institutions, but having higher average test scores—as noted above—does not necessarily result in a class of students who are better prepared for or more likely to succeed in higher education.

How Effective Are Standardized Tests in Predicting Performance?

The predictive validity of standardized tests may be assessed by comparing test scores to at least two criteria of interest. The first, more common method is to assess how well test scores predict student academic performance following admission. In the case of health professions education, for example, students' test performance may be used to predict cumulate grade point average at the end of the first or second year of training. A second, but no less important, criterion of interest is students' subsequent clinical and professional performance, which may be assessed by comparing students' pass/fail rates on professional licensure exams, clinical clerkship or internship grades, or other measures of professional performance. In general, studies indicate that standardized tests are better predictors of the former criterion, that is, academic performance, particularly in the early years of training (e.g., first- or second-year grades), than in predicting the latter criteria (e.g., professional skill or competence).

When used appropriately, standardized test scores—assessed in conjunction with other data—have proven useful in assisting admissions committees to predict which students are likely to succeed in a given educational context, and which are not likely to succeed. Several decades of research demonstrates that undergraduate admissions tests (i.e., SAT or ACT) have an average correlation with first-year college grades that ranges from .45 to .55, indicating that such tests explain approximately 25 percent of the variance in predicted grades (National Research Council, 1999). The predictive power of standardized tests improves when used in conjunction with prior grades, and therefore most undergraduate admissions offices rely on a combination of high school grade point average and standardized test scores to assess applicants' academic potential, although in many cases prior grades are a more powerful predictor of future academic performance than standardized tests (Bowen and Bok, 1998).

Similarly, standardized tests used in graduate health professions training program admissions have moderately strong correlations with early academic performance in these settings. The MCAT, for example, has been found to have a moderately strong correlation ($r = .59$) with medical students' first- and second-year grades, but this prediction improves when test scores are used in combination with undergraduate grade point average (Association of American Medical Colleges, 2000). The predictive power of both the MCAT and undergraduate grades declines slightly when third-year grades or cumulative medical school grades are the criterion. When grades and test scores are used in combination, both undergraduate grades and MCAT scores are strong predictors of student performance on the U.S. Medical Licensing Exam (USMLE) Steps I–III, with coefficients ranging from .72 for Step I, .63 for Step II, and .65 for Step III (Association of American Medical Colleges, 2000).

As with the MCAT, the Graduate Record Examination (GRE) has modest value in predicting students' academic performance in graduate school, particularly in the early years of graduate study. Yet the predictive power of the test falls precipitously as students advance in graduate training. Sternberg and Williams (1997) found that the median correlation of overall GRE scores with graduate psychology students' first-year academic performance was .17, while the GRE Advanced test in psychology correlated more strongly with first-year performance (.37). Neither the GRE overall score nor the Advanced test in psychology, however, were significant predictors of second-year performance among psychology graduate students, with correlation coefficients of .10 and .02, respectively (Sternberg and Williams, 1997).

Graduate test scores are generally less effective in predicting expected outcomes of graduate training, such as the clinical performance of physicians, or research and analytic abilities of doctoral-level psychologists. Silver and Hodgson (1997), for example, found that undergraduate grade point average and MCAT scores were only moderately predictive of students' scores on the National Board of Medical Examiners (NBME) Part I (grades and MCAT scores predicted only about one-third of the variance in NBME scores). These same predictors, however, were unrelated to clinical performance, as measured by clerkship grades (Silver and Hodgson, 1997). Similarly, Sternberg and Williams (1997) found that the GRE was not a significant predictor of graduate psychology students' analytical, creative, practical, research, and teaching abilities, as assessed by students' primary advisors. The GRE Analytical scale, however, was moderately predictive of students' dissertation scores (as assessed by dissertation committee members), analytic abilities, and creativity, with correlation coefficients ranging from .16 to .24 on these measures—but only for male students.

Given that standardized tests are good, but not entirely consistent or strong predictors of students' future academic or career performance, some scholars have sought to better understand how standardized tests can be supplemented and/or more appropriately used in the admissions process.

Robert Sternberg and his colleagues at Yale University's PACE Center, for example, are developing an assessment instrument that, drawing on Sternberg's theory of "successful intelligence,"[1] provides a supplementary test of analytic skills, as well as practical and creative skills, to improve prediction of undergraduate students' academic performance when used in conjunction with SAT scores (Sternberg et al., in review). In addition, some admissions committees have sought to better understand how standardized test data can be used as an initial "screen," allowing committees to winnow applicants who are unlikely to succeed academically in health professions educational settings based on poor test performance, while retaining applicants for consideration whose scores suggest that they are able to manage the academic rigors of health professions education. Some admissions committees have identified a cut-off "range" of scores, below which students are unlikely to succeed academically (Garcia et al., 2003). In this model, applicants whose test scores fall above the cut-off range are retained for consideration, but other "qualitative" attributes of applicants are assigned greater weight in an attempt to identify students whose personal characteristics and diverse experiences are predictive of success as health professionals (see below for more discussion of model admissions practices).

Evaluating the Predictive Validity of Standardized Test Scores for Diverse Applicants

While standardized tests have been found to be a useful tool when used in conjunction with prior grades and other information in predicting applicants' future (particularly short-term) academic performance, the predictive power of standardized tests has been found to vary by test takers' race and ethnicity. URM students tend to perform more poorly relative to white students than would be predicted by standardized test scores. That is, URM students with the same standardized test scores as whites tend to receive lower grades than these white students, a phenomenon that is termed "underperformance" by some scholars (e.g., Bowen and Bok, 1998), or "overprediction" by others (e.g., Wightman, 2003). Overprediction occurs when test takers' performance on the criterion of interest (typically first-year grades following admission) is lower, on average, than would be predicted by these individuals' standardized test scores (Wightman, 2003).

---

[1]Successful intelligence is defined as the ability to achieve success in life in terms of one's own personal standards—within one's socioeconomic context—while capitalizing on strengths or compensating for weaknesses; balancing skills in order to adapt to, shape, and select environments; and balance analytic, practical, and creative skills. The theory of successful intelligence suggests that prediction of applicants' future academic performance can be improved by broadening the range of skills assessed (Sternberg et al., in review).

While the differential predictive validity of admissions tests has largely been assessed using undergraduate admissions test data and freshman grades, the phenomenon also extends to graduate health professions training settings. Koenig, Sireci, and Wiley (1998), for example, in a study of the relationship between medical students' MCAT scores and cumulative medical school grade point average, found that whites' MCAT scores tended to under-predict their performance (although the magnitude of this underprediction was small), while the test scores of African American, Hispanic, and Asian American students tended to overpredict their medical school performance (for the latter two minority groups, this overprediction was statistically significant).

The tendency of URM students to perform academically at lower levels than their standardized tests would suggest, does not, in itself, indicate that tests are systematically biased against minority students. Little is known about why tests tend to overpredict academic performance among minorities, and inferences about bias based on the differential validity of tests are difficult to draw unless the criteria (grades) are assumed to be unbiased (Wightman, 2003). The trend toward test overprediction among minorities, however, suggests that admissions committees must be aware of special considerations in evaluating minority applicants' test performance and likely academic potential. Potential reasons for minority "underperformance" are explored below, following a review of group differences in standardized test performance.

Group Differences in Standardized Test Performance

Underrepresented minority students, on average, perform poorly relative to whites and Asian Americans on standardized admissions tests. These differences are consistent across a range of tests, with the largest gaps found between white and African American test-takers, followed by gaps between whites and Hispanics. Asian-American test-takers' mean test scores are similar to those of whites, with some exceptions. Group means for three commonly used admissions tests (SAT I, GRE, and MCAT) are displayed in Figures 2-1, 2-2, and 2-3.

Scholastic Aptitude Test

The College Board's Scholastic Aptitude Test is the most commonly used undergraduate admissions test for selective public and private colleges. As such, it is the "gateway" examination for most students interested in pursuing health professions careers. SAT I verbal and math scores range from 200 to 800, with a standard deviation of 111 to 112. As shown in Figure 2-1, whites achieve, on average, the highest scores on both scales,

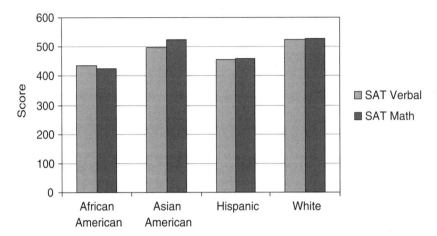

FIGURE 2-1 Group means on Scholastic Aptitude Test (SAT) performance by ethnicity and race.
SOURCE: Camara and Schmidt, 1999.

with a mean SAT verbal score of 526 and a mean SAT math score of 528. African American test-takers score nearly a full standard deviation unit lower than whites on the SAT verbal and math scales (standardized difference[2] [SD] = .83 and .92, respectively), while Hispanics score about three-fifths of a standard deviation unit lower than whites on both scales. Asian American test-takers perform nearly identically to whites on the SAT math scale, but about one-quarter standard deviation unit lower than whites on the SAT verbal scale (Camara and Schmidt, 1999).

Graduate Record Examination

The Graduate Record Examination Verbal, Quantitative, and Analytic scales range from 200 to 800, with a standard deviation of 108 for the Verbal scale and 127 for both the Quantitative and Analytic scales. The GRE is commonly used for admission to selective graduate (e.g., Ph.D.) programs in a range of academic fields, including most "scientist-practitioner" clinical psychology programs (many programs typically also require applicants to take a subject-area examination). Group differences in performance on the GRE are displayed in Figure 2-2. As with the SAT, white test-

---

[2]Standardized differences are computed by subtracting the average score for each racial and ethnic minority group from the average score of the reference group (whites), and dividing this figure by the overall test standard deviation.

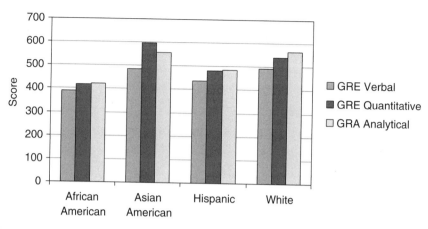

FIGURE 2-2 Group means on Graduate Record Examinations (GRE) Performance by ethnicity and race.
SOURCE: Camara and Schmidt, 1999.

takers typically score higher than other racial and ethnic groups, with the exception of the GRE Quantitative, where Asian Americans score nearly a half-standard deviation unit (SD = .46) higher than whites. African Americans score, on average, one full standard deviation unit below whites on all three scales, while Hispanic test-takers score approximately half to three-fifths of a standard deviation unit below whites on all scales (ranging from .46 on the Quantitative scale to .62 on the Analytical scale; Camara and Schmidt, 1999).

Medical College Admissions Test

The Medical College Admissions Test Verbal Reasoning, Physical Sciences, and Biological Sciences scales range from 1 to 15, with a standard deviation of 2.4 for all scales in 1998 (Camara and Schmidt, 1999). Group differences in performance on the MCAT are displayed in Figure 2-3. As is the case with the GRE and SAT, African American and Hispanic test-takers score lower than whites and Asian Americans, who tend to perform at similar levels on this test. African American and Hispanic test-takers score approximately 1 full standard deviation unit lower than white test-takers on all three scales; this difference ranges from .96 to 1.08 on all scales for African Americans and from .88 to 1.00 on all scales for Hispanics. Asian American test-takers score .29 of a standard deviation unit lower than whites on the Verbal Reasoning scale, perform slightly higher on the Physi-

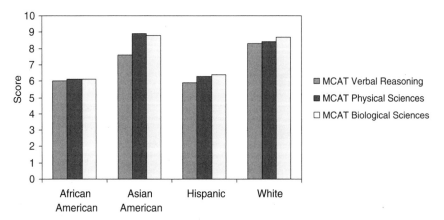

FIGURE 2-3 Group means on Medical College Admissions Test (MCAT) performance by ethnicity and race.
SOURCE: Camara and Schmidt, 1999.

cal Sciences (.21) scale, and score equivalently on the Biological Sciences scale (Camara and Schmidt, 1999).

What Causes Group Differences in Standardized Test and Academic Performance?

The causes of the persistent gap in test performance between URM and non-URM students have been the subject of hotly contested debate, with explanations ranging from accusations of test bias to assertions of genetic differences in intellectual ability among racial and ethnic groups (e.g., Hernnstein and Murray, 1999). A growing plurality of social scientists, however, agree that historic and contemporary social and economic forces and discrimination play a powerful role in shaping differences in racial and ethnic groups' educational opportunities and life experiences that affect test performance (American Sociological Association, 2003).

Bowen and Bok (1998), in their seminal research on the academic performance of African American and white students who attended selective U.S. colleges and universities, suggest two sets of factors that may contribute to poorer URM performance on standardized tests, as well as their tendency to perform at lower levels academically than non-URM students who achieve the same standardized test scores. The first set of factors refers to pre-college influences, such as the quality of prior academic preparation and family influences on educational preparation. The second set of factors emerges from experiences in higher education settings (and in this instance, health professions education institutions [HPEIs]).

Pre-College Influences on Educational Preparation

In the United States, educational opportunities are unevenly distributed by race and ethnicity. Racial and ethnic minority students are far more likely than white students to attend majority-minority schools, even when the former group of students is from middle- and upper-income families (Orfield, 2001). For example, more than 70 percent of African American students and 76 percent of Latino children attend schools that are majority non-white (American Sociological Association, 2003). Such schools tend to be characterized by fewer academic and financial resources, fewer credentialed teachers, fewer advanced placement courses, and higher dropout rates, even when in similar neighborhoods as predominantly white schools (American Sociological Association, 2003). Students in higher-income, predominantly white schools, in contrast, are exposed to more rigorous coursework, take more courses, and have greater exposure to college preparatory and advanced placement coursework (Camara and Schmidt, 1999). Such students are also more likely to take test preparation courses outside of regular coursework. Even among racial and ethnic minority students who attend integrated schools, segregation within schools in common; African American and other URM students are more likely to be "tracked" into vocational or lower-level academic programs, which offer little or no college preparatory content (Camara and Schmidt, 1999).

To a great extent, school-based inequities reflect patterns of racial housing segregation and inequities among localities in school funding (American Sociological Association, 2003). African American and Hispanic students, particularly those in inner-city and rural communities, are more likely to live in neighborhoods characterized by high poverty rates and few local resources for schools. Not surprisingly, average per-pupil expenditures for these schools are in some cases one-half to two-thirds lower than per-pupil expenditures in some of the wealthiest public school districts, resulting in inequities in teaching resources, teacher pay and qualifications, and physical accommodations (Orfield, 2001). As Camara and Schmidt (1999) note:

> The stark differences across [standardized test] assessments and other measures collectively illustrate the inequities minorities have suffered through inadequate academic preparation, poverty, and discrimination; years of tracking into dead-end educational programs; lack of advanced and rigorous courses in inner-city schools, or lack of access to such programs when available; threadbare facilities and overcrowding; teachers in critical need of professional development; less family support and experience in higher education; and low expectation (p. 13).

In addition to inequality of educational opportunities, differences in family influences may be associated with poorer URM academic performance. Bowen and Bok (1998) note that despite their efforts to account statistically for racial and ethnic differences in family socioeconomic background, students' academic performance is likely to be affected by family attributes that are difficult to measure. "College grades," they write, "may well be less affected by family income and parental education . . . than they are by the number of books at home, opportunities to travel, better secondary schooling, the nature of the conversation around the dinner table, and more generally, parental involvement in their children's education" (Bowen and Bok, 1998, p. 80). Students from higher socioeconomic backgrounds, more often non-URM students, benefit disproportionately from these influences.

Experiences in Higher Education Institutions and HPEIs

In addition to educational and socioeconomic inequities between United States racial and ethnic groups, the poorer performance of minority students on standardized tests, and their lower academic performance than would be expected on the basis of these tests, may also be traced to experiences of URM students in higher education and HPEI settings. Bowen and Bok (1998) note that these explanations "range from . . . psychological theories to assertions about discrimination by faculty members, low motivation on the part of [URM] students, special problems of adjusting to predominantly white environments, and poorly conceived institutional policies that at best accept and at worse encourage lower academic aspirations by [URM] students" (Bowen and Bok, 1998, p. 81).

URM students, particularly those that are a visible yet small minority on college and HPEI campuses, may experience academic pressure or feelings of insecurity, and especially so in contexts where URM students have been historically excluded. Pressures to perform as well as non-URM students and manage stress stemming from campus racial tensions have been found to be negatively associated with URM undergraduate students' academic performance, after controlling for standardized test scores and prior academic performance in college (Smedley et al., 1993). Other researchers suggest that peer group influences, particularly within African American peer groups, may cause minority students to be less invested in academic performance and to "experience inordinate ambivalence and affective dissonance in regard to academic effort and success" (Fordham and Ogbu, 1986, p. 177).

Among the most extensively studied social and psychological factors affecting URM academic and test-taking performance is research on "stereotype threat." Beginning with the work of Claude Steele and colleagues (Steele, 1997; Steele and Aronson, 1995), psychologists have found that African Americans and other groups whose intellectual abilities are stigmatized by widely held societal stereotypes (e.g., women undertaking mathematical problems) may respond to these stereotypes by performing poorly relative to their actual abilities. This tendency, termed *stereotype threat*, presents an additional emotional and cognitive burden for individuals who are members of the group for which the stereotype might apply. Stereotype threat exerts its influence in the form of performance-disruptive anxiety and apprehension about the possibility of confirming the stereotypes' validity in the eyes of others or for the individual affected by the stereotype. This threat applies to those who are aware of the stereotype and value high academic performance, as is the case for most African American students in higher education settings. African Americans and others affected by stereotype threat need not believe in the stereotype's validity to be affected by their consequences, given the widespread nature of many stereotypes about minority intellectual ability.[3] Rather, it is the students' concern about disproving the stereotype that confers anxiety and affects academic performance (Aronson et al., 2001; Steele, 1997; Steele and Aronson, 1995).

The impact of stereotypes on URM students' test performance has been demonstrated in a number of laboratory studies. Steele and Aronson (1995), for example, administered difficult GRE-type verbal questions to a sample of African American and white Stanford University undergraduates. In one condition, students were told that their performance on the test items was diagnostic of their intellectual abilities, while in another condition, students were told that their performance was nondiagnostic (i.e., the investigators were merely interested in how students solve problems, and their performance was unrelated to ability). After controlling for students' initial skills (as measured by SAT verbal scores), the investigators found that African American students performed significantly worse than their white peers in the "diagnostic" condition, but equaled the performance of whites in the "nondiagnostic" condition. To further assess this phenomenon, the investigators asked students in both the diagnostic and nondiagnostic conditions to complete word fragments, some of which were symbolic of African American stereotypes and self-doubt. African American students in the diagnostic condition, who were expecting to take an ability-diagnostic test, completed more stereotyping word fragments and self-doubt words compared to African American students in the nondiagnostic condition or whites in either condition, indicating that the former group of students were more

---

[3]Survey research indicates that despite the trend over the past several decades toward more egalitarian and nonracist attitudes among the American public, a majority of Americans (53 percent) believe that African Americans are intellectually inferior to whites (Bobo, 2001) . An even larger number may implicitly hold such stereotypes (Devine, 1989).

aware of and concerned about stereotypes of black academic performance. When the same students were asked to list their race on the exam, all of the African Americans in the nondiagnostic condition and whites in both conditions complied, whereas only 25 percent of African American students in the diagnostic condition did so, further indicating anxiety about test performance being viewed as confirming racial stereotypes (Steele, 1997).

What Are the Consequences of Heavy Reliance on Quantitative Measures in Admissions Processes?

Given that URM students tend to perform poorly relative to their white and Asian American peers on standardized tests, and that social and psychological factors may contribute to poorer test performance among URM students and other stigmatized groups, it is not surprising that admissions models that weigh quantitative data more heavily in admissions decisions often fail to achieve a racially and ethnically diverse class of students. Evidence, from both hypothetical analyses and policy changes in several states, suggests that absent admissions policies that allow for the consideration of applicants' race or ethnicity, URM student participation in health professions will drop precipitously.

What Would Happen to URM Enrollment in Medical Schools Without Race-Conscious Admissions?

Were medical school admissions committees to drop any consideration of race or ethnicity in admissions, URM students would find difficulty gaining admission in U.S. medical schools. Cohen (2003) reports on an exercise, based on data from URM and non-URM applicants to medical schools in 2001, in which researchers used an algorithm to calculate the numbers of students that would gain admission based on undergraduate grades and MCAT scores. This analysis assumes that all other differences between URM and non-URM students are held constant, including industriousness, leadership, or other qualities that medical schools might consider in the admissions process. Using data from all applicants to 119 nonminority medical schools (excluding historically African American and Puerto Rican medical schools), this analysis revealed that only 513 URM students would have gained admission, a figure that is 70 percent lower than the actual number (1,697) of URM students that gained admission in 2001. These 513 students would have constituted approximately 3 percent of all medical students, levels that have not been seen since the early 1960s.

Effect of "Race-Neutral" Admissions on URM Participation in Higher Education in California, Texas, and Florida

In response to public referenda, judicial decisions, and lawsuits challenging affirmative action policies in 1995, 1996, and 1997 (notably, the Fifth District Court of Appeals finding in *Hopwood v. University of Texas*, and the California Regents decision to ban race or gender-based preferences in admissions), three states—California, Texas, and Florida—developed "race-neutral" undergraduate admissions policies that guaranteed admission to the state university system to applicants who graduated within the top tiers of their high school class. In Texas, the state legislature passed legislation that guaranteed admission to the state institution of choice for applicants who graduated in the top 10 percent of their high school class. Under this plan, qualifying applicants must complete an application for admission and provide standardized admission test scores, but test scores are not considered in admissions decisions. In California, the University of California (UC) Board of Regents approved a plan to confer eligibility for admission to the UC system to the top 12.5 percent of the state's high school graduates, as well the top 4 percent of graduates from each high school. The latter pool of students (termed "eligibility in the local context" [ELC]) includes several hundred students who are at the top of low performing schools and thus would not qualify as being in the top 12.5 percent statewide. The vast majority of students in the top 4 percent of their class also qualify on statewide criteria, however. Because URMs are disproportionately from low performing schools, the ELC program tends to increase the number of URMs eligible for admission. Students who clear the eligibility hurdle are admitted to the University of California, but not necessarily to the campus or major of their choice. Similarly, Florida adopted a "percent plan" admissions policy when the state's governor, in an attempt to preempt a statewide referendum similar to that passed in California, approved a plan to guarantee admission to the University of Florida system to the top 20 percent of the state's high school graduates.

Conservative critics of these plans have charged that percent plans are merely affirmative action plans under a different name, given that the plans' proponents argue that the plans will maintain racial and ethnic diversity while eliminating the explicit consideration of race and ethnicity in the admissions process. In addition, these critics charge, guaranteeing admission to even the narrowest top percentage of high school graduates threatens to weaken state university admission standards, and that because of the relatively poorer academic resources of majority-minority high schools, even top minority graduates who gain admission will be poorly prepared for the academic rigors of selective state universities (Horn and Flores, 2003). Progressive advocates are similarly dismayed by percentage plans.

They charge that the plans are perversely dependent upon racial segregation in high schools (given that the racial and ethnic diversity that the plans' proponents expect depends largely on the assumption that top graduates of majority-minority high schools will matriculate within the state university system); that the plans are likely to miss many high-achieving minority applicants who do not graduate within the top percentage of "automatic" admits; that a guarantee of admission only within state systems does not prevent the possibility that minority admits will be "clustered" in lower tiered schools within state systems; and that, for purposes of enhancing student diversity in public institutions, such plans are an inadequate substitute for the explicit consideration of applicants' race and ethnicity (Horn and Flores, 2003).

Several major studies have been conducted to evaluate the impact of percentage plans on undergraduate student diversity in the three states (Tienda et al., 2003; Horn and Flores, 2003; Marin and Lee, 2003). Each concludes that while most students eligible for admission to state universities under the percentage plans would also have been admitted under previous admissions policies, percent plans have largely failed to restore minority enrollments to levels seen prior to the ban on the consideration of applicants' race or ethnicity imposed in each state (Horn and Flores, 2003).

Texas' "Top 10 Percent" Plan

Marta Tienda and colleagues (Tienda et al., 2003) evaluated trends in admission and enrollment of African American and Latino students at the University of Texas' flagship public institutions, the University of Texas (UT) and Texas A&M University (A&M), before and after implementation of the "Top 10 Percent" plan, and found that while some minority students who graduated among the top 10 percent of their high school class gained admission to UT and A&M under this plan (students who might previously have been rejected because of low standardized test scores or poor essays) the plan has resulted in lower minority admissions and matriculation rates for African American and Latino students than during the pre-*Hopwood* era. Post-*Hopwood*, for example, African American students constituted only 2.4 percent of enrollees at A&M, a decline from 3.7 percent prior to the ruling. Hispanic student representation similarly declined, from 12.6 percent pre-*Hopwood* to 9.2 percent following the ruling. Similar, but less striking trends were observed at UT, where African American and Hispanic students declined from nearly 20 percent prior to the *Hopwood* ruling to less than 17 percent of the undergraduate population post-*Hopwood*. More importantly, the probability of admission to the two flagship institutions for Asian American and white students *increased* following implementation of the "Top 10 percent" plan, while this probability declined for African

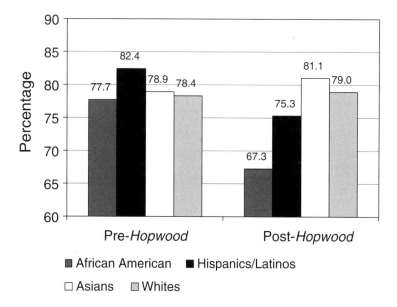

FIGURE 2-4 Probability of admission pre- and post-*Hopwood* by race and Hispanic origin: Texas public flagship.
SOURCE: Tienda et al., 2003.

American and Hispanic students (see Figure 2-4). Tienda and colleagues note that while the decline in URM representation at Texas' flagship institutions was not as dramatic as some critics had predicted (due in large part to the heavy weight placed on high school grades and class rank in UT undergraduate admissions prior to the *Hopwood* decision), the decline is particularly disturbing given the fact that Texas' "minority" population will soon become a demographic majority (Tienda et al., 2003).

University of California

As with the Texas percent plan, the UC admissions plan guarantees admission to the state system to the states' top high school graduates but differs from the Texas plan in that eligible applicants are not guaranteed admission to the campus of their choice. While data are incomplete because of California's relatively recent (1999) move toward a "percent" admissions plan, preliminary data indicate that minority admission and matriculation in the UC system has declined and that this decline was sharpest shortly after the California Regents' decision to eliminate the consideration of race and ethnicity in admissions. As shown in Figure 2-5, both African

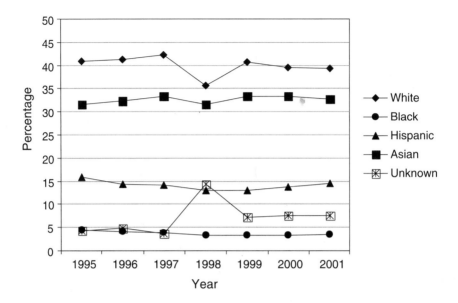

FIGURE 2-5 University of California system-wide Fall state resident freshman admissions offers, by race/ethnicity, 1995–2001.
SOURCE: UC Office of the President, Student Academic Services, OA&SA, REG004/006, January 2002, http://www.ucop.edu.news.studstaff.html.

American and Hispanic freshman admissions dropped significantly from 1995, when African Americans and Hispanics represented 4.4 percent and 15.8 percent of freshman admissions, respectively, to 1998, when African American admissions fell to 3.2 percent, while Hispanic admissions fell to 12.9 percent of the freshman class (Horn and Flores, 2003). By 2001 URM representation among freshmen in the UC system increased slightly to 3.4 percent African American and 14.6 percent Hispanic students, but these percentages are still below the levels attained prior to the Regents' decision. The decline in URM representation was more profound at the state's flagship institutions, the University of California at Los Angeles and the University of California at Berkeley. African American freshman admissions offers at UC Berkeley declined from 7.3 percent in 1995 to 3.2 percent in 1998 and 4.1 percent in 2001, and from 6.7 percent in 1995 to 3.3. percent in 2001 at UCLA. Similarly, Hispanic freshman admissions offers declined from 1995 (18.5 percent and 20.1 percent at Berkeley and UCLA, respectively) to 2001 (12.5 percent at Berkeley and 12.7 percent at UCLA), with these percentages dwindling to under half their 1995 levels in 1998 at both campuses (Horn and Flores, 2003).

In light of these data, Horn and Flores (2003) conclude that " . . . in all three states, the gap between the racial distribution of college-freshman-age population and that of the applications, admissions, and enrollments to the states' university systems and to their premier campuses is substantial and has grown even as the states have become more diverse. . . . [I]n California in particular, proportional representation of applied, admitted, and enrolled blacks and Hispanics on the flagship campuses has decreased since the end of race-conscious policies" (p. 50).

ALTERNATIVE ADMISSIONS MODELS

Given the barriers that "race-neutral" and heavily quantitatively weighted admissions policies pose to achieving racially and ethnically diverse classes, many leaders in the academic health professions have begun to reconceptualize admissions policies and practices in an attempt to enhance both the diversity and quality of admitted students. Increasingly, these needs are seen as linked. As Edwards, Elam, and Wagoner (2001) note:

> Complex societal issues affect medical education and thus require new approaches from medical school admission officers. One of these issues—the recognition that the attributes of good doctors include character qualities such as compassion, altruism, respect, and integrity—has resulted in the recent focus on the greater use of qualitative variables, such as those just stated, for selected candidates . . . [t]he second and more contentious issue concerns the system used to admit white and minority applicants. Emphasizing character qualities of physicians in the admission criteria and selection process involves a paradigm shift that could serve to resolve both issues (p. 1207).

The trend toward emphasizing professionalism and "humanistic" factors is also reflected in recent efforts by licensing and accreditation bodies to assess these qualities among both trainees and training institutions (see also chapter on accreditation and diversity). The Liaison Committee on Medical Education, for example, is reviewing efforts by medical schools to teach professionalism and demonstrate the effectiveness of these efforts. Similarly, the NBME will require that examinees pass measures of professionalism, communication, and interpersonal skills, while the Accreditation Council on Graduate Medical Education and the American Board of Medical Specialties have defined several areas of professional competency that include among them communication and interpersonal skills and understanding and sensitivity to diversity. Specialty groups such as the American Board of Internal Medicine (ABIM) are adapting similar approaches; ABIM now requires physicians seeking board certification to demonstrate integrity, respect, and compassion in their relationships with patients and their families. These trends place greater responsibility and pressure on health professions training programs to screen applicants for humanistic attributes and enhance training to help students further develop these skills (Edwards et al., 2001).

Efforts to identify and assess important qualitative attributes of applicants to health professions training programs are not without challenges. As noted above, screening and interviewing applicants for admission to health profession training programs is a labor- and time-intensive, expensive process. Assessing applicants' qualitative attributes often requires more of an admissions committee's time and energy than simply reviewing quantitative data (e.g., grades and test scores), as committee members must glean this information from essays, letters of recommendation, and personal interviews. In addition, while most health professions training faculty agree on the core humanistic attributes that ideal applicants should possess (e.g., compassion, sensitivity, commitment to service), there is not always agreement on the full range of important attributes that should be assessed, or how these attributes should be assessed. Moreover, admissions committees often respond—sometimes consciously, while in other cases unconsciously—to external pressures that discourage the broader use of qualitative data in the application process. These include, as noted above, the pressure to admit applicants with higher test scores, given that some in the media and in health professions fields will misinterpret the average test scores of admitted students as an indication of institutional "selectivity," and the fear that the institution will be less able to defend admissions decisions that consider qualitative data in the face of lawsuits filed on behalf of rejected applicants (Edwards et al., 2001).

Despite these challenges, many institutions, recognizing the need for an admissions "paradigm shift" advocated by Edwards and colleagues (Edwards et al., 2001), have begun to devise new admissions models that balance consideration of applicants' quantitative and qualitative information in an effort to achieve both quality and diversity in assembling a student body.

Conforming Admissions Policies to the Institutional Mission

A fundamental paradigm shift in health professions training programs' admissions policies and practices begins with an assessment of whether admissions process and practices conform to the institutional mission. Examples of innovative admissions practices examined by the study committee suggest that this is an important first step that is not consistently addressed by many institutions. The Texas A&M College of Medicine, for example, began its reconsideration of its admissions policies and practices in the wake of the 1997 *Hopwood* decision with "a mindfulness of the vision and mission of the institution in assessing and selecting students" (Maldonado, 2001). Similarly, Stanford University's School of Medicine restructured its admissions process by emphasizing the need for a "mission-oriented" review of each applicant, which emphasizes an assessment of applicants based on the institution's mission statement and goals (e.g., categorizing and ranking applicants' skills and attributes in a manner that reflects the institution's educational goals; Garcia et al., 2003). Examples of how the institutional mission helped to shape new admissions practices at these schools are described below. In both cases, a review of the institutional mission suggested that medical student diversity is critically important to achieving these institutions' goals of expanding research and service to underserved communities and improving the health of individuals in the region and nation.

Training and Composing Admissions Committees

Another important step toward a fundamental paradigm shift in health professions training programs' admissions policies and practices involves an assessment of the admissions committee itself, including giving careful consideration to issues such as who should serve on the committee, how will committee service be rewarded, and how should committee members be trained.

Demographic Characteristics of Admissions Committees

Little empirical research sheds light on the demographic composition of admissions committees for health professions education programs. Anecdotal evidence suggests that the vast majority of health professions training programs tend to appoint senior faculty (who tend to be predominantly white and male) to admissions committees and occasionally include representation from one or more students. Rarely are communities affected by admissions decisions, including members of communities served by teaching hospitals and community-based training institutions, represented on admissions committees.

Kondo and Judd (2000), in one of the few empirical studies of the demographic composition of admissions committees, surveyed deans or directors of admission at 85 U.S. medical schools to assess the presence of women and racial and ethnic minorities on medical school admissions committees. The results confirmed many of the anecdotal observations noted above: medical school admissions committees were largely male (the overall ratio of men to women was 1.77 to 1.0) and predominantly white (on average, 16 percent of committee members were from URM groups, only half of the URM members were physicians, and over half of the schools surveyed reported that their admissions committees had no or only one URM physician). While 74 percent of committees had at least one medical student representative, medical students constituted only 15 percent of total admissions committee members. In addition, over nine of ten admissions committees operated on a volunteer basis (Kondo and Judd, 2000).

These data suggest that admissions committees have a great deal of room for improvement with regard to representation of diverse groups. This is not to suggest that racial and ethnic minorities or women should be expected to advocate for URM candidates, or that admissions committees should be "stacked" with individuals who might be more sympathetic to URM applicants. Rather, it suggests that admissions committees can improve on their ability to incorporate the perspectives of diverse groups that contribute to the educational experience on health professions education campuses. Racial and ethnic minority members of admissions committees might be better able to understand and contextualize the life circumstances and experiences of URM applicants and help other admissions committee members to understand a URM applicant's abilities. Furthermore, racial and ethnic minority members of admissions committees may be well-positioned to assess URM applicants' academic and nonacademic accomplishments, and commitment to service in racial and ethnic minority communities.

Unfortunately, because of the lack of URM faculty in many health professions training programs, the few that are present are often "pulled" in many directions and pressed into service on admissions committees and other important institutional committees. Kondo and Judd's (2000) finding that service on the vast majority of medical school admissions committees is voluntary suggests that few rewards (e.g., consideration of committee service during promotion review) are provided for those faculty who serve in this capacity. And because minority faculty often face additional demands such as mentoring and recruiting URM students, service on institutional committees can present additional pressures that compete with teaching, research, and other work important for promotion. Service on important institutional committees, such as admissions committees, should be more appropriately rewarded to encourage the participation of URM faculty and staff.

Training of Admissions Committee Members

Another important component of fundamental change in the admission process involves training of admissions committee members. Several examples of innovative training programs are described below, including national training efforts of the Association of American Medical Colleges

(AAMC). Common attributes of admissions committee training programs include skills and knowledge development in areas such as:

- How to assess qualitative attributes of applicants;
- How to interpret the academic and standardized test performance of URM students, whose performance may be influenced by a range of factors, such as poor prior academic training and psychosocial factors (e.g., stereotype threat);
- How to assess the academic and nonacademic achievements of URM students, whose life circumstances and experiences may differ from non-URM students; and
- Interviewing skills, to identify ways to better elicit and manage information from applicants.

These skills and areas of knowledge are increasingly important for admissions committee members, who, as a result of the Supreme Court decision in the *Grutter v. Bollinger* case, may be asked to provide comprehensive reviews of applicants' files and reduce dependence upon standardized test data as a means of winnowing applications.

AAMC Expanded Minority Admissions Exercise

In 1970, the AAMC began exploring new approaches to medical school admissions that consider strategies to balance applicants' "noncognitive" qualities with other traditional predictors of medical school performance (e.g., MCAT scores, undergraduate science curriculum, and grades) in an effort to increase minority admissions. Beginning with the Simulated Minority Admissions Exercise in 1970, AAMC developed a program of case studies and training for medical school admissions officers that is designed to enhance these officers' understanding of the importance of "noncognitive" factors (such as altruism, leadership, commitment to service, and empathy), to foster an appreciation of cultural diversity in medical training, and to model interviewing skills (Cleveland, 2003). In its current iteration, the Expanded Minority Admissions Exercise (EMAE) uses case studies of actual medical school applicants and videotaped admissions interviews to help admissions officials compare their assessment of applicants and with applicants' actual admissions outcomes. Workshops are held at 28 medical schools and emphasize such strategies as:

- Reconceptualizing the initial review of applicant files to assess whether applicants have the academic skills to succeed in medical school (as assessed by MCAT scores and grades), while considering other relevant factors, such as educational and socioeconomic barriers that applicants have overcome;

• Evaluating candidates' skills and experiences, if they meet basic academic requirements in the initial review, such as clinical and health-care experiences, volunteer activities, research experiences, work activities, and leadership; and

• Better assessing applicants' personal qualities in the admissions interview.

A new edition of EMAE will focus on helping admissions committee members to evaluate personal characteristics more effectively and efficiently, to understand how admissions processes relate to the development of medical students' cultural competency and care-giving skills, and to develop a greater appreciation of the different forms of "intelligence" (e.g., analytic, creative, and practice intelligence) that applicants may possess (Cleveland, 2003).

Examples of Admissions Practices That Attempt to Increase URM Admissions

Several HPEIs have developed innovative admissions strategies that utilize one or more of the concepts discussed above in an attempt to better assess attributes of applicants that are consistent with the institutional mission, as well as to increase URM admissions. Two such examples, drawing on admissions strategies at Texas A&M and Stanford Medical Schools, are offered here. These examples are not intended to suggest that these strategies represent the best efforts in the field, not are they offered as models that must be replicated at other HPEIs. In addition, the description of these institutions' efforts should not suggest that innovative admissions strategies are being developed only in medical schools. Rather, they reflect innovative adaptations of these unique institutions to particular circumstances and policy contexts: one, at a state institution that faced a court-mandated ban on the consideration of applicants' race or ethnicity in the admissions process, and the other, at a prestigious, well-funded private institution that, like many other similar institutions, did not have an impressive record of inclusion of underrepresented groups. The effectiveness of these strategies in increasing URM admissions has not been rigorously evaluated; data presented below suggest that the institutions' efforts are likely to result in increases in URM admits, but future research should more thoroughly assess the long-term effect of these strategies on URM admission rate. For other examples of admissions policies and practices that endeavor to increase racial and ethnic diversity across a range of health professions and types of institutions, see the contribution by Garcia, Nation, and Parker in this volume.

The Texas A&M Medical School Experience

Prior to the Supreme Court ruling in *Grutter v. Bollinger*, the decision by the U.S. Fifth Circuit Court in the *Hopwood v. University of Texas* suit created a mandate that all public higher education institutions in Texas (as well as other states in the Fifth Circuit) abandon the consideration of applicants' race or ethnicity in the admissions process. In response, the Texas A&M Medical School, like other institutions in the state, attempted to develop a "race-neutral" admissions process that would allow the institution to continue to admit and enroll URM students. As a first step, the admissions committee considered the Health Sciences Center and College of Medicine's (COM) mission and institutional goals to reassess the admissions process and, in particular, reconsider the weights placed on applicants' MCAT scores, academic records, and personal and experiential qualities. The COM's mission and institutional goals "became the philosophy by which the admissions committee guided and directed the admissions process" (Maldonado, 2001, p. 314). Texas A&M's new admissions plan called for:

- "A mindfulness of the vision and mission of the institution in assessing and selecting students;
- A more inclusive approach to assessing cognitive abilities;
- A broad-minded scrutiny of applicant's noncognitive characteristics at the pre-interview and interview phases of the evaluation process;
- Enhanced interview techniques;
- Improved protocol for admissions committee deliberations; and
- Frequent self-monitoring" (Maldonado, 2001, p. 314).

Subsequently, COM admissions officials decided to widen the pool of applicants to be interviewed by carefully analyzing the distribution of academic scores (i.e., a combination of MCAT scores and undergraduate grade point average) of applicants. A top tier of applicants was identified with superior academic scores and were considered "automatic" interviews. These applicants, approximately 20 percent of the applicant pool, tended to be less racially and ethnically diverse, but also were less likely to enroll in the medical school if admitted (less than one in five accepted offers of admission). The admissions committee identified a middle group of applicants whose academic scores were considered acceptable (average MCAT scores and GPA of this group were 26 and 3.45, respectively) and indicative that the applicant could complete the medical school curriculum, if admitted. This middle pool included a broader representation of "underrepresented and disadvantaged" applicants and tended to be more likely to accept offers of admission to the medical school than the top pool of applicants. Finally, the admissions committee identified a pool of applicants that were considered "high-risk" on the basis of academic scores. Applicants in this pool were not considered for interviews unless they self-identified as "disadvantaged" (Maldonado, 2001).

The Stanford University Model

The Stanford University School of Medicine has adopted a model of medical school admissions that reflects the institution's mission, which includes recognition that racial and ethnic diversity in the medical school is essential to achieving the institution's educational goals. This commitment to diversity begins with strong leadership from the university president and others who have articulated clear diversity goals and strongly support diversity as central to the institution's mission (Garcia et al., 2003). The admissions process is driven by the institutional mission and includes:

• Training of admissions committee members, who are taught about the impact of "stereotype threat" on minority test performance and other contextual factors that are important for assessing minority applicants, such as the role of cultural and language barriers, family background, and the educational "distance traveled" (e.g., the impact of prior experiences of prejudice or discrimination, the greater likelihood that minority students must work during college to meet financial obligations);
• A "mission-oriented" file review, which emphasizes assessment of applicants based on the institution's mission statement and goals (e.g., categorizing and ranking applicants' skills and attributes in a manner that reflects the institution's educational goals); and
• Developing partnerships with undergraduate faculty and advising staff of undergraduate colleges to support the admissions process.

Stanford's admissions committee has developed extensive barometers for assessing applicants' qualitative attributes. For example, candidates' success as a role model for others is assessed by looking for evidence that the applicant has participated in activities that are visible and are intended to influence members of the community in a positive manner. Similarly, applicants' commitment to service is assessed by evidence of community involvement, volunteer service, and other activities. Applicants' degree of engagement in these activities is assessed by evidence of participation, particularly over a long period of time; assuming a leadership role; advocacy on behalf of the organization or issue; programmatic innovation; and, perhaps more importantly, evidence that the applicant has left a legacy or lasting impact in the community served.

MCAT data are considered early in the admissions process as an initial "screen" to identify applicants who are not likely to be able to manage the medical school curriculum. A range of scores has been identified as a "qualifying range," based on the admissions committee's prior experience and knowledge of the curriculum. Applicants who perform at or above the cutoff range are likely to possess the academic skills and background to pass the school's core curricula. When the admissions committee makes final decisions, quantitative variables are not considered as "individual items of great importance" (Garcia et al., 2003), but rather, the committee attempts to answer two questions:

- "How will this candidate contribute to and benefit from the learning climate at [the] institution?; [and]
- Will accepting this candidate be in line with the mission and values of the school?" (Garcia et al., 2003).

Stanford has achieved significant success in recruiting and admitting URM students (over 20 percent of the medical students in 2002–2003 were African American, Hispanic, or Native American). Of these, nearly three in five (57 percent) are involved in scholarly research through the institution's Medical Scholars Program, a rate that is comparable to participation in research among Stanford's non-URM students. Stanford's success with URM students is providing longer-term benefits: follow-up data reveal that 18 percent of the school's URM graduates have a full-time career in academic medicine (Garcia et al., 2003).

The institution supports its admissions efforts by extending academic and social support to URM students and assesses its progress in attracting and retaining URM students. The Early Matriculation Program (EMP), in particular, offers URM and non-URM students a summer premedical curriculum that provides an early introduction to the culture of the medical school, builds student confidence and leadership skills, and promotes scholarship. Follow-up data reveal that EMP participants have a slightly higher than average rate of receipt of Stanford Medical Student Scholar awards, have a lower rate of attrition, and have published at slightly higher levels (22 percent, or nearly one in four) than other Stanford Medical School students (Garcia et al., 2003).

SUMMARY AND RECOMMENDATIONS

This chapter has reviewed typical admissions policies and practices of health professions educational programs, with particular attention to the role of standardized tests in the admissions process. Standardized test scores are generally good predictors of subsequent academic performance, but they have been used—in some cases inappropriately—as a barometer of applicants' academic "merit," often to the detriment of URM students. URM students often score lower than their white or Asian American peers on a range of standardized tests, including the SAT, GRE, and MCAT. This disparity occurs for a variety of reasons, principally because of poorer educational opportunities afforded to African American, Latino, and American Indian/Alaska Native students. These students are more likely than non-URM students to attend racially and economically segregated, poorly funded schools that offer few (if any) advanced placement and college preparatory classes, have fewer credentialed teachers, and suffer from a climate of low expectations. Standardized test performance is variable and may be improved significantly through costly private test preparation classes. Moreover, even among those URM students who are invested in high academic performance, social and psychological factors, such as the pressure to perform above levels suggested by stereotypes of low minority academic ability, may serve to suppress their test performance.

When quantitative variables such as standardized test scores are weighted heavily in the admissions process, URM applicants, because of their generally poorer academic preparation and test performance, are less successful in gaining admission than non-URM applicants. Absent admissions practices that allow applicants' race or ethnicity to be considered along with other personal characteristics of applicants, URM student participation in health professions education is likely to decline sharply. States that have implemented "percent solution" admissions strategies (i.e., where a top percentage of high school graduates are guaranteed admission to the state university system) have found that URM admissions have generally declined. In California, even when URM students gain admission, these students are not guaranteed a seat at the university of their choice, which may result in URM students disproportionately matriculating in "lower-tier" campuses within the University of California system.

These barriers to URM admission have led some organizations and institutions to reconceptualize their admissions policies and practices to place greater weight on applicants' qualitative attributes, such as leadership, commitment to service, community orientation, experience with diverse groups, and other factors. This shift of emphasis to professional and "humanistic" factors is also consistent with a growing recognition in health professions fields that these attributes must receive greater attention in the admissions process to maintain professional quality, to ensure that future health professionals are prepared to address societal needs, and to maintain the public's trust in the integrity and skill of health professionals. Anecdotally, evidence suggests that this shift may also reduce barriers to admission of qualified URM applicants, thereby achieving the dual goals of improving both the quality and diversity of health professions students.

Recommendation 2-1: HPEIs[4] should develop, disseminate, and utilize a clear statement of mission that recognizes the value of diversity in enhancing its mission and that of the relevant health care professions. The mission statement should identify the stakeholders (e.g., the community or public served) to whom the institution is accountable as well as (where applicable) state, regional, or national health workforce goals.

Recommendation 2-2: HPEIs should establish explicit policies regarding the value and importance the institution places on the teaching and provision of culturally competent care and the role of institutional diversity in achieving this goal.

Recommendation 2-3: Admissions should be based on a comprehensive review of each applicant. Admissions committees should determine which attributes of applicants best support the mission of the institution and assess these attributes as part of the admissions process. Such attributes include, but are not limited to, applicants' race or ethnicity, socioeconomic background, cross-cultural experience, life choices, multilingual abilities, interpersonal skills, cultural competence, leadership qualities, barriers the applicant has overcome, and other attributes that reflect the institutional mission. Admissions models should balance quantitative data (i.e., prior grades and standardized test scores) with these qualitative characteristics.

Recommendation 2-4: Admissions committees should include voting representation from underrepresented groups, including, but not limited to, racial/ethnic minorities, and should reflect the geographic and socioeconomic diversity of the communities served by the institution. In addition, health professions education institutions should provide special incentives to faculty for participation on admissions committees (e.g., by providing additional weight or consideration for service during promotion review) and provide training for committee members on the importance of diversity efforts and means to improve diversity within the committee purview.

---

[4]Recommendations regarding admissions policies and practices are intended to apply to health professions educational institutions, whether free-standing or affiliated with a university or embedded in another institution.

REFERENCES

American Sociological Association. 2003. *Brief of the American Sociological Association et al., as Amicus Curiae in Support of Respondents.* Merritt DJ, Lee BL, Attorneys for Amici Curiae. Washington, DC: American Sociological Association.

Aronson J, Fried CB, Good C. 2001. Reducing the effects of stereotype threat on African American college students by shaping theories of intelligence. *Journal of Experimental Social Psychology* 38(2):113–125.

Association of American Medical Colleges (AAMC). 2000. The predictive validity of the Medical College Admission Test. *Contemporary Issues in Medical Education* 3(2):1–2.

Bobo LD. 2001. Racial attitudes and relations at the close of the twentieth century. In: Smelser NJ, Wilson WJ, Mitchell F, eds. *America Becoming: Racial Trends and Their Consequences.* Vol.1. Washington, DC: National Academy Press. Pp. 264–301.

Bowen WG, Bok D. 1998. *The Shape of the River: Long-Term Consequences of Considering Race in College and University Admissions.* Princeton, NJ: Princeton University Press.

Calvin A. 2000. Use of standardized tests in admissions in postsecondary institutions of higher education. *Psychology, Public Policy, and Law* 6(1):20–32.

Camara WJ, Schmidt AE. 1999. *Group Differences in Standardized Testing and Social Stratification.* College Board Report No. 99-5. New York: College Board Publications. Pp. 1–18.

Cleveland E. 2003. *AAMC's Expanded Minority Admissions Exercise.* Presentation to IOM Committee on Institutional and Policy-Level Strategies to Increase the Diversity of the U.S. Health Care Workforce, April 9, 2003, Washington, DC.

Cohen JJ. 2003. The consequences of premature abandonment of affirmative action in medical school admissions. *Journal of the American Medical Association* 289(9):1143–1149.

Devine PG. 1989. Stereotypes and prejudice: Their automatic and controlled components. *Journal of Personality and Social Psychology* 56:5–18.

Edwards JC, Elam CL, Wagoner NE. 2001. An admission model for medical schools. *Academic Medicine* 76(12):1207–1212.

Fordham S, Ogbu JU. 1986. Black students' school success: Coping with the burden of "acting white." *Urban Review* 18(3):176–206.

Garcia G, Nation CL, Parker NH. This volume. Increasing diversity in the health professions: A look at best practices in admissions. In Smedley BD, Stith-Butler A, Bristow LR, eds. *In the Nation's Compelling Interest: Ensuring Diversity in the Health-Care Workforce.* Washington, DC: The National Academies Press.

Garcia JA, Paterniti DA, Romano PS, Kravitz RL. 2003. Patient preferences for physician characteristics in university-based primary clinics. *Ethnicity & Disease* 13:259–267.

Gould SJ. 1996. *The Mismeasure of Man.* New York: W.W. Norton.

Herrnstein RJ, Murray C. 1999. *The Bell Curve: Intelligence and Class Structure in American Life.* New York: Free Press.

Horn CL, Flores SM. 2003. *Percent Plans in College Admissions: A Comparison of Three States' Experiences.* Cambridge, MA: The Civil Rights Project, Harvard University.

Koenig JA, Sireci SG, Wiley A. 1998. Evaluating the predictive validity of MCAT scores across diverse applicant groups. *Academic Medicine* 73(10):1095–1106.

Kondo DG, Judd VE. 2000. Demographic characteristics of U.S. medical school admission committees. *Journal of the American Medical Association* 284(9):1111–1113.

Maldonado F. 2001. Rethinking the admissions process: Evaluation techniques that promote inclusiveness in admissions decisions. In: Smedley BD, Stith AY, Colburn L, Evans CH eds. *The Right Thing to Do, The Smart Thing to Do: Enhancing Diversity in Health Professions.* Washington, DC: National Academy Press.

Marin P, Lee EK. 2003. Appearance and reality in the Sunshine State: The Talented 20 Program in Florida. Cambridge, MA: The Civil Rights Project, Harvard University.

Matherlee K. This volume. The Role of Public Financing in Improving Diversity in Health Professions. In Smedley BD, Stith-Butler A, Bristow LR, eds. *In the Nation's Compelling Interest: Ensuring Diversity in the Health-Care Workforce*. Washington, DC: The National Academies Press.

McGaghie WC. 2002. Assessing readiness for medical education: Evolution of the Medical College Admission Test. *Journal of the American Medical Association* 288(9):1085–1090.

National Research Council. 1999. *Myths and Tradeoffs: The Role of Tests in Undergraduate Admissions*. Beatty A, Greenwood MRC, Linn RL, eds. Washington, DC: National Academy Press.

Orfield G. 2001. *Schools More Separate: Consequences of a Decade of Resegregation*. Cambridge, MA: The Civil Rights Project, Harvard University.

Silver B, Hodgson CS. 1997. Evaluating GPAs and MCAT scores as predictors of NBMEI and clerkship performances based on students' data from one undergraduate institution. *Academic Medicine* 72(5):394–396.

Smedley BD, Myers HF, Harrell SP. 1993. Minority-status stresses and the college adjustment of ethnic minority freshmen. *The Journal of Higher Education* 64(4):434–452.

Steele CM. 1997. A threat in the air: How stereotypes shape intellectual identity and performance. *American Psychologist* 52(6):613–629.

Steele CM, Aronson J. 1995. Stereotype threat and the intellectual test performance of African Americans. *Journal of Personality and Social Psychology* 69(5):797–811.

Sternberg RJ, Williams WM. 1997. Does the Graduate Record Examination predict meaningful success in the graduate training of psychologists? A case study. *American Psychologist* 52(6):630–641.

Sternberg RJ and the Rainbow Project Collaborators. In review. The Rainbow Project: Enhancing the SAT through assessments of analytical, practical, and creative skills.

Tienda M, Leicht KT, Sullivan T, Maltese M, Lloyd K. 2003. Closing the Gap?: Admissions & Enrollments at the Texas Public Flagship Before and After Affirmative Action. [Online]. Available: http://www.texastop10.princeton.edu/publications/tienda012103.pdf [accessed January 15, 2004].

Wightman LF. 2003. Standardized testing and equal access: A tutorial. In: Chang M, Witt D, Jones J, Hakuta K, eds. *Compelling Interest: Examining the Evidence on Racial Dynamics in Higher Education*. Stanford, CA: Stanford University Press.

3

Costs and Financing of Health Professions Education

The costs associated with health professions education pose a considerable barrier for many underrepresented minority (URM) students, whose economic resources are, on average, more limited compared to their majority counterparts. URM students, in particular, may be discouraged from entering health professions training programs when faced with the prospect of high debt. Some health professions leaders have therefore called for a reexamination of the costs and financing of health professions training to significantly reduce or eliminate many training costs, particularly for those students whose service in the public sector is likely to increase access to care for medically underserved populations.

While URM students are more likely than non-URM students to come from low-income families, most low-income students are white. Policies that solely target financial support to low-income students may or may not successfully help URM students to access and succeed in health professions training programs. Therefore, it is important for financial strategies to be implemented in conjunction with other "race-conscious" interventions targeting, for example, admissions and accreditation policies.

A number of public and private initiatives have been established to assist URM students finance the costs of their education and training. Some provide direct financial assistance to students and others indirectly support URM students through funding provided to institutions for diversity activities. All, however, provide support to increase URM participation in health professions and reduce financial barriers, directly or indirectly, for students who experience difficulty financing their training. This chapter will provide an overview of the financial status of URM families, assess the costs of training, and show the negative impact of these costs on URM students' pursuit of education. In addition, the chapter will assess the role of private and public sources of funding for health professions students, and examine issues regarding the financing of education. For a detailed review of publicly funded health professions programs that support URM students, the reader is referred to the commissioned paper, *Public Financing of the Health Professions: Levers for Change*, prepared by Karen Matherlee, which appears as an appendix of this report.

For purposes of this report, the study committee defines health professions educational costs as a formulation involving total educational and living expenses: including tuition and fees (which vary considerably across institutions, particularly between public and private health professions education institutions [HPEIs]); other educational expenses (including books, equipment, supplies, etc.); the number of years to degree completion; living costs (including rent, utilities, and other living expenses); and the costs of any specialized, prerequisite post-high school or post-baccalaureate preparation. The other side of this equation—financing of health professions training—can be described as a student's financial resources (both personally and nonpersonally derived), as well as scholarships, loans, and other forms of financial assistance. Unmet financial need is therefore total health professions educational costs, minus student financial resources. This chapter attempts to describe educational costs, sources of financing of training, and unmet financial need, and how these factors affect URM participation in health professions education. This analysis is severely limited, however, by a lack of data regarding these factors, particularly in disciplines other than medical education, where financing issues are more thoroughly documented. This absence of data prevents a comparison of financing issues across health professions disciplines, because the factors identified above, such as tuition, fees, number of years to degree completion, and sources of financial aid, vary considerably across disciplines. The most useful perspective is therefore to examine the financial obstacles within each profession, rather than across professions.

FINANCIAL STATUS OF UNDERREPRESENTED
MINORITY FAMILIES

Census figures indicate a large disparity in family income among various racial and ethnic groups in the United States (Figure 3-1) (U.S. Census Bureau, 2002a). Households headed by black and Hispanic individuals earn significantly less than either white non-Hispanic or Asian and Pacific Islander householders. In 2001, the median income for black and Hispanic families was approximately $34,000 and $35,000, respectively. In com-

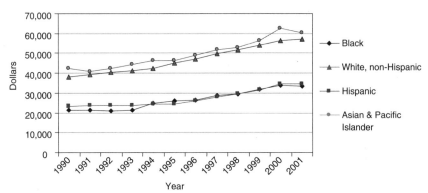

Year

FIGURE 3-1 Race and Hispanic origin of householder: families by median income, 1990–2001.
SOURCE. U.S. Census Bureau, *Historical Income Tables—Families, 2002.*

parison, white families had a median income of $57,000 and Asian/Pacific Islander families had a median income of $60,000. American Indian and Alaska Native families were not included in these census figures; however other census data indicate that the three-year average median income for 1999–2001 was $32,116 for American Indian and Alaska Native households, which was higher than the median income of black households and similar to the median income of Hispanic households during this time period (U.S. Census Bureau, 2002b). Thus, as URM students prepare for higher education, they are more likely to face difficulties financing their education.

In addition to disparities in household income, data indicate large racial and ethnic differences in wealth (Figure 3-2). On average, white families are wealthier than black or Hispanic households, even after controlling for income and demographic variables (Choudhury, 2002). Housing equity is fairly equally distributed across racial and ethnic groups, although rates of homeownership are greater for whites. Nonhousing equity (e.g., liquid assets, stocks, bonds, IRAs, vehicle and business equity) varies more widely between racial and ethnic groups as income increases, with whites holding larger sums of nonhousing equity.

COSTS OF UNDERGRADUATE EDUCATION: EFFECTS ON ACCESS AND COMPLETION

Much of the available data regarding the impact of the high costs of education relates to college access and degree attainment. These findings have implications for health professions education and strategies that may be employed to reduce financial barriers for URM students entering these fields.

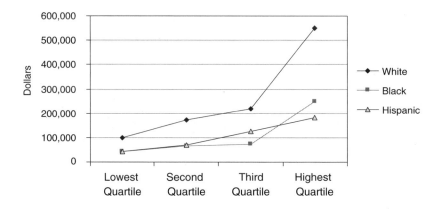

FIGURE 3-2 Mean net worth for households by race, ethnicity, and income quartile.
NOTE: Cutoff points for income quartiles, in 1992 dollars: $23,460; $41,900; $66,900.
SOURCE: *Health and Retirement Study Wave 1* (1992) as cited in Choudhury, 2002.

The Advisory Committee on Student Financial Assistance reports that ". . . financial barriers to a college education have risen sharply due to shifts in policies and priorities at the federal, state, and institutional levels, resulting in a shortage of student aid, and in particular need-based grant aid, as well as rising college tuition" (Advisory Committee on Student Financial Assistance, 2002, p. v). The Advisory Committee estimated that these financial barriers prohibit 48 percent of low-income students who are academically qualified for college from attending a four-year institution. The lowest achieving, highest socioeconomic status (SES) students attend college at approximately the same rate as the highest achieving, lowest SES students, at 77 percent and 78 percent, respectively (Advisory Committee on Student Financial Assistance, 2002). Because URM families earn less, on average, than their white or Asian/Pacific Islander counterparts, they may face greater difficulty in financing their children's undergraduate education. Estimates from the 1999–2000 academic year indicate that among full-time undergraduate students who were financially dependant on their families, black, Hispanic, Asian, and those students who indicated more than one race were more likely to be from low-income families (Figure 3-3; U.S. Department of Education, 2003b). White, Pacific Islander, and American Indian students were more likely to come from high-income families.

While rates of tuition have climbed steadily, sources of grant aid have

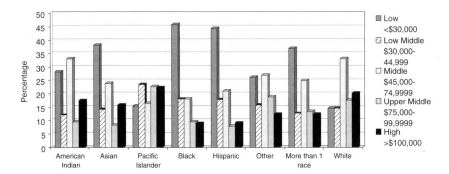

FIGURE 3-3 Percentage distribution of full-time, full-year dependent undergraduates according to family income, 1999–2000, by race and ethnicity.
SOURCE: U.S. Department of Education, National Center for Education Statistics, 2003b.

decreased. At the federal level, the maximum awards provided by Pell grants, awarded to help low-income students attend college, have decreased significantly relative to the cost of attendance. The maximum award decreased from 84 percent of public 4-year costs during the 1975–1976 academic year to 39 percent of costs during the 1999–2000 academic year (College Board, 2000, and U.S. Department of Education, 2000b, as cited in Advisory Committee on Student Financial Assistance, 2001). At the state level, more new grants are merit-based rather than need-based. In 1982, 9.6 percent of grants were merit-based compared to 18.6 percent in 1998 (Heller, in press, as cited in Advisory Committee on Student Financial Assistance, 2001). Similarly, higher education institutions are increasing merit-based awards. At private institutions, grants for middle-income students have exceeded grants for low-income students (McPherson and Shapiro, in press, as cited in Advisory Committee on Student Financial Assistance, 2001).

Increased tuition costs and decreased need-based aid have resulted in higher levels of unmet need for lower income students (Figure 3-4). Unmet financial need is calculated as the total cost of education minus expected family contribution minus aid (U.S. Department of Education, 2003a). In 1995–1996, students from the lowest income families faced $3,800 in unmet need for a public 4-year college and $6,200 for private 4-year colleges. For middle-income students, whose family income was between $25,000 and $49,000, average unmet need was $3,000 for public and $4,900 for private college. In comparison, those students from the highest SES level faced $400 in need for public college and $3,000 for private institutions (U.S.

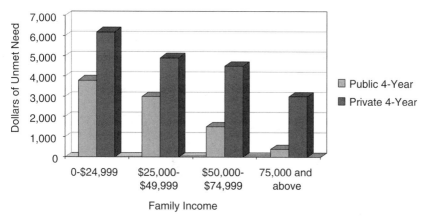

FIGURE 3-4 Average annual unmet need of high school graduates, by family income and type of institution.
SOURCE: Advisory Committee on Student Financial Assistance, 2002.

Department of Education, 1999). Between 1992 and 1999, average annual borrowing by low-income students with high unmet need increased from $1,812 to $2,982 at public 4-year colleges (Advisory Committee on Student Financial Assistance, 2002). At private colleges borrowing increased from $2,935 to $4,130 (Advisory Committee on Student Financial Assistance, 2002). Thus, a 4-year baccalaureate degree can result in over $16,000 of debt for low-income students.

The impact of high unmet need can be considerable on low-income students, even those who are academically prepared for the challenges of higher education. Low-income students with high unmet need are significantly less likely than high-income students with low unmet need to expect to finish college; plan to attend a 4-year college after graduating from high school; take entrance exams; and apply, enroll, and persist to degree completion (Figure 3-5) (Advisory Committee on Student Financial Assistance, 2002). Students who have sufficient funds for college enjoy enhanced academic performance and social integration on campus and are more likely to persist to graduation (Nora and Cabrera, 1996).

In an investigation of the influence of race and gender on the awarding of financial aid, Heller (2000), using data from the National Postsecondary Student Aid Studies, found that while there were variations in financial aid by geographic region and type of institution, in general, African American students were more likely to receive nonneed grants (based on merit or other circumstance not related to financial need, such as academic, artistic, or athletic merit), particularly those students attending public institutions. Hispanic students were less likely to receive nonneed grants. The author

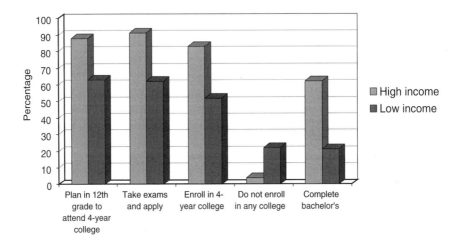

FIGURE 3-5 College access process for high- and low-income college-qualified high school graduates.
SOURCE: Advisory Committee on Student Financial Assistance, 2002.

speculates that since academic achievement and other institutional and student characteristics served as controls, the effect of race on receiving nonneed aid was the result of institutional financial aid policies and that African American students were specifically targeted for financial aid compared with white students (Heller, 2000).

Several studies have examined the impact of financial barriers and the effect of financial aid on student enrollment. An investigation of racial differences in high school students' access to postsecondary education found that low-income, black, and Hispanic high school graduates were less likely to be academically prepared for a 4-year college and that among those who were prepared, low-income and Hispanic students were less likely to take entrance exams and apply for admissions (U.S. Department of Education, 1997). However, differences in enrollment rates between college-qualified low- and middle-income students were eliminated among those students who took college entrance exams and completed the admissions application. Similarly, differences in enrollment between college-qualified students of varying race and ethnicity (black, Hispanic, Asian, and white) were also eliminated among those who took entrance exams and completed an application. This study also found that "the more sources of information they had obtained, and the more people with whom they had discussed financial aid, the more likely college-qualified low- and middle-income, black, and Hispanic students were to take college entrance exams and apply for admission to a four-year college" (U.S. Department of Education, 1997, p. 60). However, a causal relationship between college attendance and information-seeking could not be established. It may be that students who intended to attend sought more information.

The type of aid received by students also may influence college attendance. In a review of evidence of financial aid's impact on college entry and retention, Grumbach et al. (2002) reported that grants had a large effect on increasing attendance for students in the lowest income category. In contrast, loans were not associated with enrollment rates for this group of students. For middle-income students, both grants and loans were associated with increased attendance (St. John, 1994; Grumbach et al., 2002).

Grumbach and colleagues also noted that differences in how far low-income students advance in their education are not only a function of the ability to pay. Low socioeconomic status is associated with a range of factors that may affect college access and success, including attendance at primary and secondary schools with few resources and having few family members who have attended college (and therefore know what the experience is like and can help navigate the application process). As mentioned in the outset of this chapter, providing financial aid alone is unlikely to remove all barriers to higher education for URM students.

In light of trends in tuition costs, educational organizations have called for changes in policies for the provision of financial aid to low-income students. Recently, the College Board urged the government to raise the maximum awards for Pell Grants to cover the average cost of tuition, fees, room, and board, which was estimated to be $9,000 for the 2002–2003 academic year, and to expand loan forgiveness for students who enter and stay in occupations that serve high-need areas (College Board, 2003). In addition, the Board urged the federal government to partner with states, colleges, universities, and the private sector and to take the lead in developing programs to encourage investment in need-based aid. Specific recommendations included:

- ". . . Loan forgiveness for students who enter and remain in certain key occupations and those who serve in high-need areas should be supported and expanded. . ." (College Board, 2003, p. 6).
- ". . . The federal government should also increase its level of support directly to institutions that serve large percentages of high-need students . . ." (College Board, 2003, p. 7).
- ". . . Colleges and universities should reaffirm their commitment to need-based aid, striving to enroll larger numbers of students from low-income and underrepresented backgrounds" (College Board, 2003, p. 7).
- "The federal government and the states should explore ways of more closely linking increases in tuition to increases in need-based aid, to insulate

financially needy student from effects of economic downturns. . ." (College Board, 2003, p. 8).

In summary, the financial burdens imposed by undergraduate education are a significant factor for low-income students who wish to attend college. A student's ability or academic readiness does not make them immune to these difficulties. These impediments may continue for those who continue their studies at the graduate level.

COSTS OF HEALTH PROFESSIONS EDUCATION: TUITION AND STUDENT DEBT

By the time students with high unmet need complete college, they may have debts of $10,000 to $15,000 or more. As students consider obtaining degrees in one of the health professions, they must contemplate the even higher costs of these degrees. There is some evidence to suggest that low-income students who graduate from college are less likely than their higher income peers to continue on to graduate education (Grumbach et al., 2002). This section will review trends in costs of health professions education and debt incurred by students.

Dental Education

In 1999, the average first-year resident tuition for dentistry schools was $15,653 (Figure 3-6), compared to $7,086 in 1985 (Valachovic et al., 2001). The fees at public schools were $9,354 while private school tuition and fees totaled $30,208, resulting in costs ranging from $37,000 to $120,000 at the end of four years. Moreover, the average debt of dental students has significantly increased in the past 20 years (see Figure 3-7) (Hardigan, 1999). The average rate of increase for all schools between 1991–1992 and 1997–1998 was 84.6 percent. The increase was greatest at public schools (94.5 percent).

Medical Education

For medical students, average tuition and debt are similarly high. During the 2001–2002 academic year, mean tuition and fees for residents at public medical schools were $12,970. Fees for nonresidents were more than double this figure (Figure 3-8) (AAMC, 2003).

In 2001, approximately 75 percent of URM graduates had received scholarships during medical school, with average scholarship awards of $46,383 for private school graduates and $25,184 for public school graduates (AAMC, 2002). By comparison, nearly 50 percent of non-URM stu-

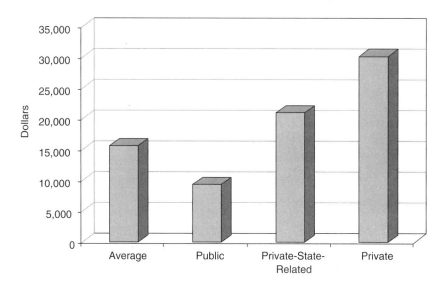

FIGURE 3-6 Average first year resident tuition and fees at U.S. dental schools, 1999.
SOURCE: Valachovic et al., 2001. Reprinted, with permission, from the American Dental Education Association, 2004. Copyright 2004 by ADEA.

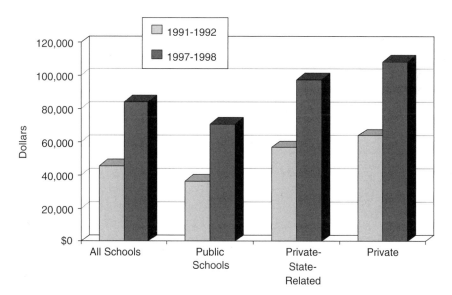

FIGURE 3-7 Average debt of senior dental students, 1991–1992, 1997–1998.
SOURCE: Hardigan, 1999. Reprinted, with permission, from the American Dental Education Association, 2004. Copyright 2004 by ADEA.

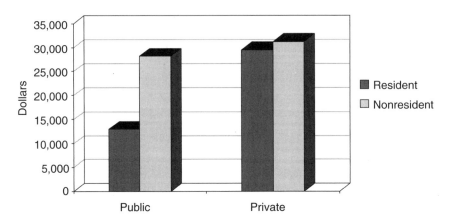

FIGURE 3-8 Tuition and fees for first year students at U.S. medical schools, 2001–2002.
SOURCE: AAMC, 2003.

dents received scholarship aid, averaging $40,197 for private school graduates and $18,134 for public school graduates.

Like dental students, medical graduates face high levels of debt, which have increased six-fold in the past 20 years. Among students who incur debt, URM and non-URM students face similar levels of total debt. However, URM graduates are twice as likely to carry some educational debt. Among 2001 private school graduates, 20.3 percent of non-URMs had no debt, as compared to 8.1 percent of URMs (AAMC, 2002). For public school graduates, 16.8 percent of non-URM students completed with no educational debt, while only 8.4 percent of URM student graduated debt free. However, for those that had debt, approximately 50 percent of all students owed more than $100,000 (AAMC, 2002).

Professional Psychology Education

The average cost of education for students in schools of psychology is less, on average, than for students in other health professions. However, these students tend to earn less once in practice than some other health professionals. During the 2001–2002 academic year, the average cost of tuition at public institutions offering graduate degree programs in psychology was $3,380 for state residents and $8,858 for state nonresidents (Figure 3-9; APA, 2003). Tuition at private institutions was approximately $17,000.

Debt for clinical and other psychology health-service areas has, like other health professions, increased in recent years (Murray, 1999). A larger

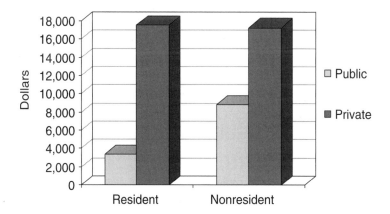

FIGURE 3-9 Median tuition in U.S. graduate departments of psychology by type of institution, 2001–2002.
SOURCE: Graduate Study in Psychology, Compiled by APA Research Office, 2003. 2001–2002 Tuition in Graduate Departments of Psychology. Adapted with permission from the American Psychological Association. Copyright 2004 by APA.

percentage of psychology Ph.D. recipients reported debt in excess of $30,000 than Ph.D. recipients in other science and engineering fields (NSF, 2000). The proportion of students in health-service provider fields with loan debt of more than $30,000 has increased from less than 20 percent in 1989 to more than 40 percent in 1996 (Murray, 1999). Thirty percent of those with Ph.D.s in clinical psychology (1993–1997) had debt exceeding $30,000 (Figure 3-10) (NSF, 2000). Of those with doctoral degrees in counseling, family and marriage, and school psychology, 17 percent carried more that $30,000 in debt. For graduates with Psy.D. degrees (whose programs focus on training for clinical practice), 55 percent had debt in excess of $30,000 (NSF, 2000).

Nursing Education

National-level data on the costs of nursing education, average levels of debt incurred by nursing students, and sources of financial aid for nursing education are not routinely collected and are therefore not as readily available as are data from other health professions. To obtain this information, the study committee contacted several major nursing organizations (e.g., National League of Nursing, the American Association of Colleges of Nurses). National-level statistics for tuition were obtained for basic registered nursing (RN) programs (Figure 3-11), but tuition data for other types

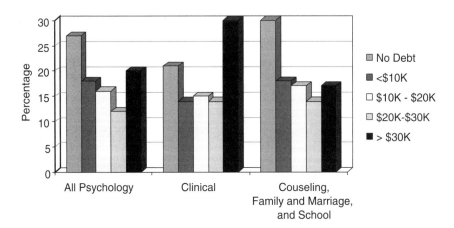

FIGURE 3-10 Percent of debt of 1993–1997 psychology Ph.D.s by field.
SOURCE: National Science Foundation, 2000.

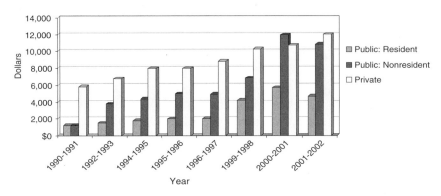

FIGURE 3-11 Estimate of mean annual tuition of full-time students in public or private basic RN programs (preliminary and unpublished data).
NOTE: Tuition data is not a required field in the annual survey.
SOURCE: National League for Nursing. Figure included with the permission of the National League for Nursing, New York, NY.

of nursing programs were not available. Data from the National League for Nursing reveal a steady increase in tuition costs for public and private RN programs from the 1990–1991 to 2001–2002 academic years. In this latter year, tuition for resident at public programs decreased by approximately $1,000.

National level data regarding debt for nursing students were not available. However, anecdotal reports suggest that nursing students experience large debt loads, as do students in other health professions. For example, at the University of Colorado Health Sciences Center, a public institution, average debt among nursing students (accumulated while attending the university) receiving degrees in 2003 ranged from $19,258 for B.S.N. students to $72,940 for N.D. students, for a total of $31,765 in debt for students receiving degrees in the school of nursing (includes B.S.N., M.S., Ph.D., N.D.) (personal communication, Marlaine Smith, professor and associate dean for academic affairs, University of Colorado Health Sciences Center School of Nursing). These figures, however, may represent a slight overestimate of debt due to a high proportion of N.D. students attending 1.5 to 2 years at N.D. degree-granting institutions and receiving graduate level loans, then transferring to B.S.N. programs (causing the B.S.N. average to be larger than if the student attended only as a B.S.N.). In addition, in many cases students receiving M.S. and or Ph.D. degrees at the school of nursing also receive other degrees at the university.

At Vanderbilt University, a private institution, master's and baccalaureate nursing students graduated with an average debt burden of $80,000 (personal communication, Colleen Conway-Welch, dean and professor, Vanderbilt University School of Nursing). While 90 percent of students at Vanderbilt qualified for financial assistance as determined by the Free Application for Federal Student Aid (FAFSA), the average scholarship was $4,000, which met 15 percent of the FAFSA need. *These examples are taken from private and selective institutions and may not generalize to the educational experiences of other nursing students.*

COSTS OF HEALTH PROFESSIONS EDUCATION: BEYOND TUITION

While much of the literature on costs is focused on tuition, it is important to note that the total costs of a health professions education are often far greater than tuition costs alone. Other costs—such as room and board, books and professional supplies and equipment, and other educational expenses—are often difficult to quantify but can be significant depending on the geographic location of the educational institution, institutional requirements for equipment and supplies, and other factors.

In addition to expenses directly related to education, other costs such as consumer debt may cause considerable burden. For example, among 2001 medical graduates, 63 percent of URM students carried consumer debt (for example, credit cards and/or auto loans), compared to 37 percent of non-URM students. However, among those with consumer debt, non-URM graduates carried an average level of $20,783 compared to $12,803 for URM graduates (AAMC, 2002).

As will be discussed in Chapter 5 ("Transforming the Institutional Climate to Enhance Diversity in Health Professions"), to the extent that students must repeat a year of training, tuition and other costs will increase accordingly. These costs, as noted above, disproportionately burden URM students, who have fewer resources, on average, than non-URM students. More research is needed to assess these costs, the impact of educational and noneducational costs on URM students' decisions to pursue health professions careers, the availability of financial resources (both scholarship and loan) to address unmet financial need, and the impact of these factors on URM student completion of training, graduation rates, and choice of practice location and specialty.

IMPACT OF COSTS AND DEBT

The impact of education costs and debt on students can be quite substantial, affecting persistence, career choices, job satisfaction, and lifestyle. The 2002 National Student Loan Survey (of Nellie Mae subsidized or unsubsidized Stafford or SLS borrowers) examined the impact of debt repayment on students paying back loans in 2002 (Baum and O'Malley, 2003). The analysis included undergraduate as well as graduate borrowers. Students from low-income families (defined as those receiving Pell Grants) reported more feelings of burden about their debt compared to other students. This is reported as a change from previous surveys where there was no significant difference in feeling of burden between low-income students and those not receiving Pell Grants. In addition, African American, Asian American, and Hispanic borrowers reported more burden than white borrowers, after controlling for other factors. The association was strongest for Hispanics, but also significant for African American borrowers. The authors suggest that "socioeconomic and racial background are correlated with perceptions of debt burden, with low-income and minority students perceiving greater hardship than other borrowers with given amounts of debt and current income levels" (Baum and O'Malley, 2003, p. 22).

In a study of debt and persistence among dental students, an analysis of the 1993 National Postsecondary Student Aid Study (DeAngelis, 2000) revealed that receiving financial aid of any type promoted within-year persistence. However, when taking tuition, financial aid received, and debt into account, debt was the only variable found to significantly influence persistence. For every $1,000 in debt, students were 5.76 percentage points less likely to persist to their next semester. The authors conclude that while financial aid meets immediate needs, the accumulation of debt may significantly and negatively affect persistence and that there may be a limit to the amount of debt students are willing to amass.

Most evidence of the effect of debt on career choice is found in the medical literature. There have been two hypotheses regarding the effect of debt on physicians' choice of primary care practice versus other specialties (Colquitt et al., 1996). One is that students with high levels of debt chose primary care careers because the training period is shorter and they can begin earning a physician's salary sooner. The other posits that students with high debt choose specialty fields other than primary care because the salaries are higher and therefore allow them to pay off debt sooner. Several studies have examined the effect of debt on career choice (Baker and Barker, 1997; Brotherton, 1995; Colquitt et al., 1996; Rosenthal et al., 1996). While some evidence suggests that debt has little influence on choice of general or specialty careers (Brotherton, 1995), others have suggested that debt does, in fact, independently contribute to the selection of career specialty. Rosenthal and colleagues (1996) found that debt above a certain threshold (at least $75,000) was an independent predictor of career choice away from family practice. Colquitt and colleagues (1996) suggest that the relationship between debt and career choice is a complex one and that it is important to assess the context, particular groups of students, which specialties are being considered, and how the impact of debt changes over time. In their study, the effect of debt on preferences for family medicine, general internal medicine, and general pediatrics varied, for example, by how much income medical school graduates expected to earn, the level of debt they incurred, how much debt was from subsidized loans, and in which geographic location graduates expected to practice. The researchers concluded that debt was an important factor in specialty choice, driven by a variety of issues. Rico and Stagnaro-Green (1997) reported similar results in a study examining the relationship between debt and career choice in URM and non-URM students placed in residencies at Mount Sinai School of Medicine. While mean debt levels were similar for URM and non-URM graduates, half of URMs had debt in excess of $75,000 compared to 37 percent of non-URMs. Overall, fewer URM graduates chose primary care fields (37.5 percent vs. 46.6 percent). When examining career choices by level of debt, the investigators found that among students with more than $75,000 of debt, 31 percent of URM chose primary care fields, compared to 49 percent of non-URMs. However, among those with debt levels under $75,000, choices for primary care were similar (40 percent URM, 48 percent non-URM). The authors conclude from their preliminary findings that high debt may influence choices for URM students.

The relationship between debt and career satisfaction has also been investigated. Results from a study of nearly 5,000 physicians that examined characteristics of those having second thoughts about their decision to pursue a career in medicine suggests that financial debt may contribute to feelings of dissatisfaction (Hadley et al., 1992). Results revealed that those most likely to have second thoughts were white women, blacks, and Hispanics, all of whom reported lower incomes, higher debt, and higher patient loads. The authors suggest a reexamination of the reliance of medical students, particularly minorities, on loans to finance their education.

Another important impact of student debt that may be overlooked is the effect on graduates' lifestyle once they are in the workforce. Repayment is made with after-tax dollars and graduates must earn more than what is owed. While debt levels have grown, resident salaries have remained relatively stable (*American Medical News*, as cited in Johnson, 2002b). Based on the average house staff salary (1999–2000) of $36,928 in the northeast United States, a URM medical student with $105,136 in school debt would have only $737 per month left to cover living and other expenses after making the monthly loan payment. Six years post graduation with an annual salary of $43,045, a URM student with the same level of debt would have $1,079.25 left after making the monthly payment. Consolidating and extending payments 20 years would leave $1,490.78 (Johnson, 2002b). It is important to note that women, who constitute half of the physician workforce, make less, on average, than men. In 1998 the median net earnings for women was $123,390 compared to $171,800 for men (Johnson, 2002b). Thus, women may have more difficulty managing debt.

Students in other disciplines, such as dentistry, face similar circumstances. For example, in 1995 the average student loan debt of dental students (from private and public institutions) was $67,772. If these were all Federal Stafford Loans with relatively low interest rate of 7.66 percent (at that time), students would need an annual income of $121,554 to manage this debt (Myers and Zwemer, 1998). While debt has increased at a rate greater than the growth of the economy, income of dental practitioners has increased at a level lower than the growth of the economy (Myers and Zwemer, 1998). The authors suggest that students will need to have successful practices early on to manage their repayment and that debt can make it difficult for students to consider careers in education because of the salaries of starting faculty.

It has been reported that many students do not think about or plan for debt management (Johnson, 2002b; Lofton, 2002; Zeigler, 2003). Students are encouraged to adjust their lifestyles to help ensure that they can manage their debt once they enter practice. Strategies include keeping spending at a minimum, understanding the consequences of delinquent payments and default, understanding terms of grace periods and methods for deferment, understanding choices for repayment, keeping good financial records, seeking professional financial help if needed, and maintaining a good credit report (Johnson, 2002a). The impact of debt can be quite substantial in the short and long term. Students should be encouraged to plan carefully when financing their education and to consider a range of options that are available for paying these sizeable costs.

SOURCES OF FINANCIAL ASSISTANCE FOR STUDENTS PURSUING EDUCATION BEYOND COLLEGE

Like students entering college, most students who pursue education beyond the college level rely on grants and loans to finance their education. Among students making choices about attending graduate school, URM students were more likely to have borrowed to finance their undergraduate education (Heller, 2001) and to face unpaid debts related to undergraduate education while in graduate school. Nettles (1990) estimated that 46 percent of African American and 43 percent of Hispanic graduate students had unpaid undergraduate student loans compared to 36 percent of white students.

Millet and MacKenzie (1995) investigated the role of financial aid in the education of minority doctoral students using a subset of the 1989–1990 National Postsecondary Student Aid Survey. Results indicate that minority students were more likely to take out loans and receive fellowships than nonminority students. However, minorities were less likely to receive administrative assistantships. This latter finding is a significant area of concern, as Nettles (1990) and others suggested that assistantships may be particularly important for student integration, socialization, and persistence.

National-level data indicate that students who pursue their education beyond the college level tend to rely heavily on loans. Data from the 1999–2000 National Postsecondary Student Aid Study report on the financing used by 2.7 million masters, doctoral (Ph.D., Ed.D., Doctor of Business Administration [D.B.A.], Doctor of Public Administration [D.P.A.], and Doctor of Fine Arts [D.F.A.]), and professional (allopathic medicine, osteopathic medicine, dentistry, law, optometry, pharmacy, podiatry, veterinary medicine, chiropractic, theology) students across the country. Among the 2.7 million students, 12 percent were full-time professional students (of these, 27 percent were in medicine, and 29 percent were in dentistry and other health fields) and 13 percent were enrolled full-time in doctoral programs (U.S. Department of Education, 2002). Figures indicate that among full-time, full-year doctoral students, African American and Hispanic students were slightly more likely to receive any source of aid (Figure 3-12). Hispanic students received more grants and African American students took out more loans than students of other races or ethnicities. Figures were not available for American Indian, Alaska Native, Native Hawaiian, and other Pacific Islander populations.

Among professional students in the U.S. Department of Education survey (2002), African American, Hispanics, and those indicating their race as "other" received more loans, on average, than students of other racial and ethnic groups (Figure 3-13). Hispanic and those indicating "other race"

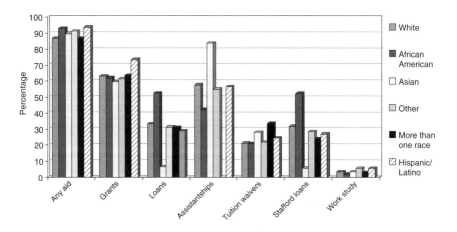

FIGURE 3-12 Percent of full-time, full-year doctoral students who received financial aid, by type of aid, race, and ethnicity.
SOURCE: *Student Financing of Graduate and First-Professional Education, 1999-2000.* U.S. Department of Education, 2002.

were also more likely to receive grants. Only a minority of all students received assistantships, tuition waivers, and work study.

FINANCING OF HEALTH PROFESSION EDUCATION

Financial Assistance for URM Students

Low-income URM individuals considering health professions education face increasing tuition and other costs, on top of the undergraduate debt they have likely accrued. The thought of accumulating debt in excess of $100,000 can be daunting and serve as a barrier for prospective students. There are several programs that provide financial assistance for students indirectly by giving funds to institutions to recruit URM students. A handful of programs provide assistance directly to students through scholarships, loans, or loan repayment programs.

Financial assistance for health professions students is provided by the federal government, states, and private sources. The paper prepared by Matherlee (this volume) provides a more detailed review of many of these federal and state programs. This section discusses a sample of public and private initiatives that seek to improve the representation of URM students in health professions education through the provision of financial assistance. This section is not meant to represent a comprehensive inventory of

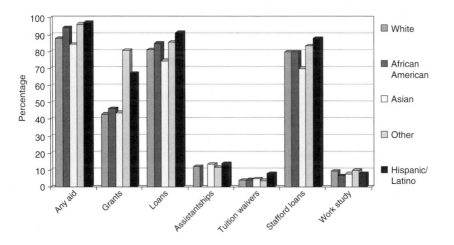

FIGURE 3-13 Percent of full-time, full-year first-professional students who received financial aid, by type of aid, race, and ethnicity.
SOURCE: *Student Financing of Graduate and First-Professional Education, 1999–2000.* U.S. Department of Education, 2002.

these mechanisms; rather, it highlights some prominent examples of efforts to provide financial aid.

Federal Sources of Financial Assistance

Table 3-1 lists some of the largest federal health professions training programs that focus on increasing racial and ethnic diversity. At the federal level, the Health Resources and Services Administration (HRSA) is the primary funder for health professions programs that either target or predominantly include URM students, practitioners, and/or faculty. HRSA is charged with administering Title VII and Title VIII of the Public Health Service Act. These titles authorize funding, through a variety of programs for students and institutions, in order to increase the quality of the education and training of the primary care provider workforce, including the geographic, racial and ethnic diversity of the United States health-care workforce. Title VII applies to medicine and dentistry (and in many cases mental health), while Title VIII pertains to nursing.

Within HRSA's *Bureau of Health Professionals (BHPr)*, the Division of Health Careers Diversity and Development administers Title VII programs. *The Health Careers Opportunities Program (HCOP)* (http://bhpr.hrsa.gov/diversity/hcop/default.htm) is the most extensive of the division's programs.

TABLE 3-1 Examples of Federal Funding for Health Professions
Programs with the Goal of Increasing Diversity

Agency	Division	Program	Funding provided to:
HRSA, BHPr	Division of Health Professions Diversity	Centers of Excellence (COE)	Institutions
		Health Careers Opportunities Program (HCOP)	Institutions
		Minority Faculty Fellowship Program	Institutions
	Division of Nursing	Nursing Workforce Diversity Program	Institutions
	Division of Health Careers Diversity and Development	Scholarships for Disadvantaged Students	Institutions
		Loans for Disadvantaged Students	Institutions
		Disadvantaged Faculty Loan Repayment	Individuals
	National Health Service Corps (NHSC)	Scholarship	Individuals
		Loan repayment program	Individuals
Indian Health Service		Health Professions Scholarship Program	Individuals
NIMH & SAMHSA		Minority Fellowship Program	Institutions

Purpose	Disciplines included	Funding
Improve ability of schools to train URM students	Medicine, Dentistry, Psychology, among others	$32.7 mil (2002)
Increase number of professionals from disadvantaged backgrounds to meet needs of the underserved	Psychology, Dentistry, Medicine, among others	$34.6 mil (2002)
Matching funds to award fellowships to URM faculty	Dentistry, Medicine, among others	$280,857 (2002)
Academic preparation activities, retention efforts, student stipends	Nursing	$6.2 mil (2002)
Scholarship awarded to students based on financial need	Nursing, Dentistry, Medicine, Psychology, among others	$46.2 mil (2002)
Loans awarded to students based on financial need	Medicine, Dentistry, among others	$16.2 mil (2002)
Faculty serve at eligible health professions programs in exchange for loan repayment	Psychology, Dentistry, Nursing, Medicine, among others	$1.3 mil (2002)
Students compete for educational scholarships and in return for this support they must agree to practice in high-need communities	Dentistry, Nursing, Medicine, Psychology, among others	$46.2 mil (2002)
Professionals with qualifying educational loans compete for repayment. Clinicians also receive salary and some tax relief benefits	Nursing, Medicine, Psychology, Dentistry, among others	
Scholarship support in exchange for service after graduation	Medicine, Dentistry, Psychology, Nursing, among others	$9.75 mil (grants) (2002)
Scholarship awarded to students	Psychology, Nursing, Medicine (psychiatry), among others	$3 mil (2001)

Its purpose is to increase the number of health and allied health profession-als from disadvantaged backgrounds. Medicine, dentistry, and clinical psychology are among the many professions targeted. Institutions receiving funds recruit individuals; provide counseling, mentoring, and other services to help retain students; publicize financial aid information; and engage in pipeline initiatives. *The Centers of Excellence (COE)* (http://bhpr.hrsa.gov/diversity/coe/default.htm) awards are designed to improve health professions schools' ability to train underrepresented minority students. These grants provide funds to health professions schools with URM enrollments above the national average. Schools of dentistry, psychology, and medicine are included among eligible disciplines. Activities include minority faculty development, information resources, faculty and student research, and additional support for students in the form of stipends. The COE institutions also engage in a number of pipeline efforts. Another of the Division's programs is the *Minority Faculty Fellowships Program* (http://bhpr.hrsa.gov/diversity/mffp/default.htm), whose goal is to increase the number of URM faculty at awardee institutions. The program awards 50 percent of salary funds, with the institution matching funds. Fellows are prepared to assume tenured faculty positions at the institution and also provide services in underserved areas.

Under Title VIII, *The Division of Nursing, Nursing Workforce Diversity Program* (http://bhpr.hrsa.gov/nursing) awards grants to institutions to increase the number of nurses from disadvantaged groups. Eligible institutions receive funds to support a variety of activities. In addition to pipeline efforts (for example, pre-entry preparations), activities include scholarships and retention activities, such as counseling, mentoring, and licensure preparation.

The BHPr also administers the *National Health Service Corps (NHSC)* (http://nhsc.bhpr.hrsa.gov), whose mission is to improve health care for medically underserved communities. NHSC has supported more than 2,700 clinicians and health care professionals who provide primary health care in medically underserved communities. The NHSC recruits nurse practitioners, certified nurse-midwives, dentists, mental and behavioral health providers, and primary care physicians, among others. A portion of HRSA's funding is reserved to recruit professionals from disadvantaged backgrounds into the corps. Both scholarship and loan repayment programs are offered.

Other HRSA programs that provide funding include three within the Division of Health Careers Diversity and Development, Student Assistance Programs, which provide loans and scholarships to individuals from disadvantaged backgrounds. HRSA funds a variety of other programs, such as the Area Health Education Centers, Health Education and Training Centers, and Kids into Health Careers, that primarily target students before they reach health professions institutions.

The *Indian Health Service (IHS)* offers *Scholarships for Health Professions Students* (http://www.ihs.gov/JobsCareerDevelop/DHPS/Scholarships/ Section_104.asp). Priority is given to graduate students and junior and senior students who are no more than four years away from completing their degree. Among the list of eligible disciplines, psychology, nursing, dentistry, and medicine are included. In exchange for scholarship awards, recipients are required to pay back one year of service for each year of support received. Service is provided to the IHS or in other designated communities and areas of need.

The *National Institutes of Health* and *Substance Abuse and Mental Health Services Administration* sponsor the *Minority Fellowship Program,* which supports the training and research of minority students in psychology and other disciplines. The primary goal of the program is to identify, select, and support the training of doctoral-level ethnic minority students and postdoctoral trainees in psychology, nursing, social work, and psychiatry who will make significant contributions to the mental health needs of ethnic and racial minorities. Psychology fellowships are administered by the *American Psychological Association.* (http://www.apa.org/mfp/pprograms. html). Programs are sponsored by the National Institutes of Mental Health (NIMH), National Institute on Aging (NIA), National Institute of Drug Abuse (NIDA), and the Substance Abuse and Mental Health Services Administration (SAMSHA). The program provides stipend support, ancillary training experiences, mentoring and career guidance, and access to a network of professional contacts. The amount of support varies, depending on federal allocations to the program and on cost-sharing arrangements that the program negotiates with universities.

Private Sources of Financial Assistance

Most funding available to URM students pursuing health professions education is provided by federal sources. A small amount comes from state, local, and private entities. This section reviews a sample of private sources providing funds to students, organizations, and institutions to increase the number of minorities in a variety of health professions (see Table 3-2). It was beyond the scope of the committee's charge to provide an exhaustive list of private sources of student financial aid. Rather, several examples of these initiatives are presented here.

National Medical Fellowships, Inc. (NMF) (http://www.nmf-online.org) is a nonprofit organization dedicated to improving the health of underserved communities. They seek to increase the representation of minority physicians, educators, researchers, and policy makers in the United States and to train URM minority medical students to address the special needs of their

TABLE 3-2 Examples of Private Funding for Health Professions Programs with the Goal of Increasing Diversity

Source	Program	Funds provided to:	Purpose/ Activities	Disciplines Included
National Medical Fellowships, Inc.		Students	Scholarships provided on a need-basis	Medicine
California Endowment	Administered by Health Professions Education Foundation	Students	Scholarships and loan repayment	Unspecified health professions
California Wellness Foundation		Organizations	Scholarships, mentoring to support minorities	Unspecified health professions
W.K. Kellogg Foundation	Administered by the American Dental Education Association	Institutions	Scholarships and financial aid; postdoctoral and fellowship support; faculty, student, and campus development	Dentistry
Ford Foundation	Administered by the National Research Council Ford Foundation Fellowships for Minorities	Students	Stipends for predoctoral fellows and dissertation fellows	Psychology

communities. NMF provides funding to students in the form of need-based scholarships to first- and second-year medical students. Fellowship programs provide training opportunities in substance abuse research and treatment, HIV/AIDS care, violence prevention, biomedical research, community-based primary care, and health services research. A recent initiative, the NMF Fellows Academy, open to current NMF Scholars, provides programs to develop leadership skills, prepare for residency and careers, and expose fellows to role models and mentors who help guide their professional development.

The California Endowment (http://www.calendow.org), a statewide health foundation, awards grants to organizations that engage in activities directly benefiting the health and well-being of the people of California. The mission of the California Endowment is to expand access to affordable, quality health care for underserved individuals and communities, and to promote fundamental improvements in the health status of all Californians. The Endowment recently provided a 3-year $500,000 grant to the *Health Professions Education Foundation* (http://www.healthprofessions. ca.gov), a nonprofit public benefit corporation established to provide financial assistance to health professional students throughout California who are willing to practice in medically underserved areas. The Foundation oversees the administration of two funds established by state legislation, the Health Professions Education Fund and the Registered Nurse Education Fund, and closely coordinates its programs with the Office of Statewide Health Planning and Development and its health professional education programs.

The funding received from the California Endowment will support up to 20 scholarships and loan repayment grants annually to underrepresented and economically disadvantaged health professions students who will practice in underserved areas of California. The Foundation offers a variety of other financial assistance programs, including the Associate Degree Nursing Pilot Scholarship Program (ADN), Registered Nurse Education Scholarship Program (BSN), and Registered Nurse Education Loan Repayment Program (LRP). Over the last nine years, the Foundation has given out scholarship and loan repayment awards totaling nearly $4.9 million dollars. The awards have helped approximately 1,100 economically disadvantaged and demographically underrepresented students pursue a career in the health professions.

The California Wellness Foundation (http://www.tcwf.org) has established as its mission to improve the health of the people of California by making grants for health promotion, wellness education, and disease prevention. Through its grants, the Foundation addresses the health needs of traditionally underserved populations, including low-income individuals, people of color, youth, and residents of rural areas.

Grants are provided that address diversity in the health professions workforce. Awards are commonly given to organizations that provide fellowships to support pipeline programs, scholarships, mentoring programs, internships and fellowships that support and advance career opportunities for people of color in the health professions, including allied health and public health professions. Organizations that support URM students in the health professions through strategic partnerships, leadership development, continuing education, and networking activities are also eligible for funding. In addition, the Foundation funds organizations that educate policy makers about public and institutional policies that promote diversity in the health professions. The Foundation's *Diversity in the Health Professions Priority Area Grants* provide academic enhancement, financial support,

professional opportunities, and psychosocial support for those in nonspeci-
fied health professions.

The *W.K. Kellogg Foundation* (http://www.wkkf.org), a nonprofit organization whose mission is to apply knowledge to solve the problems of
people, provides grants in several areas including health, higher education
and efforts to capitalize on diversity. In 2001, the Foundation awarded a $1
million grant to the American Dental Education Association (ADEA) to
help increase the number of minority students and faculty in the country's
dental schools. The ADEA awards grants to schools that distribute funds to
students and faculty in the form of scholarships and financial aid, postdoctoral and fellowship support, or faculty, student, and campus development. Students may receive up to $5,000 per academic year.

The *National Research Council Ford Foundation Pre-doctoral and Dissertation Fellowships for Minorities* (http://www7.nationalacademies.org/
fellowships/fordpredoc.html) seeks to increase the presence of underrepresented minorities on college and university faculties. The program is funded
by the Ford Foundation and administered by the National Research Council of the National Academy of Sciences. The predoctoral fellowship provides support for 3 years in research-based programs in social and behavioral sciences, among other disciplines. Fellows receive stipend and funding
toward tuition and fees. Dissertation fellows receive stipends. In 2002, the
program made awards to 60 beginning graduate students, 41 students writing dissertations, and 29 recent Ph.D. recipients.

Broader Public Funding of Health Professions Training and Education

The federal health professions training programs described above are
funded via discretionary funds and are therefore subject to annual appropriations struggles. One of the primary financing mechanisms for health
professions education and training, funded via nondiscretionary funds, is
Medicare Graduate Medical Education (GME), which is administered by
the Center for Medicare and Medicaid Services (CMS) within the Department of Health and Human Services. Because educational activities enhance the quality of patient care, they are considered a part of the cost of
patient care and are paid for, in part, by insurance programs. Medicare
GME provides a significant source of funding for the costs of educating
physicians and other health professionals. The large majority of this funding goes to hospitals for the training of physicians, with training of nursing
diploma program graduates, dental professionals, and allied health professionals constituting a relatively minor role. Payments are made by commercial insurance and managed care companies, government programs such as
Medicare and Medicaid, and other state and local appropriations (Knapp,
2002). Funds are paid to over 1,000 teaching hospitals. Direct GME funds

provide medical and dental resident salaries and benefits, hospital overhead related to training, and salaries and benefits of faculty who supervise residents. Indirect payments refer to those costs that are incurred by teaching hospitals as a result of teaching activities and are calculated through statistical analysis. Teaching hospitals receive an additional payment for each Medicare inpatient treated. In the past several years, issues regarding the needs of the workforce and the role of Medicare GME have been the subject of discussion by the Council on Graduate Medical Education (COGME) among others.

In contrast to medical education, dental schools and graduate programs in psychology are largely responsible for financing their clinical programs. As discussed in the previous section, tuition rates have increased substantially in the past 10 to 20 years as federal and state support for education has declined. For example, in 1973, the federal government provided support for 30 percent of dental education. However by 1997, the government supported only 0.9 percent of the dental enterprise (Hardigan, 1999). Expenses of running these programs have continued to exceed revenues. In order to compensate for these losses, dental schools have increased clinic income and tuition (Myers and Zwemer, 1998).

Do These Programs Increase URM Participation in Health Professions Education?

The critical question regarding these targeted public and private programs is whether they are, in fact, successful at significantly increasing the numbers of URMs in the health professions workforce. Does financial assistance provided to students allow them to succeed in completing their education and training? Evidence from college financial aid strategies suggests that the receipt of financial aid is important in determining whether low-income students will attend school. High college costs may reduce the retention of lower-income students, and those who are offered aid may be more likely to apply to college. Some evidence suggests that aid, particularly the receipt of grants, is an important predictor of attendance for students in the lowest income groups. While these issues have not been extensively examined among health professions students, recently researchers have attempted to evaluate components of public programs.

Two studies are cited by Grumbach and colleagues (2002) that attempted to evaluate BHPr programs. The first, an assessment of minority and disadvantaged programs, was conducted in 1994 by Houston Associates. Data collected by HCOP grantees, however, was inconsistent across programs, incomplete, or not able to be used, so that a useful assessment could not be made. The authors of this review offer several recommendations regarding effective ways to collect data so that the program's activities could be monitored and evaluated. Subsequently, an evaluation of COE awardees between 1993 and 1999 was conducted by Carline and colleagues (1999). Again, a meaningful assessment was not possible because of inconsistent data collection. To address this deficiency, Carline and colleagues developed a data collection system, including narrative and other objective evidence, such as number of applicants, enrollees, and graduates; demographic characteristics of students; sponsored faculty; amount and dispersment of funding; and research and other activities and experiences of COE faculty and students. While a rigorous evaluation was prohibited by the lack of baseline data and comparison groups, results suggested that many of the COE objectives had been met.

While this chapter has focused on HRSA programs that target minority and disadvantaged students, HRSA's Title VII, Section 747 programs, which focus on the education and training of the primary care provider workforce more generally, have increased the number of graduates who practice in underserved communities and who are members of racial and ethnic minority groups (Advisory Committee on Training in Primary Care Medicine and Dentistry, 2001). In a report to the Department of Health and Human Services (HHS) and Congress, the Advisory Committee reported that graduates of these programs (in family medicine residency, general dentistry, physician assistant, and general internal medicine/pediatric residency programs) are three to ten times more likely to practice in medically underserved communities. In addition, these programs graduate two to five times the number of minority and disadvantaged students than other programs.

The BHPr also employs funding factors that increase the likelihood that its grants will be awarded to programs that enroll significant numbers of students from minority and disadvantaged backgrounds. While these are not direct strategies to increase diversity, they may indirectly achieve this goal. As with other BHPr activities, it is difficult to assess the impact of such strategies. Grumbach and colleagues (2002) speculate that these strategies may be less effective for increasing the overall pool of URMs in health professions when employed for funding of residency training, since these programs are competing for a finite pool of URM students already enrolled in schools. Rather, funding factors may be more effective for predoctoral education, but the authors note that the amount of funding is not large enough to make a substantial change. It has also been suggested that while requirements for BHPr programs to collect data on race and ethnicity of students and trainees are important in measuring efforts to increase diversity, there is no evidence that collecting this data encourages institutions to improve recruitment efforts (Matherlee, this volume).

The General Accounting Office (GAO) provided an assessment of Titles VII and VIII programs and provided testimony for congressional reauthorization of the programs in 1997 (GAO, 1997). The office concurred with other assessments that the effectiveness of these programs is difficult to evaluate. The GAO found that Titles VII and VIII supported a wide range of objectives without common goals, outcome measures, and reporting requirements and noted that HHS was not required to evaluate their programs. Furthermore, GAO noted that the programs were not linked to improvements in the supply, distribution, and minority of health professionals. Evaluations of some of the programs measured outcomes for particular institutions as opposed to the national impact. Some institutions receiving grants reported on program process as opposed to outcomes (for example, a report was provided on how the institution established recruitment strategies and not the number of students recruited through the activity). The GAO report concluded by stating that "if these programs are to specifically improve supply, distribution, and minority representation for health professionals, federal efforts need to be directed to activities that clearly support those goals and whose results can be measured and reported in terms of those goals. . . . [O]nce goals are defined, performance measures and targets are critical to determine when federal intervention is no longer required, or when federal strategies are not successful and should be redirected" (GAO, 1997, pp. 6–7).

Another concern critics have raised regarding some of the BHPr's programs is that program payback requirements often "track" students into specialty areas without the flexibility to expand or change these areas. This may dissuade some students from participating in these programs. It may be beneficial to explore potential options for increasing flexibility of HRSA programs to allow students to explore more specialty options.

In summary, little is known about the efficacy of financial aid programs in increasing URM participation in health professions. Evidence suggests that components of BHPr activities may meet program goals. However, comparisons of programs and knowledge of best practices are lacking. Policy makers have a substantial need to obtain data to evaluate how well various programs that provide financial assistance to students succeed in recruiting *and* retaining URM students. The National Center for Health Workforce Analysis and its regional centers, which collect and analyze health profession data and evaluate health professions training programs, among other efforts, have made a significant step toward collecting data at the state level (Matherlee, this volume).

Recommendation 3-1: HRSA's health professions programs should be evaluated to assess their effectiveness in increasing numbers of URM students enrolling and graduating from HPEIs to ensure that they maximize URM participation.

THREATS TO HEALTH PROFESSIONS FINANCING

In the current environment of federal, state, and local budget deficits and reduced endowments of many foundations, programs that support URM access to and success in health professions education programs may be threatened. Matherlee (this volume) cites seven factors that may impede public efforts to increase diversity in the workforce via financing of training and education at the institutional and policy level:

1. Much of the emphasis of programs and funding of educational efforts is on increasing the pipeline of URM students, rather than supporting students in higher education.

2. Most federal health professions training funds rely on discretionary funding, making them vulnerable to cuts.

3. Discretionary funds are "siloed" in various agencies and division within the government, making coordination of funding and communication about the shared goal more difficult. This may also reduce the ability of students to become familiar with career options and paths across disciplines and limit student awareness of varied funding opportunities.

4. The Medicare GME program lacks workforce goals regarding URM participation.

5. There is considerable variation among states in the use of funds to increase URM participation in the workforce.

6. High debt incurred by health professions students may disproportionately hurt URM participation.

7. Policy makers are reluctant to fund new URM initiatives because of federal and state budget deficits.

Several avenues have been discussed for using financial incentives to increase URM participation in health professions education, including the collection of data on various programs and efforts, the use of Medicare GME to develop new policy approaches, and expansion of the NHSC. Evidence from undergraduate education suggests that students may benefit from increased knowledge about the various sources of financial assistance and the provision of grant-based aid rather than loans.

Recommendation 3-2: Congress should increase levels of funding for diversity programs and strategies shown to be effective in ensuring diversity within the National Health Service Corps and Titles VII and VIII of the Public Health Service Act. Furthermore, Congress should develop other financial mechanisms to enhance the diversity of the health-care workforce. This may include exploring changes in Medicare GME to increase URM participation in medicine, psychology, dentistry, and nursing.

RETHINKING THE FINANCING OF
HEALTH PROFESSION EDUCATION

The large variety and scope of public and private efforts for funding URM students in health profession education programs make it difficult to assess if and how well funding programs work together and complement one another to expand opportunities for URM participation. While there are many programs targeting URM students who are entering graduate education, many of these same programs as well as a host of others also engage in pipeline enhancement efforts. Grumbach and colleagues note that the result of this compilation of programs is "a discontinuity of interventions across regions and across stages of the educational pipeline, making it difficult to sustain gains from one educational stage to the next" (Grumbach et al., 2002, p. 71). They conclude that coordination and communication among various programs will assist funders to better plan their own efforts and determine additional needs, and that the formation of coalitions of funders may facilitate these goals.

Another area of need identified by Grumbach et al. (2002) is the relative amounts of funding for various health professions disciplines. For example, in FY 2003, Title VII programs received $308.4 million and Title VIII programs received $112.8 million. As discussed in Chapter 1, the nursing profession has reached a critical shortage in its workforce.

An area in need of further exploration in terms of URM student participation in health profession education is the impact of institutional funding programs, policies, and perspectives dealing with URM access. At the institutional level, many students are funded based on need alone and many URM students are funded based on need and ethnicity. The effect of these funding policies on URM student access is an important area that should be investigated further.

While there are barriers for financial aid programs due to larger scale funding or political priorities, some public and private entities have developed innovative ways of using financing as a lever to increase the number of URMs in health professions programs. One new model for education funding is through a unique public–private partnership. The *University of Colorado Health Sciences School of Dentistry* has partnered with the *Orthodontic Education Company (OEC)* to establish a new dental center that they hope will address the shortage of orthodontists and provide low-cost care to children in underserved areas (see Box 3-1). The OEC provides scholarships and stipends in exchange for service in OEC private or group practices following graduation. The University of Colorado will establish and administer the program, which will involve the investment of almost $100 million by the OEC. This type of partnership may be an innovative way to deal with an anticipated shortage of orthodontists as well as a variety of other health professionals in the next decade and finance education while reducing the burden on taxpayers, students, and parents.

A second program at the University of Colorado, legislated by the state, provides community-based learning experiences for students. The *Advanced Clinical Training and Service Program,* treats the oral health needs of disadvantaged citizens of Colorado (Box 3-2). The program may help to increase diversity by not only generating, among youth served, interest in dental careers, but drawing prospective health professions students through the availability of community-based learning.

As an example from the field of pharmacy, *CVS* provides a *Scholarship of Excellence*, a program in which CVS interns apply to receive $5,000 per academic year for a maximum of 4 years. For each year the scholarship is received, students commit to work full-time for 1 year as a CVS registered pharmacist.

In other efforts, *New York State* has initiated the *Minority Participation in Medical Education Grant Program*, which provides funds to institutions to enhance minority recruitment and retention, develop minority student mentoring programs, develop medical career pathways for minority

---

BOX 3-1
University of Colorado Dental School and Orthodontic Education Company Partnership

In January 2003, the School of Dentistry at the University of Colorado and the Orthodontic Education Company (OEC) initiated a 30-year business partnership with a $3 million gift and $92.7 million commitment from OEC to build the Lazzara Center for Oral–Facial Health and establish a training program in orthodontia.

The partnership will help to address the anticipated shortage of orthodontists and help to provide low-cost care for low-income, minority, and underserved children in the state of Colorado. It is hoped that qualified students from diverse and economically disadvantaged backgrounds, for whom costs of dental education may be prohibitive, will consider dental specialties as a result of the scholarships. It is also hoped the program will have an indirect benefit of increasing diversity in dentistry by exposing underserved children to the profession through the program's services.

Each year, the OEC will sponsor 12 of the 16 students that the Center will train. These students will receive a $30,000 salary, benefits, malpractice insurance, tuition, and additional funds for instruments and computers. In exchange for sponsorship the students will commit to practice for 7 years postgraduation at OEC sites throughout the country, earning a salary of $150,000 per year.

The school will establish admission criteria, curriculum, and academic standards for graduation. Selected residents will have to meet criteria established by the admissions and chair of orthodontics. In addition, the school will follow accreditation procedures set for by the Commission on Dental Accreditation for a specialty program in orthodontics (Landesman, 2003).

BOX 3-2
University of Colorado Dental School Advanced Clinical
Training and Service Program

The Advanced Clinical Training and Service (ACTS) program at the University of Colorado School of Dentistry is a community-based service learning program. This program was legislated by the state of Colorado. Students perform the equivalent of one academic year of direct service, under supervision, to underserved communities in Colorado. Training sites include community health clinics, hospital-based practices, and private practices. Supervision is provided by community dentists who are also faculty members (Landesman, 2003).

There are two required rotations for the program. The first, Integrated Care Clinics, provides treatment for older adults and those with HIV or who are mentally and physically challenged. The second rotation involves service provision in rural dental practices. Students choose other rotations in clinics for underserved populations across the state (University of Colorado School of Dentistry, 2003).

These experiences in underserved communities help students to increase self-confidence in their clinical skills, promote greater independence, and enhance students' sense of personal responsibility. As with the university's business partnership with OEC, it is hoped that ACTS will help to promote diversity in the health professions by drawing students who are interested in serving disadvantaged populations and exposing those who receive the services to the field of dentistry.

students, and develop minority faculty role models (New York State Office of the Governor, 2002; Stoll, 2003). Funds were provided to seven institutions across the state. There have been no published reports assessing the program's results or whether certain approaches have been successful in recruiting and retaining minority students. However, the state announced in 2002 that over 155 minority students participated in medical school and residency programs sponsored by the programs in the previous year.

Programs such as the ones outlined in this section may serve as models for ways to use public and private funds to increase diversity of the health-care workforce. While much of the funding for health profession education is from public sources, private sources can also contribute and have much to gain by investing in diversity. Joint investments made by business, states, the federal government, foundations, and institutions will be crucial in this effort.

Recommendation 3-3: State and local entities, working where appropriate with HPEIs, should increase support for diversity efforts. This may be accomplished via a variety of mechanisms in programs committed to diversity, such as loan forgiveness, tuition reimbursement, loan repayment, GME, and supportive affiliations with community-based providers.

Recommendation 3-4: Private entities should be encouraged to collaborate through business partnerships and other entrepreneurial relationships with HPEIs to support the common goal of developing a more diverse health-care workforce.

SUMMARY

URM students may face sizeable financial barriers as they consider health professions education. The disparity between URM and non-URM family incomes is significant, leaving minority students with fewer financial resources to attend college and health profession schools. The costs of both college and health professions education have increased sharply, while the availability of sufficient need-based aid has decreased, leaving students with higher unmet need and record levels of debt. College tuition trends have prompted the College Board to call for colleges and universities to reaffirm their commitment to need-based aid and for the federal government to increase support to institutions that serve large percentages of high-need students.

While the impact of financial barriers has not been well studied among health professions students, evidence from undergraduate education reveals that low-income students and some URM students may be less likely to apply to college and that aid, particularly grants, may be associated with increased attendance for low-income students.

There are a variety of public and private sources of financial assistance for health professions students, through the provision of scholarships, loans, and loan repayment programs. Most provide funds to institutions that, in turn, make awards to students. The distribution of these funds vary across disciplines, with nursing Title VIII programs receiving significantly less funding than Title VII programs. In addition, these federal programs are funded via discretionary funding and are vulnerable to cuts. It is difficult to assess the impact of these programs on increasing diversity in the health professions workforce, as the scopes of the programs are broad, outcome measures are not clearly specified, and evaluation is not required. The primary source of funding, provided for with mandatory funds, is Medicare Graduate Medical Education (GME). GME dollars have not been tied to efforts to increase the representation of URMs in the health-care workforce.

The high debt incurred by health professions students, reliance on discretionary funding for minority programs, lack of coordination and communication among funding sources, and lack of workforce goals in Medicare GME are among the barriers for the use of financing to increase diversity in the health professions workforce. In addition to a reexamination of existing programs, new and innovative strategies are necessary. Recent efforts have included, for example, partnerships between institutions and private business, which reduce the burden on taxpayers and families. Reexamining the structure of financing programs, systematically measuring outcomes, and exploring new ways to help URM students finance their education will be crucial in increasing diversity in the health professions workforce.

REFERENCES

Advisory Committee on Student Financial Assistance. 2001. *Access Denied: Restoring the Nation's Commitment to Equal Educational Opportunity.* Washington, DC: Advisory Committee on Student Financial Assistance.

Advisory Committee on Student Financial Assistance. 2002. *Empty Promises: The Myth of College Access in America.* Washington, DC: Advisory Committee on Student Financial Assistance.

Advisory Committee on Training in Primary Care Medicine and Dentistry. 2001. *Comprehensive Review and Recommendations: Title VII, Section 747 of the Public Health Service Act.* Report to Secretary of the U.S. Department of Health and Human Services and Congress. [Online]. Available: http://bhpr.hrsa.gov/medicine-dentistry/actpcmd1.htm [accessed October 1, 2002].

American Psychological Association (APA) Research Office. 2001. *Analysis of Data from Graduate Study in Psychology: 1999–2000.* By WE Pate II. [Online]. Available: http://research.apa.org/grad00contents.html [accessed August 5, 2003].

Association of American Medical Colleges (AAMC). 2002. *Minority Students in Medical Education: Facts and Figures XII.* Washington, DC: Association of American Medical Colleges Division of Community and Minority Programs.

Association of American Medical Colleges (AAMC). 2003. *Tuition and Student Fees Reports.* [Online]. Available: https://services.aamc.org/tsf/TSF_Report/report_intro.cfm [accessed August 5, 2003].

Baker LC, Barker DC. 1997. Factors associated with the perception that debt influences physician's specialty choices. *Academic Medicine* 72(12):1088–1096.

Baum S, O'Malley M. 2002. *College on Credit: How Borrowers Perceive Their Education Debt. Results of the 2002 National Student Loan Survey.* Braintree, MA: Nellie Mae Corporation.

Brotherton SE. 1995. The relationship of indebtedness, race, and gender to the choice of general or subspecialty pediatrics. *Academic Medicine* 70(2):149–151.

Carline JD, Patterson D, Mandel L. 1999. *Methodology Development and Assessment of the Impact of the Centers of Excellence Program.* Prepared for the Division of Disadvantaged Assistance, Bureau of Health Professions, Health Resources and Services Administration, Public Health Service, HRSA 240-91-0045.

Choudhury S. 2002. *Racial and Ethnic Differences in Wealth and Asset Choices.* Social Security Bulletin 64(4). [Online]. Available: http://www.ssa.gov/policy/docs/ssb/v64n4/v64n4p1.pdf [accessed October 2, 2003].

College Board. 2000. *Trends in College Pricing.* Washington, DC: College Board.

College Board. 2003. *Challenging Times, Clear Choices: An Action Agenda for College Access and Success. Investing More Equitably and Efficiently in Higher Education, Creating Value for America.* Washington, DC: College Board.

Colquitt WL, Zeh MC, Killian CD, Cultice JM. 1996. Effect of debt on U.S. medical school graduates' preferences for family medicine, general internal medicine, and general pediatrics. *Academic Medicine* 71(4):400–411.

DeAngelis SL. 2000. Tuition, financial aid, debt, and dental student attrition. *Journal of Student Financial Aid* 30(2):7–21.

General Accounting Office (GAO). 1997. *Health Professions Education: Clarifying the Role of Title VII and VIII Programs Could Improve Accountability.* Testimony by Bernice Steinhardt, Director Health Services Quality and Public Health Issues Health, Education, and Human Services Division before the Subcommittee on Public Health and Safety, Committee on Labor and Human Resources, U.S. Senate. GAO/T-HEHS-97-117. [Online]. Available: http://www.gao.gov/archive/1997/he97117t.pdf [accessed September 5, 2003].

Georges A. 1999. Keeping what we've got: The impact of financial aid on minority retention in engineering. *National Action Council for Minorities in Engineering Research Letter* 9(1):1–20.

Grumbach K, Coffman J, Muñoz C, Rosenoff E, Gándara P, Sepulveda E. 2002. *Strategies for Improving the Diversity of the Health Professions.* University of California, San Francisco: Center for California Health Workforce Studies.

Hadley J, Cantor JC, Willke RJ, Feder J, Cohen AB. 1992. Young physicians most and least likely to have second thoughts about a career in medicine. *Academic Medicine* 67(3):180–190.

Hardigan, J. 1999. The costs and financing of dental education. *Journal of Dental Education* 63(12):873–881.

Heller D. 2000. *The Role of Race and Gender in the Awarding of Institutional Financial Aid.* Paper presented at the Annual Meeting of the American Educational Research Association. New Orleans.

Heller D. 2001. Debts and decisions: Student loans and their relationship to graduate school and career choice. Lumina Foundation for Education. *New Agenda Series* 3(4):2–50.

Heller DE. In press. *State Student Aid. The Condition of Access.* Washington, DC: Advisory Committee on Student Financial Assistance.

Houston Associates. 1994. *Evaluation of the Health Careers Opportunity Program Summer Programs Final Report.* Silver Spring, MD: Health Resources and Services Administration, Division of Disadvantaged Assistance.

Johnson L. 2002a. Financial planning for residency: Part 2. *Journal for Minority Medical Students* 14(3):17–20.

Johnson L. 2002b. Planning for residency: First do no harm. *Journal for Minority Medical Students* 14(2):40–46.

Knapp RM. 2002. Complexity and uncertainty in financing graduate medical education. *Academic Medicine* 77(11):1076–1083.

Landesman HM. 2003. *Potential of Three Colorado Programs to Increase Access to and Interest in Dental Careers among Underrepresented Minorities.* Presentation to Committee on Institutional and Policy-Level Strategies for Increasing the Diversity of the U.S. Health Care Workforce, June 30, Washington, DC.

Lofton K. 2002. How med students' indebtedness influences career choices. *Journal for Minority Medical Students* 14(2):47–48.

McPherson MS, Schapiro MO. In press. *Institutional Student Aid: The Condition of Access.* Washington, DC: Advisory Committee on Student Financial Assistance.

Millet C, MacKenzie S. 1995. *An Exploratory Study of the Role of Financial Aid in Minority Doctoral Education.* Paper presented at the Annual Meeting of the Association for the Study of Higher Education, Orlando, FL.

Mullan F. 1997. The National Health Service Corps and inner-city hospitals. *Health Affairs* 336(22):1601–1603.

Murray B. 1999. Some clinical psychology students' growing debt burden triggers response from training programs. *American Psychological Association Monitor Online* 30(2). [Online]. Available: http://www.apa.org/monitor/feb99/debt.html [accessed August 18, 2003].

Myers DR, Zwemer JD. 1998. Cost of dental education and student debt. *Journal of Dental Education* 62(5):354–360.

National Science Foundation (NSF). 2000. *Psychology Doctorate Recipients: How Much Financial Debt at Graduation?* By AI Rapoport, J Kohout, M Wicherski. [Online]. Available: http://www.nsf.gov/sbe/srs/issuebrf/sib00321.htm [accessed August 18, 2003].

Nettles M. 1990. *Black, Hispanic, and White Doctoral Students: Before, During and After Enrolling in Graduate School.* Princeton, NJ: Educational Testing Service.

New York State Office of the Governor. 2002. Nearly $1 Million to Boost Minority Physician Training. Press Release April 19, 2002. [Online]. Available: http://www.state.ny.us/governor/press/year02/april19_1_02.htm [accessed January 16, 2004].

Nora A, Cabrera AF. 1996. The role of perceptions in prejudice and discrimination and the adjustment of minority students to college. *Journal of Higher Education* 67(2):119–148.

Rico M, Stagnaro-Green A. 1997. Debt and career choices of underrepresented minorities. *Academic Medicine* 72(8):657–658.

Rosenthal MP, Marquette PA, Diamond JJ. 1996. Trends along the debt-income axis: Implications for medical students' selections of family practice careers. *Academic Medicine* 71(6):675–677.

St. John EP. 1994. Prices, productivity, and investment: Assessing financial strategies in higher education. *ERIC Digest.* EDO-HE-94-3.

Stoll B. 2003. *Overview of the New York State Council on Graduate Medical Education.* Boston, MA: Community Catalyst.

University of Colorado School of Dentistry. 2003. Advanced Clinical Training and Service Program. [Online]. Available: http://www.uchsc.edu/sd/sd/advanced.html [accessed September 5, 2003].

U.S. Census Bureau. 2002a. *Historical Income Tables—Families.* [Online]. Available: http://www.census.gov/hhes/income/histinc/f05.html [accessed August 14, 2003].

U.S. Census Bureau. 2002b. *Money Income in the United States: 2001. Current Population Reports, P60-218.* Washington, DC: U.S. Government Printing Office. [Online]. Available: http://www.census.gov/prod/2002pubs/p60-218.pdf [accessed September 3, 2001].

U.S. Department of Education. National Center for Education Statistics. 1997. *Access to Postsecondary Education for the 1992 High School Graduates.* NCES 98-105. By L Berkner, L Chavez. Project Officer CD Carroll. Washington, DC: U.S. Department of Education.

U.S. Department of Education, National Center for Education Statistics. 1999. *College Access and Affordability. Findings from The Condition of Education 1998.* NCES 1999-108. Washington, DC: U.S. Department of Education.

U.S. Department of Education, National Center for Education Statistics. 2000a. *1999–2000 National Postsecondary Student Aid Study (NPSAS: 2000).* Washington, DC: U.S. Department of Education.

U.S. Department of Education, National Center for Education Statistics. 2000b. *Digest of Education Statistics, 1999.* NCES 2000-031. Washington, DC: U.S. Department of Education.

U.S. Department of Education, National Center for Education Statistics. 2002. Student Financing of Graduate and First-Professional Education, 1999–2000. *Profiles of Students in Selected Degree Programs and Their Use of Assistantships.* NCES 2002-166. By SP Choy, S Geis. Project Officer: AG Malizio. Washington, DC: U.S. Department of Education.

U.S. Department of Education, National Center for Education Statistics. 2003a. *Characteristics of Undergraduate Borrowers: 1999–2000.* NCES 2003-155. By ME Clinedinst, AF Cunningham, JP Merisotis. Project Officer: CD Carroll. Washington, DC: U.S. Department of Education.

U.S. Department of Education, National Center for Education Statistics. 2003b. *How Families of Low-and Middle-Income Undergraduates Pay for College: Full-Time Dependent Students in 1999–2000.* NCES 2003-162. By SP Choy, AM Berker. Project Officer: CD Carroll. Washington, DC: U.S. Department of Education.

Valachovic RW, Weaver RG, Sinkford JC, Haden NK. 2001. Trends in dentistry and dental education. *Journal of Dental Education* 65(6):539–561.

Zeigler J. 2003. As tuitions rise, medical students struggle with excessive loans. *New Physician* 52(6):15–23.

4

Accreditation and Diversity in Health Professions

Accreditation is the process by which nongovernmental organizations set standards for and monitor the quality of educational programs provided by member institutions. Accreditation is a voluntary process of institutional self-regulation, often conducted within the broad framework of standards established by the U.S. Department of Education and the Council for Higher Education Accreditation (CHEA). By setting standards for educational programs and methods for institutional peer review, accrediting bodies advance academic quality, ensure accountability to the public, encourage institutional progress and improvement, and provide a mechanism for continual assessment of broad educational goals for higher education. As such, accreditation is an important vehicle for institutional change and a potential means to enhance diversity in health professions.

Despite the potential for accreditation standards to play a role in enhancing diversity in health professions, its application must be considered with an appropriate degree of caution. Accreditation standards adopted by the majority of health professions' standard-setting bodies should and do attempt to balance "prescriptive" standards that mandate institutional compliance in core areas with more general goals that take into account variations in institutional mission and educational objectives. In addition, most accreditation standards acknowledge the importance of preserving academic freedom, which is critical to curriculum innovation. Uniformity of educational programs is not a goal of the accreditation process and is discouraged by most accreditation bodies (CDA, 2002). Flexibility (within limits) is therefore a core component of most accreditation processes, and standard-setting bodies and their member institutions are unlikely to retreat from this goal.

Most health professions education accreditation bodies must also comply with broad regulations established by the U.S. Department of Education, which is required by law to recognize accrediting agencies that the Secretary approves as "reliable authorities as to the quality of education provided by higher education institutions" (U.S. Department of Education, 2003). Accrediting bodies seeking national recognition must meet the Secretary's procedures and criteria, as published in the *Federal Register*. In addition to recognition by the Department of Education, most higher education accrediting bodies seek recognition from CHEA, a nongovernmental coordinating agency for accreditation. CHEA serves to facilitate the role of accrediting agencies in promoting and ensuring the quality and diversity of postsecondary education. Accrediting organizations must therefore meet procedures and criteria established by these groups as they establish standards for diversity.

The following chapter reviews the accreditation standards adopted by the major accrediting bodies that oversee nursing, dental, professional psychology, and medical education and assesses the potential for these standards to stimulate more intensive diversity efforts on the part of health professions training programs.

THE STANDARDS OF PROFESSIONAL ACCREDITING BODIES RELATED TO DIVERSITY

National League for Nursing Accreditation Commission

The National League for Nursing Accreditation Commission (NLNAC), established in 1997, accredits 1,500 of the nation's nursing education programs granting degrees at the master's, baccalaureate, associate, diploma, and practical nursing levels. Its goals are to:

- Promulgate a common core of standards and criteria for the accreditation of nursing programs found to meet those standards and criteria;
- Strengthen educational quality through assistance to associated programs and schools, and evaluation processes, functions, publications, and research;
- Advocate self-regulation in nursing education;
- Promote peer review;
- Foster educational equity, access, opportunity, and mobility, and preparation for employment based upon type of nursing education; and
- Serve as gatekeeper to Higher Education Act Title IV programs for which NLNAC is the accrediting agency (NLNAC, 2002).

NLNAC is recognized by the U.S. Department of Education and CHEA, among other national and international organizations, as an accrediting body for a range of nursing education programs. NLNAC assesses academic quality relative to seven standards (i.e., rules established for the measurement of quantity, quality, extent, and value of educational programs), which determine:

- Institutional Mission/Governance—whether the program has a clear and publicly stated mission and/or philosophy and purposes appropriate to postsecondary or higher education in nursing;
- Faculty—whether the program has quality and credentialed faculty appropriate to accomplish its purposes and strengthen its educational effectiveness;
- Students—whether the program has ensured teaching and learning environments conducive to student academic achievement and life-long learning;
- Curriculum and Instruction—whether the program accomplishes its educational and related purposes;
- Resources—whether the program has effectively organized processes and human, fiscal, and physical resources;
- Educational Effectiveness—whether the program has an identified plan for systematic evaluation and assessment of educational outcomes; and
- Integrity—whether the program demonstrates integrity in its practices and relationships.

Of these, only the first standard ("mission and governance") specifically addresses diversity, in stating that nursing education programs must "demonstrate commitment to the cultural, racial, and ethnic diversity of the community in which the institution and the nursing education unit exist" (Grumet, 2003). Other standards that are related to diversity include criteria regarding student policies ("student policies [must be] . . . non-discriminatory").

As a broad set of objectives, NLNAC endorses the PEW Health Commission's *Competencies for 2005* and the 21 *Competencies for the Twenty-First Century*. Among these competencies is the objective that practitioners must "participate in a racially and culturally diverse society, appreciate the growing diversity of the population and the need to understand health status and health care through differing cultural values, [and] provide culturally sensitive care to a diverse society" (NLNAC, 2002, p. 107).

NLNAC is purposefully nonprescriptive with regard to student and nursing faculty diversity, according to Barbara Grumet, NLNAC's Executive Director. NLNAC "does not require schools to practice affirmative action," according to Grumet. At the same time, NLNAC sees its role as that of a "bully pulpit," urging its institutions to recruit and retain a diverse student body (Grumet, 2003).

Commission on Collegiate Nursing Education

The Commission on Collegiate Nursing Education (CCNE) accredits baccalaureate and graduate nursing degree programs located in regionally accredited colleges and universities in the United States. CCNE is recognized by the U.S. Department of Education and CHEA and is a member of the Association of Specialized and Professional Accreditors. CCNE accredits 438 nursing programs at 278 institutions and reviews 75–90 program each year that seek renewal of their accreditation.

CCNE's goals are to:

• Hold nursing programs accountable to the "community of interest" (i.e., the nursing profession, consumers, employers, higher education, students and their families) by "ensuring that these programs have mission statements, goals, and outcomes that are appropriate for programs preparing individuals to enter the field of nursing" (CCNE, 2002);
• Evaluate the success of nursing programs in achieving their mission, goals, and outcomes;
• Assess the extent to which nursing programs meet accreditation standards;
• Inform the public of the purposes and values of accreditation; and
• Foster continuing improvement in nursing education programs.

The values upon which CCNE accreditation activities are premised include:

• Trust, integrity, life-long learning, review and oversight by peers, innovation, and accountability; and
• Inclusiveness in the implementation of CCNE's activities and an openness to the "diverse institutional and individual issues and opinions of the interested community" (CCNE, 2002).

CCNE's accreditation standards are focused on both nursing education program quality and effectiveness. With regard to program quality, standards address institutional mission and governance (i.e., "the mission, philosophy, and goals/objectives of the program should be congruent with those of the parent institution, should reflect professional nursing standards and guidelines, and should consider the needs and expectations of the community of interest"), institutional commitment and resources (i.e., "the parent institution demonstrates ongoing commitment and support [and] makes available resources to enable the program to achieve its mission, philosophy, goals/objectives and expected results"), and curriculum and teaching-learning practices (i.e., "the curriculum is developed in accordance with clear statements of expected results derived from the mission, philosophy, and goals/objectives of the program with clear congruence between the teaching-learning experiences and expected results") [CCNE, 2002]. With regard to program effectiveness, CCNE standards address student performance and faculty accomplishments (e.g., accomplishments in teaching, scholarship).

CCNE's program standards do not specifically refer to racial and ethnic diversity among nursing program students and faculty. However, according to Charlotte Beason, chair of the CCNE Board of Commissioners, each nursing program is expected to define and achieve program goals that are consistent with the expectations of the program's community of interest, which includes health-care consumers.

Commission on Dental Accreditation

The Commission on Dental Accreditation (CDA) "serves the public by establishing, maintaining and applying standards that ensure the quality and continuous improvement of dental and dental-related education and reflect the evolving practice of dentistry" (CDA, 2002, p. 2). CDA accredits over 1,350 dental, advanced dental, and allied dental education programs, 56 of which are D.D.S. or D.M.D. programs. CDA is recognized by the U.S. Department of Education as the sole accreditation agency for dental education programs.

CDA's *Accreditation Standards for Dental Education Programs* have been developed to:

- Protect the public welfare;
- Guide institutions in developing their academic programs;
- Provide a vehicle for site visit teams to make judgments as to the quality of the program; and
- Provide students with reasonable assurance that the program is meeting its stated objectives.

In addition, CDA's standards were designed to:

- Improve the assessment of quality in dental education programs;
- Streamline the accreditation process by including only standards critical to the evaluation of the quality of the educational program;

- Increase the focus on competency statements in curriculum-related standards; and
- Emphasize educational goals to ensure that graduates are life-long learners.

CDA assesses dental program quality relative to six overarching standards: institutional effectiveness; educational programs (including admissions, instruction, curriculum management, biomedical sciences, behavioral sciences, practice management, ethics and professionalism, information management and critical thinking, and clinical sciences); faculty and staff; educational support services (including facilities and resources, student services, student financial aid, and health services); patient care services; and research programs.

Of these, two standards explicitly address diversity concerns. Standard 2-2 (Educational Program) mandates efforts to recruit and retain a diverse dental student body:

"Admissions policies and procedures **must** be designed to include recruitment and admission of a diverse student population" (CDA, 2002; emphasis in text).

Standard 2-17 mandates that dental graduates must possess the skills and competencies to serve a racially and ethnically diverse patient population:

"Graduates **must** be competent in managing a diverse patient population and have the interpersonal and communications skills to function successfully in a multicultural work environment" (CDA, 2002; emphasis in text).

Dental programs have been successful in meeting these standards. According to Karen Hart, director of the CDA, all 46 doctoral-level dental programs have been found to be in compliance with Standard 2-2, with 13 programs receiving commendations regarding their efforts to recruit and retain a diverse student body. Similarly, all 46 programs have been found to be in compliance with Standard 2-17, with two receiving commendations for their efforts to ensure that dental graduates possess multicultural competencies (Hart, 2003).

Hart noted that CDA is assessing whether the diversity standard has proven effective in encouraging dental programs to increase the percentage of qualified URM admissions and matriculants to dental programs. While the current CDA standards have been in place only since 1998, preliminary data suggest that the answer to this question is a "qualified maybe," according to Hart. URM enrollment in U.S. dental programs has increased slightly since 1998 (see Chapter 1), but this increase may also be attributable to other efforts that the profession has undertaken to increase URM admission and enrollment (Hart, 2003).

Liaison Committee on Medical Education

The Liaison Committee on Medical Education (LCME) accredits 142 medical education programs in the United States and Canada (the latter in conjunction with the Committee on Accreditation of Canadian Medical Schools). The LCME is recognized by the U.S. Department of Education as an accrediting agency for medical education programs, but not as an institutional accrediting agency. Therefore, LCME requires medical schools to attain institutional accreditation from a regional accrediting body if not already a component of a regionally accredited institution.

LCME standards are organized to reflect five broad standards:

• Institutional Setting (with criteria related to governance and administration and academic environment);
• Educational Programs (with criteria related to educational objectives, structure, teaching and evaluation, curriculum management, and evaluation of program effectiveness);
• Medical Students (with criteria related to admissions policies and practices, student services, and the learning environment);
• Faculty (with criteria related to number, qualifications, and functions, personnel policies, and governance); and
• Educational Resources (with criteria related to finances, general facilities, clinical teaching faculties, and information resources and library services).

LCME standards, like those of many of the other professional accrediting bodies, are specific with regard to the use of language and the level of effort that medical schools are required to demonstrate in order to achieve compliance with the standards. In particular, LCME standards use the words "must" and "should" to reflect different areas of emphasis in program standards. "Use of the word 'must' indicates that the LCME considers meeting the standard to be absolutely necessary for the achievement and maintenance of accreditation. Use of the word 'should' indicates that compliance with the standard is expected unless these are extraordinary any justifiable circumstances that preclude full compliance" (LCME, 2002, p. ii).

Three LCME standards are directly related to student diversity and multicultural education and training. With regard to admissions policies,

Standard MS-8 states, "Each medical school should have policies and practices ensuring the gender, racial, cultural, and economic diversity of its
students" (LCME, 2002, p. 18). In a discussion of LCME intent for this
standard, the committee notes, "The standard requires that each school's
student body exhibit diversity in the dimensions noted. The extent of diversity needed will depend on the school's missions, goals, and educational
objectives, expectations of the community in which it operates, and its
implied or explicit social contract at the local, state, and national levels"
(LCME, 2002, p. 18).

Regarding cultural competence, LCME standard ED-21 states, "The
faculty and students must demonstrate an understanding of the manner in
which people of diverse cultures and belief systems perceive health and
illness and respond to various symptoms, diseases, and treatments" (LCME,
2002, p. 12). LCME further explicates this standard by noting that:

> All instruction should stress the need for students to be concerned with
> the total medical needs of their patients and the effects that social and
> cultural circumstances have on their health. To demonstrate compliance
> with this standard, schools should be able to document objectives relating
> to the development of skills in cultural competence, indicate where in the
> curriculum students are exposed to such material, and demonstrate the
> extent to which the objectives are being achieved (LCME, 2002, p. 12).

One outcome of such training might be to address racial and ethnic
biases that may affect medical care (Institute of Medicine, 2003). LCME
standard ED-22 requires that medical students "learn to recognize and
appropriately address gender and cultural biases in themselves and others,
and in the process of healthcare delivery" (LCME, 2002, p. 12). LCME
intends that the objectives of such training "include student understanding
of demographic influences on health care quality and effectiveness, such as
racial and ethnic disparities in the diagnosis and treatment of diseases. The
objectives should also address the need for self-awareness among students
regarding any personal biases in their approach to health care delivery"
(LCME, 2002, p. 12).

According to David Stevens, secretary of the LCME, the appropriate
role of the LCME in promoting diversity is to "advocate for the improvement of medical education and health care—including establishing expectations that lead to diversity in the physician workforce," and to "work in
every context to achieve this goal" (Stevens, 2003).

Similarly, the Accreditation Council for Graduate Medical Education
(ACGME), which accredits residency education programs, has established
general competencies in graduate medical education, including standards
with regard to patient care, medical knowledge, practice-based learning
and improvement, interpersonal and communication skills, professionalism, and systems-based practice. Of these general competencies, only the

professionalism standard specifically addresses diversity concerns, noting that professionalism is "manifested through a commitment to carrying out professional responsibilities, adherence to ethical principles, and sensitivity to a diverse patient population" (ACGME, 2003).

Committee on Accreditation, American Psychological Association

The Committee on Accreditation of the American Psychological Association (APA) accredits doctoral-level education and training in professional psychology (i.e., clinical, counseling, and school psychology), including internship programs and postdoctoral residency programs. APA accredits more than 300 doctoral programs in over 190 institutions of higher education, as well as more than 400 internship and postdoctoral residency programs.

More so than the other health professions noted above, APA's accreditation standards reflect considerable attention to the role of diversity in psychology education and program quality. According to Susan Zlotlow, director of the APA Office of Program Consultation and Accreditation, the APA Committee on Accreditation debated whether to address student and faculty diversity standards as a single, separate domain or to infuse diversity issues throughout the guidelines. The committee elected to adopt both approaches—diversity is addressed across several domains, as well as in a separate domain focused on cultural and individual differences and diversity (Zlotlow, 2003). "Cultural and individual diversity" in APA's standards refers to diversity with regard to individual personal and demographic characteristics. These include, but are not limited to "age, color, disabilities, ethnicity, gender, language, national origin, race, religion, sexual orientation, and socioeconomic status" (APA Committee on Accreditation, 2003, p. 5).

APA's standards begin with explicit guidelines for the composition of the Committee on Accreditation. While graduate educators hold the largest share of seats on the committee, seats are reserved for "representation of the general public's interest by persons outside the profession who have an informed, broad-gauged community perspective about matters of higher education" (APA Committee on Accreditation, 2002, p. v). In addition, appointments to the committee "shall reflect the individual and cultural diversity within our society among psychologists, and the breadth of psychology as a discipline" (APA Committee on Accreditation, 2002, p. v).

APA has established eight domains of accreditation standards: Eligibility (the educational program's purpose must be consistent with the scope of the accreditation body and the goal of training students in professional psychology); program philosophy, objectives, and curriculum plan (the program must have a clearly specific philosophy of education and training consistent with the science and practice of psychology); program resources (the program must demonstrate that it has sufficient resources to meet educational objectives); cultural and individual differences in psychology (the program recognizes the importance of cultural and individual differences and diversity in the training of psychologists); student–faculty relations (the programs' educational, training, and socialization opportunities are characterized by mutual respect and courtesy and facilitates students' learning experiences); program self-assessment and quality enhancement (the program demonstrates a commitment to excellence through self-study); public disclosure (the program appropriately represents itself to the public); and relationship with accrediting body (the program demonstrates its commitment to the accreditation process).

Within these domains, specific criteria relevant to racial, ethnic, and cultural diversity serve as benchmarks:

• Domain A (Eligibility). "The program engages in actions that indicate respect for and understanding of cultural and individual diversity. . . . Respect for and understanding of cultural and individual diversity is reflected in the program's policies for the recruitment, retention, and development of faculty and students, and in its curriculum and field placements. The program has nondiscriminatory policies and operating conditions, and it avoids any actions that would restrict program access or completion on grounds that are irrelevant to success in graduate training or the profession" (APA Committee on Accreditation, 2002, p. 5).

• Domain B (Program Philosophy, Objective, and Curriculum Plan). The program implements a clear and coherent curriculum plan that enables students to acquire and demonstrate competence in scientific psychology (including research methods), scientific and theoretical foundations for professional practice, diagnosis and assessment, and implementing intervention plans. "Issues of cultural and individual diversity that are relevant to all of the above" must be integrated into the curriculum plan (APA Committee on Accreditation, 2002, p. 7).

• Domain D (Cultural and Individual Differences and Diversity). Specific criteria within this standard mandate that:

> The program has made systematic, coherent, and long-term efforts to attract and retain students and faculty from differing ethnic, racial, and personal backgrounds into the program. Consistent with such efforts, it acts to ensure a supportive and encouraging learning environment appropriate for the training of diverse individuals and the provision of training opportunities for a broad spectrum of individuals. Further, the program avoids any actions that would restrict program access on grounds that are irrelevant to success in graduate training.

> The program has and implements a thoughtful and coherent plan to pro-

vide students with relevant knowledge and experiences about the role of cultural and individual diversity in psychological phenomena as they relate to the science and practice of professional psychology. The avenues by which these goals are achieved are to be developed by the program (APA Committee on Accreditation, 2002, p. 9).

- Domain E (Student–Faculty Relations). This criterion mandates that training programs must "show respect for cultural and individual diversity among their students" by treating them in accordance with the above standards (APA Committee on Accreditation, 2002).

In evaluating how training programs perform relative to diversity standards, the APA Committee on Accreditation focuses on the *effort* that programs display, according to Zlotlow. Recruitment and retention plans, for example, must be systematic, coherent, and long-term, and "not a one-year effort prior to completing the self-study" (Zlotlow, 2003). Programs are asked to evaluate the success of the plan as part of overall efforts at self-assessment and enhancement. Should training programs fail to meet the standard, the Committee on Accreditation offers "multiple levels of encouragement," according to Zlotlow. These include:

- annual report response—the program is asked to provide additional information in an annual report to the committee to document its steps toward remedying problems;
- "flag" response—programs found to have continued deficiencies are required to respond to specific issues for review by the committee, which may then either deem the response to be adequate, request additional information, or request an invitation for a special site visit;
- years of accreditation—the committee may elect to award a shorter period of accredited status (minimally, 3 years, or a maximum of 6 years) to programs with a history of not improving in any area of the guidelines; or
- adverse decision—programs that fail to improve after increasing sanctions (above) may be placed on probation (Zlotlow, 2003).

APA's accreditation standards have contributed to an increased level of attention and effort among psychology education and training constituencies in addressing diversity concerns, according to Zlotlow. New websites devoted to promoting and enhancing diversity-related institutional policies and curriculum have been developed, and the standards have promoted greater sharing among training programs regarding strategies to improve minority recruitment and retention efforts. This change has been slow, Zlotlow notes, given that APA's approach is developmental in nature (i.e., the Committee on Accreditation seeks to promote incentives for change and is willing to work with training programs over time to foster the long-term enhancement of diversity efforts). Once in place, however, "recruitment efforts have longer term dividends and the training curriculum generally is a more permanent part of the educational program," according to Zlotlow (2003).

THE POTENTIAL OF ACCREDITATION TO ENHANCE DIVERSITY IN HEALTH PROFESSIONS

Accreditation and the U.S. Department of Education

As noted earlier in this chapter, the U.S. Department of Education is charged with recognizing national accrediting agencies that the secretary determines to be reliable authorities as to the quality of education or training provided by institutions of higher education. An accrediting body seeking national recognition by the secretary must meet the procedures and criteria established by the department for the recognition of accrediting agencies. These procedures and criteria include organizational and administrative requirements, operating policies and procedures, and required standards and their application. Among the required standards, an accrediting body must demonstrate that it has standards for accreditation "that are sufficiently rigorous to ensure that the agency is a reliable authority regarding the quality of the education or training provided by the institutions or programs it accredits" (U.S. Department of Education, 2003, accessed from Internet website http://www.ed.gov). An accrediting agency meets this requirement if its standards effectively address the quality of the institution or program in areas such as:

- "success with respect to student achievement in relation to the institution's mission, including, as appropriate, consideration of course completion, State licensing examination, and job placement rates" (U.S. Department of Education, 2003, accessed from Internet website http://www.ed.gov);
- curriculum;
- faculty;
- student support services;
- recruiting and admissions practices; and other relevant program areas.

The department therefore exerts broad influence over the scope and tenor of accrediting bodies' standards and can play a significant role in encouraging accreditation bodies to adopt diversity-related standards. Because the department's standards are not (and must not be) proscriptive with regard to specific standards of accreditation bodies, the department can encourage the development of diversity-related standards by raising awareness among accrediting bodies of the value of diversity in health professions education and the role of diversity in increasing Americans' access to culturally competent care. In addition, the department could identify "best practices" regarding diversity-related standards and promulgate these among health professions education accrediting bodies.

Recommendation 4-1: The U.S. Department of Education should strongly encourage accreditation bodies to be more aggressive in formulating and enforcing standards that result in a critical mass of URMs throughout the health professions.

The increasing diversity of the U.S. population requires that accreditation bodies be responsive to demographic changes and develop and enforce standards that ensure that health professionals are prepared to serve diverse segments of the population. As one accreditation official noted during a public workshop hosted by the study committee, "Our role is to serve the public." Given that almost all accreditation bodies view public service and accountability as central to their mission, establishing and monitoring goals related to diversity among health-care professions can be unambiguously viewed as an important aspect of this effort.

Accreditation bodies may take varying approaches in efforts to accomplish these goals. First, accrediting bodies must accept diversity as a core component of high-quality health professions education and care giving. Subsequently, a number of strategies may be adopted to stimulate institutional diversity efforts. The standards and practices adopted by the APA are instructive and offer several approaches for accreditation standards to address diversity concerns:

1. *Develop a plan to achieve diversity, consistent with the institutional mission, and demonstrate efforts to reach diversity goals.* APA's standards emphasize that programs should develop a plan and demonstrate *effort* toward recruiting and retaining a diverse faculty and student body. The plan should be consistent with the institutional mission and should articulate a rationale for how and why diversity is important to the mission (e.g., research-oriented training programs should consider how diversity may enhance the range and scope of research at the institution).

2. *Develop standards that encourage the development and infusion of diversity-related curricula throughout the training program.*

3. *Regularly monitor and evaluate the efforts of accredited institutions in achieving their diversity goals.* APA's Committee on Accreditation seeks annual reports from institutions, particularly to document steps toward remedying any problems in achieving accreditation goals. Educational programs found to be deficient in meeting diversity standards may face addi-

tional site visits on a yearly basis to ascertain progress toward meeting the standards.

4. *Use graduated sanctions and reinforcement from the accrediting body to help "shape" appropriate diversity efforts.* APA's Committee on Accreditation works collaboratively with institutions to help them reach their diversity goals. Sanctions for failure to achieve diversity standards are graduated, such that first-time or isolated infractions result in institutions being asked to report to the committee the steps planned to rectify the infraction. Repeated instances of failure to meet standards are met with increasing sanctions.

5. *Seek community representation on standard-setting bodies.* APA's Committee on Accreditation reserves seats for nonprofessional community members, who often bring a broader perspective to accreditation efforts. Their presence on the committee also helps to ensure pubic accountability and transparency.

6. *Seek diverse representation on peer review teams.* Anecdotally, the study committee is aware of instances in which peer review teams have lacked significant racial and ethnic diversity. Even in the face of strong accreditation standards related to diversity, the absence of racial and ethnic diversity on peer review teams can send a signal that may undermine the accreditation body's intent. Peer review teams should reflect the same goals and objectives that the accrediting body adopts, including in areas of diversity.

Many of the standards and practices adopted by the APA are also reflected in diversity-related standards of the other health professions accrediting bodies reviewed here. In particular, the CDA's requirement that dental schools develop admissions policies and procedures that attend to recruitment and admission of a diverse student population and its mandate that dental graduates must possess the skills and competencies to serve a racially and ethnically diverse patient population are consistent with the goal of encouraging student diversity and diversity-related curriculum. In addition, CDA's efforts to assess the impact of accreditation standards on dental school student diversity are an important to evaluate the effectiveness of program standards. Similarly, LCME's standards require attention to diversity in recruitment and retention of students, as well as in curriculum to improve students' cross-cultural competencies and reduce individual biases.

> **Recommendation 4-2:** Health professions education accreditation bodies should develop explicit policies articulating the value and importance of providing culturally competent health care and the role it sees for racial and ethnic diversity among health professionals in achieving this goal.

> **Recommendation 4-3:** Health professions education accreditation bod-

ies should develop standards and criteria that more effectively encourage health professions schools to recruit URM students and faculty, to develop cultural competence curricula, and to develop an institutional climate that encourages and sustains the development of a critical mass of diversity.

Recommendation 4-4: Accreditation standards should require HPEIs to collect and report data relevant to diversity criteria. Data should include the number and percentage of URM candidates, students admitted and graduated, time to degree, and number and level of URM faculty.

Recommendation 4-5: Accreditation-related advisory boards and accreditation bodies should include URMs and other individuals with expertise in diversity and cultural competence.

Recommendation 4-6: If diversity-related standards are not met, the institution should be required to declare formally what steps will be put in place to address the deficiencies. Repeated deficiencies should result in accreditation-related sanctions.

REFERENCES

Accrediation Council for Graduate Medical Education (ACGME). 2003. ACGME Outcome Project. [Online]. Available: http://www.acgme.org/Outcome/ [accessed October 13, 2003].

American Psychological Association (APA) Committee on Accreditation. 2002. *Guidelines and Principles for Accreditation of Programs in Professional Psychology.* Washington, DC: American Psychological Association.

Commission on Collegiate Nursing Education (CCNE). 2002. *Standards for Accreditation of Baccalaureate and Graduate Nursing Education Programs.* Washington, DC: Commission on Collegiate Nursing Education.

Commission on Dental Accreditation (CDA). 2002. *Accreditation Standards for Dental Education Programs.* Chicago: Commission on Dental Accreditation.

Grumet B. 2003. *Strategies for Increasing the Diversity of the U.S. Health Care Workforce.* Presentation before IOM Committee on Institutional and Policy-Level Strategies for Increasing the Diversity of the U.S. Health Care Workforce. April 9, 2003, Washington, DC.

Hart K. 2003. *Diversity and Cross-Cultural Training: Accreditation Standards for Dental Education.* Presentation before IOM Committee on Institutional and Policy-Level Strategies for Increasing the Diversity of the U.S. Health Care Workforce. April 9, 2003, Washington, DC.

Institute of Medicine. 2003. *Unequal Treatment: Confronting Racial and Ethnic Disparities in Health Care.* BD Smedley, AY Stith, AR Nelson, eds. Washington, DC: The National Academies Press.

Liaison Committee on Medical Education (LCME). 2002. *Functions and Structure of a Medical School: Standards for Accreditation of Medical Programs Leading to the M.D. Degree.* Washington, DC, and Chicago: Liaison Committee on Medical Education.

National League for Nursing Accreditation Commission (NLNAC). 2002. *Accreditation Manual*. [Online]. Available: http://www.nlnac.org [accessed October 30, 2002].

Stevens D. 2003. *Diversity and the LCME*. Presentation before IOM Committee on Institutional and Policy-Level Strategies for Increasing the Diversity of the U.S. Health Care Workforce. April 9, 2003, Washington, DC.

U.S. Department of Education. 2003. Overview of Accreditation. [Online]. Available: www.ed.gov [accessed April 13, 2003].

Zlotlow S. 2003. *Committee on Accreditation of the American Psychological Association: Efforts to Promote Diversity*. Presentation before IOM Committee on Institutional and Policy-Level Strategies for Increasing the Diversity of the U.S. Health Care Workforce. April 9, 2003, Washington, DC.

5

Transforming the Institutional Climate to Enhance Diversity in Health Professions

The intervention strategies to increase diversity in health professions described in previous chapters all focus on improving the yield of qualified underrepresented minority (URM) students matriculating to health professions training programs. Such strategies address potential institutional and policy-level "barriers" (e.g., financial constraints, admissions practices that disadvantage URM students), as well as relatively underutilized opportunities to create institutional standards to enhance diversity (e.g., accreditation standards).

Equally important to these efforts, however, is the need to assess and improve, where necessary, the institutional climate for diversity. This includes strategies that encourage the introduction of diverse viewpoints in classroom pedagogy, attract and support URM students and faculty, and transform institutions and institutional environments to support diversity-related goals. This chapter will explore such strategies. The chapter begins by providing a framework for understanding how the institutional climate influences diversity efforts and how diversity is linked to the educational mission of health professions training institutions. Second, the chapter reviews literature that assesses the impact of racial and ethnic diversity in educational settings on student and institutional outcomes. Specific strategies to transform the institutional climate for diversity are then discussed, followed by the committee's recommendations for change.

Throughout this discussion, the committee emphasizes several conditions and characteristics of institutional change processes that must be present to ensure the success of efforts to enhance the institutional climate for diversity. These include:

• *The need for "holistic" institutional change.* Evidence suggests that efforts to enhance diversity require comprehensive, systematic changes in the ways that institutions value and respond to diversity. By themselves, "added-on" diversity programs (e.g., sensitivity training, cultural programs, and workshops) are unlikely to affect meaningful change absent systematic, integrated diversity efforts.

• *The need for strong institutional leadership.* Institutional leaders— including university presidents, deans, governance bodies, department chairs, and other administrators—must clearly articulate the importance of diversity for the institutional mission. In addition, institutional leaders must establish clear expectations for all students, faculty, and staff regarding diversity goals and the roles all members of the campus community must adopt to attain these goals.

• *The need for a long-term perspective.* Academic institutions are slow to change. In addition, the history of diversity efforts in higher education suggests that improvements are often modest and ebb and flow with changing policy contexts, social attitudes, and resource constraints. A long-term perspective is needed to maintain the institutional commitment to diversity and realize gains over time.

• *The need for adequate resources.* In the current fiscal climate, almost all academic institutions are facing tight budgets and limited resources. Institutional diversity efforts, however, cannot be developed and implemented without adequate resources to invest in programming, training, support services, and other tools that are an important aspect of a comprehensive diversity plan.

• *The need for planning and evaluation.* Institutions should develop long-range diversity plans and regularly evaluate the effectiveness of diversity efforts, with an eye toward modifying the plan where necessary.

Support for the importance of these conditions for diversity efforts is summarized in this chapter. These efforts require strong, sustained institutional commitment and support from many sectors of the university community. As will be discussed below, such changes can be expected to result in tangible benefits for training institutions and their students, including improvements in pedagogy and educational outcomes for all students, as well as better care for the patient populations that these institutions serve.

DEFINING "DIVERSITY" AND THE "INSTITUTIONAL CLIMATE"

As noted above, earlier discussions of diversity in this report have focused on efforts to improve the *structural diversity* within health professions training settings. Structural diversity is defined as the numerical and proportional representation of URM groups among students, faculty, and administrators (Hurtado et al., 1998; Gurin et al., 2002). Many higher education institutions place the largest share of emphasis on this dimension of diversity. Diversity, however, also can be conceptualized as the *diversity of interactions* that take place on campus (e.g., the quality and quantity of interactions across diverse groups and the exchange of diverse ideas), as well as *campus diversity-related initiatives and pedagogy* (e.g., the range and quality of curricula and programming pertaining to diversity, such as cultural activities and cultural awareness workshops; Milem, Dey, and White, this volume). Each of these dimensions influences the others; indeed, research evidence indicates that students' experiences with campus diversity affect the quality of their educational experiences and learning outcomes (to be reviewed later in this chapter). This evidence formed part of the basis of the University of Michigan's successful defense of its rationale for considering race and ethnicity in admissions processes in the *Grutter v. Bollinger et al.* U.S. Supreme Court case (Krislov et al., 2003).

The institutional climate for diversity is defined as the perceptions, attitudes, and expectations that define the institution, particularly as seen from the perspectives of individuals of different racial or ethnic backgrounds. The institutional climate is influenced by several elements of the institutional context (see Figure 5-1), including the degree of structural diversity, the historical legacy of inclusion or exclusion of students and faculty of color, the psychological climate (i.e., perceptions of the degree of racial tension and discrimination on campus), and the behavioral dimension (i.e., the quality and quantity of interactions across diverse groups and diversity-related pedagogy; Hurtado et al., 1999). Each of these elements influences others; an institution's historical legacy of inclusion or exclusion, for example, can affect the ability of the institution to successfully recruit URM faculty and students. The institutional history and degree of structural diversity, in turn, can influence the nature and quality of intergroup relations, classroom diversity, and individuals' perceptions of the racial climate. Perceptions of the racial climate often vary among individuals of different racial and ethnic backgrounds and campus roles (e.g., faculty, students, staff) but are significant because these perceptions are both a product of the institutional environment, as well as a significant predictor of individuals' future interactions and campus experiences (Hurtado et al., 1999). In this framework, structural diversity is an important first step toward enhancing the climate for diversity but is insufficient in and of itself to create an institutional climate that supports and values diversity as central to the educational mission.

The institutional context, in turn, is influenced by forces external to the institution (i.e., the policy context and the sociohistorical context). The

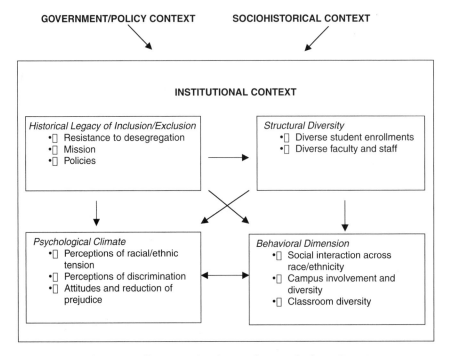

FIGURE 5-1 Elements influencing the climate for racial/ethnic diversity.
SOURCE: Hurtado et al., 1999.

governmental and policy context can powerfully affect structural dimensions of diversity, as financial aid policies and programs, state and federal policy regarding affirmative action, and court decisions related to desegregation of higher education institutions all may shape the socioeconomic and racial/ethnic diversity of the student body. Similarly, the sociohistoric context influences institutional and individual attitudes toward diversity, as social and political movements have often shaped popular opinion regarding diversity and access to higher education (Hurtado et al., 1999).

The institutional climate for diversity is therefore "conceptualized as a product of these various elements and their dynamics" (Hurtado et al., 1999, p. 6). It is distinct from the institutional "culture" (i.e., the stable norms and beliefs that may constitute an organizational system). More importantly, however, the institutional climate is malleable and can be altered through systemic intervention efforts aimed at each of the elements of the institutional context. Each of the dimensions of the institutional climate may influence diversity efforts, in both positive and negative ways.

Institutions that focus exclusively on the numeric or proportional representation of URM students on campus, have, in many cases, found that insufficient attention to other dimensions of the campus climate for diversity may pose challenges to the effective integration and retention of URM students. Greater proportions of URM students can cause conflict and resistance among students and faculty if the institution does not anticipate and take steps toward maximizing cross-racial interactions and facilitating discussions about diversity (Milem, Dey, and White, this volume). Training and educational programs, for example, to better inform students and faculty of the value of diversity in the institution can help to facilitate positive diversity interactions, while cultural exchanges and workshops may assist diverse students as they attempt to integrate into the campus environment. Attention to the structural dimensions of diversity is therefore important, but only as an initial step towards comprehensive diversity efforts (Chang, 2001).

THEORY AND RESEARCH ON DIVERSITY AND LEARNING

A growing body of research demonstrates that college students, of all racial and ethnic backgrounds, benefit from interaction with a diverse group of college student peers (see also discussion in Chapter 1). This research indicates that it is not merely the case that the presence of diverse students on campus fosters richer learning experiences. Research also indicates that student learning experiences are enhanced in proportion to the frequency and quality of students' informal interactions across racial and ethnic lines. These informal interactions, along with the discussion of racial/ethnic issues in classroom settings, confer benefits for students' academic development, as well as for their civic and community orientation. While the majority of this research has been conducted with undergraduate students, many of the principles regarding diversity's benefits extend to health professions training settings (Tedesco, 2001), as will be discussed below.

Gurin et al. (2002), in seminal research that formed the core of the social science evidence base cited by the University of Michigan in its Supreme Court defense, utilized longitudinal data from two student surveys (a survey conducted at the University of Michigan and a national survey of student collegiate experiences) to assess whether students' diversity experiences as undergraduates were related to their "learning outcomes" (defined as the use of active thinking, intellectual engagement and motivation, and academic skills) and "democracy outcomes" (i.e., citizenship engagement, belief in the compatibility of group differences and democracy, the ability to take the perspective of others, and cultural awareness and engagement). Over 11,000 white, African American, Asian American, and Latino students were among the national sample, while the Michigan sample included over 1,500 white, African American, and Asian American students, all of whom were surveyed as they entered college and again after 4 years.

Among both the Michigan and national samples of students, Gurin and colleagues found that diversity experiences were significantly related to learning outcomes upon follow-up, even after adjusting for students' academic and socioeconomic background (i.e., gender, SAT scores, high school grade point average [GPA], parents' educational level, racial composition of high school and neighborhood growing up), institutional characteristics (among the national sample), and prior scores on learning outcome measures. In the national sample, informal interactional diversity was especially significant for all four racial/ethnic groups in predicting intellectual engagement and academic skills, as was the impact of classroom diversity on these measures for white and Latino students. Among the Michigan students, both classroom diversity and campus-facilitated diversity activities (i.e., participation in multicultural events and intergroup dialogues) were significantly and positively associated with active thinking and intellectual engagement for all racial groups (Gurin et al., 2002).

Similarly, diversity experiences were found to significantly predict students' democracy outcomes, even after adjustment for students' prior academic and socioeconomic background and precollege racial exposure, as well as measures of democracy orientation upon initial assessment. For all racial groups, informal interactions across racial and ethnic lines were associated with higher levels of citizenship engagement and awareness and appreciation of racial and cultural diversity. Classroom diversity was associated with these outcomes for white, Asian American, and Latino students, again after controlling for students' prior scores on these measures. In the Michigan sample, informal cross-racial and ethnic interactions, classroom diversity, and campus-sponsored events and dialogues about multicultural issues were associated with students' belief in the compatibility of differences with democratic processes, the ability to understand the perspectives of individuals from other groups, and engagement in racial and cultural issues, while controlling for students' background characteristics and prior scores on democracy measures, although the strength of these relationships varied by racial/ethnic group (Gurin et al., 2002).

Gurin and colleagues concluded that students who were exposed to higher levels of campus diversity, experienced and discussed diversity issues in the classroom, and participated in informal discussions across racial and ethnic groups were better able to understand and consider multiple perspectives, deal with the conflicts that different perspectives sometimes create, and "appreciate the common values and integrated forces that harness differences in pursuit of the common good" (University of Michigan, 2000, p. 5). These students can best develop the capacity to understand the ideas and feelings of others in an environment characterized by a diverse study body, equality among peers, and discussion of the rules of civil discourse. Diversity experiences in college were also associated with a range of better cognitive and intellectual outcomes. Interactions with peers from diverse racial backgrounds, both in the classroom and informally, were associated with greater levels of engagement in active thinking processes, growth in intellectual engagement, and motivation and growth in intellectual and academic skills (Gurin et al., 2002).

Similarly, Chang (2001), using data from a national, longitudinal survey of college students' attitudes and experiences before, during, and after college, assessed whether the degree of racial/ethnic diversity that students experience on campus was associated with educational outcomes. Data from over 18,000 college students attending 392 4-year colleges and universities were utilized, with controls for variation in institutional size, location, type, religious affiliation, gender (coed or single-sex), and selectivity. Chang assessed whether students' self-reported experiences of having socialized with someone of a different race and having discussed racial issues while in college were associated with the degree of racial diversity at the students' institution. In addition, he assessed whether these experiences were associated with four educational outcomes (retention, satisfaction with college, intellectual self-concept, and social self-concept). Chang found that campus diversity was a small, but statistically significant, predictor of students' likelihood of forming interracial friendships and talking about race and ethnicity, even after students' background (e.g., socioeconomic status, standardized test scores) and campus environment were taken into account. In addition, Chang found that socializing with students of another racial or ethnic background had a small but significant direct effect on students' self-reported satisfaction with college and social self-concept, and discussion of racial issues similarly was a small but significant predictor of students' intellectual self-concept (Chang, 2001).

Hurtado (2001) also assessed the relationship between undergraduate students' diversity experiences and their assessments of civic, job-related, and educational outcomes. Using longitudinal data from nationwide surveys of students and faculty, Hurtado found that students who reported that they studied with someone of a different racial or ethnic background while in college were more likely upon one-year follow-up to report having greater acceptance of people of different racial/ethnic groups, greater cultural awareness, greater tolerance of people with different beliefs, a greater ability to work cooperatively with others, and greater critical thinking skills, among a range of other learning, job-related, and civic outcomes. These relationships remained significant even after controlling for institutional selectivity, students' prior academic performance, and academic habits (e.g., hours per week spent studying; Hurtado, 2001).

The finding that students benefit from diversity in the classroom and in informal interactions has been extended to health professions educational settings. Whitla and colleagues (2003), in a survey of recent Harvard and University of California, San Francisco, medical school graduates' attitudes regarding diversity in medical education, found that students reported experiencing greater levels of diversity in medical school than in their prior educational experiences, as the percentage of students reporting contact with other groups increased from 50 percent prior to college to 85 percent in medical school. These trends were true for majority group as well as URM students. Overwhelmingly, these students viewed diversity among their medical student peers as a positive; 86 percent thought that classroom diversity enhanced discussion and was more likely to foster serious discussions of alternate viewpoints. Over three-quarters of the students surveyed found that diversity helped them to rethink their viewpoints when racial conflicts occurred, and the same percentage felt that diversity provided them with a greater understanding of medical conditions and treatments. The pattern of responses did not differ by respondents' racial or ethnic group (Whitla et al., 2003). While we found no similar published surveys of dental, nursing, and professional psychology students, anecdotal evidence (Davis and David, 1998) suggests that these students may experience similar benefits.

Related research in developmental and cognitive psychology offers a theoretical framework to understand these findings. The period of late adolescence and early adulthood is characterized by significant social and emotional growth, as individuals attempt to define their personal and social identity as adults while learning about the complex social structures and communities in which they live and work. Personal and social identity develops best, according to developmental theorists, when young adults are exposed to novel situations, particularly those characterized by diversity and complexity of perspectives and experiences (Gurin et al., 2002). Residential colleges and universities provide students with an opportunity to explore ideas and perspectives that are different from their own prior experiences. In such situations, young people commonly lack a "script" to understand and predict social expectations and roles, and are therefore likely to experience uncertainty and discontinuity as they are exposed to different perspectives, experiences, and viewpoints. Research in cognitive psychology illustrates that this discontinuity is more likely to promote "active," complex thinking. This form of thinking results in new ways of processing information, promotes intellectual engagement, and reduces dependence on prior learned scripts. Exposure to racial and ethnic diversity in college settings and, more importantly, meaningful interaction across racial and ethnic lines in informal settings and in classroom discussion are experiences that improve active thinking by providing opportunities to identify discrepancies with precollege experiences and to encounter novel and unfamiliar perspectives (Gurin et al., 2002). Gurin and colleagues illustrate this phenomenon as they quote a white undergraduate student evaluating a course on intergroup relations:

> I came from a town in Michigan where everyone was white, middle-class and generally pretty closed-down to the rest of the world, although we didn't think so. It never touched us, so I never questioned the fact that we were "normal" and everyone else was "different." Listening to other students in the class, especially the African American students from Detroit and other urban areas just blew me away. We only live a few hours away and yet we live in completely separate worlds. Even more shocking was the fact that they knew about "my world" and I knew nothing about theirs. Nor did I think that this was even a problem at first. I realize now that many people like me can go through life and not have to see another point of view, that somehow we are protected from it. The beginning for me was when I realized that not everyone shares the same views as I, and that our different experiences have a lot to do with that (Gurin et al., 2002, p. 338).

Because of stark patterns of racial and ethnic residential housing segregation, most high school students entering college have limited experience with individuals from other racial, ethnic, and socioeconomic groups (Frankenberg and Lee, 2002). Very few of the freshman students matriculating at the University of Michigan, for example, have had significant contact with students from other racial and ethnic groups (see Box 5-1). As the University of Michigan, in its document *The Compelling Need for Diversity in Higher Education*, notes, "[t]he costs of this persistent and

---

BOX 5-1
Racial and Ethnic Segregation in Detroit-Area Schools

Schools in the Detroit metropolitan area are among the most segregated in the nation, although many metropolitan school districts are also characterized by high levels of segregation:

- In 60 of the 83 school districts in the three-county Detroit metropolitan area, the black student population is 3 percent or less;
- 82 percent of African American students attend schools in only three districts;
- More than 90 percent of the area's white students attend schools in districts with black student populations under 10 percent;
- Only two school districts in the area come close to reflecting the overall proportions of the Detroit metropolitan region's African American, Latino, and white students (University of Michigan, 2000).

pervasive racial separation are profound for minorities and non-minorities alike . . . [m]embers of differential racial and ethnic groups too often are denied the opportunity to benefit from all that our diverse communities have to offer" (University of Michigan, 2000, p. 4). Segregation limits opportunities for individuals to confront and correct racial stereotypes, to learn how to interact with others in an increasingly multicultural America; segregation also fosters mistrust and large gaps in the experiences, values, and viewpoints of different racial and ethnic groups. The University of Michigan determined that such segregation is detrimental to the community's best interests; moreover, the university asserts that the quality of higher education is vastly improved when the barriers of racial segregation are removed and students from diverse racial and ethnic groups are encouraged to learn from, and with, each other.

HOW CAN HEALTH PROFESSIONS TRAINING PROGRAMS ENSURE THE SUCCESS OF DIVERSITY EFFORTS?

As noted above, efforts to improve the structural diversity of higher education institutions are a positive first step, but alone they are insufficient to improve the institutional climate for diversity and ensure that diversity benefits both students and the institution. Universities must create conditions in which students from different racial and ethnic backgrounds can have meaningful, productive interactions, and maximize educational experiences. Absent these efforts, institutions that bring together diverse groups run the risk of allowing conflict, misunderstanding, and resentment to poison students' educational experiences. Fortunately, a body of theory and research has informed efforts to enhance the conditions under which diversity can provide educational benefits.

Design Principles for Improving the Campus Climate for Diversity

Building on research and theory, Hurtado et al. (1999) outline 12 strategies to achieve an improved climate for and maximize the benefits of diversity. The first four principles are "core" to any institutional efforts for change, while the remaining eight offer guidance for the development of new programmatic initiatives and policies. Hurtado and colleagues stress that these principles represent a comprehensive, "holistic" approach to institutional change and require that institutions possess strong leadership, adequate resources to support change efforts, strong planning and evaluation, and a long-term commitment. Research supporting these design principles is summarized in Hurtado et al. (1999), as well as Milem, Dey, and White (this volume).

Core principles include the need to:

1. *Affirm the goal of achieving a campus climate that supports racial and ethnic diversity as an institutional goal.* Campus leadership should be able to articulate the need for diversity and communicate institutional goals clearly. In addition, leadership must understand how diversity and educational excellence are "inseparable" (Hurtado et al., 1999, p. 71).

2. *Systematically assess the institutional climate for diversity in terms of historical legacy, structural diversity, psychological climate, and behavioral elements to understand the dimensions of the problem.* Self-appraisal of the institutional climate for diversity across a range of dimensions is critical to gather "baseline" data on how the institution is experienced by diverse groups, to identify areas of strength and weakness, and to assess the impact of diversity improvement efforts. Such self-assessment should be ongoing and should inform program changes. An example of a "cultural audit" that led to an on-going process of institutional change is provided in Box 5-2.[1]

3. *Develop a plan, guided by research, experiences at peer institutions, and results from the systematic assessment of the campus climate for diversity, for implementing constructive change that includes specific goals, timetable, and pragmatic activities.* Institutions should develop a "template" for change that is based on self-study and identifies measurable goals. This template should serve as a guiding blueprint for departmental and other programmatic activities.

4. *Implement a detailed and ongoing evaluation program to monitor the effectiveness of and build support for programmatic activities aimed at improving the campus climate for diversity.* Ongoing evaluation will help to assess the effectiveness of programs and serve as the basis for program modification. Evaluation will also serve as a mechanism for holding key elements of the university—including faculty, staff, and administrators—responsible for achieving desired outcomes.

The following eight principles are designed to help guide specific programming efforts. These principles may vary in their applicability or relevance across institutions, based on institutional history, type of control, geographic circumstances, etc. They can be tailored to meet the specific circumstances and goals of individual institutions, but they must be accompanied by the four components above—setting priorities, fact finding, es-

---

[1]Examples of institutional diversity efforts provided in this chapter are abstracted from published literature. They do not represent a systematic effort to document "best practices" or to describe the full range of diversity programs implemented in health professions education institutions (HPEIs). For a more comprehensive description of programs to improve the institutional climate for diversity, see Hurtado et al. (1999).

BOX 5-2
A "Multicultural Audit" at the University of Michigan
School of Dentistry

Early in 1994, the University of Michigan School of Dentistry, under the leadership of Dean Machen, initiated a "multicultural audit" to assess the institution's climate for diversity and develop recommendations to promote greater multicultural awareness and receptivity to diversity concerns in teaching, service delivery, and other aspects of the institution's mission. This extensive self-study process was undertaken to help students, faculty, and staff gain awareness of the different perceptions that individuals from different groups hold regarding the campus climate. Members of the school's Multicultural Initiatives Committee write, "Understanding how . . . different persons perceive and experience the particular work and learning environments and what advantages and disadvantages they have as a consequence of their social group affiliations is the main goal of the cultural audit" (Inglehart et al., 1997, p. 284).

The Michigan team conducted its audit by:

- developing a task force composed of student, faculty, and staff representatives, and that reflected the diversity of the institution;
- developing a plan for data collection, which was multimethod and included a questionnaire, focus group data, analyses of the curriculum, library resources, and records on URM recruitment, and an observational study;
- collecting and analyzing data; and
- authoring a report that outlined specific recommendations.

The audit was conducted in an open process, and members of the school population were regularly informed about ongoing activities and invited to contribute. At the conclusion of the process, the committee's report and findings were communicated to faculty, students, and staff and submitted to the dean. The report's recommendations fell into six broad areas: structuring and communicating the institution's commitment to improving the climate for diversity; changing institutional foundations to promote multiculturalism; improving academic programs; recruiting and retaining diverse students, faculty, and staff; creating a process to facilitate communication and handle grievances; and providing additional resources to promote multiculturalism and diversity.

As a result of this process, the School of Dentistry initiated a process of organizational change, with the goal of building a community of diverse students, faculty, and staff in which all members can gain awareness and skills regarding diversity issues. In addition, this process helps the school to achieve its goal of pushing dental education to be both patient-centered and culturally sensitive—in short, to achieve "excellence through diversity."

Among the "lessons learned," the Multicultural Initiatives Committee noted that the audit would not have been successful without the full support of institutional leadership, representation of diverse groups from the university committee on the audit team, efforts to inform and invite participation from the institutional community, and a commitment to a long-term process of self-assessment and institutional change (Inglehart et al., 1997).

tablishing a plan, and evaluating results—to be successful (Hurtado et al., 1999):

5. *Make a conscious effort to rid the campus of its exclusionary past and adopt proactive goals to achieve desegregation; this includes increasing opportunity for previously excluded groups.* Most predominantly white public and private higher education institutions have a history of exclusion of minority groups before the large-scale desegregation efforts of the late 1960s. Vestiges of this history may remain and influence who attends or seeks employment at the institution. Leadership should carefully assess and acknowledge how this history may affect diversity efforts and develop strategies to counter its influence.

6. *Involve faculty in efforts to increase diversity that are consistent with their roles as educators and researchers.* Faculty can have a powerful influence on students' attitudes toward diversity. Even the most experienced faculty members, however, may need assistance in appropriately harnessing classroom diversity to enhance students' learning experiences. Institutions should provide faculty with training and support to manage classroom conflict, to create opportunities for open discussion of diversity, and to become aware of their own attitudes and beliefs regarding diversity.

7. *Create collaborative and cooperative learning environments where students' learning and interaction among diverse groups can be enhanced.* Research demonstrates that cooperative learning environments can improve students' learning and enhance their diversity experiences. Institutions should provide tools and incentives to faculty for the adaptation of these pedagogical practices, which can include study groups, group projects, the creation of a community service component as an adjunct to classroom work, and other activities.

8. *Increase students' interaction with faculty outside class by incorporating students in research and teaching activities.* Contact between students and faculty outside of class is associated with higher student achievement, yet URM students report lower levels of such contact. Institutions should develop programs and incentives to encourage broad segments of students to interact formally and informally with faculty. Examples include student–faculty research projects, workshops and seminars, sharing meals, and other activities.

9. *Initiate curricular and cocurricular activities that increase dialogue and build bridges across communities of difference.* Students naturally form affinity groups and friendships based on commonality of background and experience, yet institutions can take steps to encourage meaningful intergroup interaction. These may include informal dialogue groups or sessions affiliated with formal coursework, perhaps facilitated by trained peer leaders. In addition, institutions may consider sponsoring multicultural pro-

grams that celebrate the history and cultures of different racial and ethnic groups and provide incentives for diverse participation, including among majority groups.

10. *Create a student-centered orientation among faculty and staff.* Research indicates that those institutions that are more student-centered—that is, where faculty and staff convey an interest in students' academic and personal development and where students feel valued—experience lower levels of intergroup tension and better student outcomes. Faculty and staff orientation sessions can be used to provide tools and strategies to enhance students' feelings of validation and create a welcoming environment for students of all backgrounds.

11. *Include diverse students in activities to increase students' involvement in campus life. Ensure that programming for diversity involves general support services as well as coordinated activities and support programs for URM students.* Administrators and faculty sometimes express concern, appropriately, that URM students may "self-segregate" on predominantly white campuses. They fear that racially and ethnically oriented student groups and activities, such as minority student organizations or minority peer support services, may tend to reinforce segregation from majority groups on campus. Yet research indicates that URM student involvement in such groups and activities is associated with higher social involvement, informal interactions with faculty, and use of general support services. Institutions should therefore encourage a wide range of student support services and programming, as a means to encourage URM students to take advantage of general university supports and other campus activities.

12. *Increase sensitivity and training of staff members who are likely to work with diverse student populations.* Administrators and staff can have a powerful influence in shaping students' perceptions of the campus climate for diversity. Institutions should consider offering sensitivity training and opportunities to develop cross-cultural and conflict resolution skills for those staff that work with students on a regular basis.

Institutional Leadership and Diversity

Institutional leaders—including university presidents, deans, department chairs, and other administrators—are crucial in the effort to establish and maintain a learning environment that values and is enriched by a diverse, multicultural campus community. Institutional leaders must establish expectations regarding diversity goals, "set the tone" for how diversity objectives will be met, and hold all members of the campus community accountable for achievement of these goals. Writing about the responsibility of leadership in creating multicultural dental schools, Kalkwarf (1995) notes, "it is only when [institutional leaders'] actions reinforce the concept of cultural diversity that a program of multiculturalism within an educational institution will truly be successful" (p. 1108). Kalkwarf describes several initiatives undertaken at the Dental School at the University of Texas Health Sciences Center-San Antonio that reflected institutional leaders' desire to educate faculty and students regarding the institution's diversity goals. These efforts included a faculty retreat to discuss cultural diversity goals, a perceptual survey of students and faculty to assess attitudes toward diversity and multicultural issues, and interventions—including faculty development workshops—that were developed in response to survey findings. Other intervention efforts initiated by the institutional leadership included programs to enhance multicultural understanding among staff and students (Kalkwarf, 1995).

Similarly, Monts (1995) argues that university leaders must "initiate efforts [in support of diversity and multiculturalism] that reflect both a top-down and bottom-up approach" (p. 1113), with roles for university administrators, faculty, staff, and students. Elements of this approach at the University of Michigan, according to Monts, include a strategic plan for linking academic excellence and diversity, a program of special incentives for academic units to recruit and hire women and faculty of color, and a program of self-study to assess students' expectations, perceptions, and experiences regarding diversity and multiculturalism (Monts, 1995).

Recruitment, Hiring, and Retention of Underrepresented Minority Faculty

"Psychologists . . . continue to be predominantly Caucasian; to be trained by predominantly Caucasian faculty members; and to be trained in programs in which ethnic issues are ignored, regarded as deficiencies, or included as an afterthought" (Myers et al., 1991, p. 5).

Over a decade ago, Myers, Echemendia, and Trimble (1991) observed that faculty and curricula in graduate professional psychology training programs remained homogeneous and unresponsive to the growing diversity of the U.S. population. Unfortunately, this pattern still holds true among many HPEIs (see Chapter 1 for a review of data on faculty diversity in health professions training programs). While some institutions have made great progress in recruiting URM faculty, others continue to experience difficulty in expanding diversity among faculty, despite growing evidence of its benefits. In addition to providing support for URM students as role models and mentors, racially and ethnically diverse faculty can be expected to "bring new kinds of scholarship to an institution, educate students on issues of growing importance to society, and offer links to communities not often connected to our campuses" (Smith, 2000, p. 51).

Greater diversity among faculty can also be expected to lead to important pedagogical changes. In a study to determine if faculty diversity has an impact on curriculum and teaching methods, Hurtado (2001) assessed racial/ethnic and gender-related differences in university faculty teaching and instructional methods in required undergraduate courses. Using longitudinal data from nationwide surveys of students and faculty, Hurtado found that African-American and Latino faculty were more likely than faculty of other racial/ethnic groups to utilize cooperative and "active" learning techniques,[2] while American Indian faculty were more likely to use experiential learning/field studies techniques. Female faculty were also more likely to utilize these pedagogical approaches, which in other research have been found to lead to more active learning and favorable educational outcomes than "passive" learning approaches, such as learning via lectures. Minority and female faculty were also more likely to assign readings on racial/ethnic or gender issues.

Similarly, Milem (2001), in a study of faculty attitudes and teaching, found that increased faculty diversity is associated with the use of active learning techniques and inclusion of racial/ethnic issues in the curriculum. This same study, however, found that the institutions that had made the most progress in admitting and enrolling URM students—typically, large, selective, research-intensive institutions—also were the "least flexible and least adaptive in responding to changing student needs," given that their faculty are "oriented to specialized research, not to flexible approaches to teaching" (Milem, 2001, p. 234).

Given the important benefits of faculty diversity for enhancing institutional diversity efforts, what are some successful strategies that health professions training institutions can adopt to improve faculty diversity efforts? Smith (2000) offers a series of strategies and issues for institutions to consider as they initiate faculty recruitment and hiring efforts. Smith notes that many myths about minority faculty recruitment abound and may *hinder* faculty search committees, to the extent that they believe the myths, from seriously recruiting minority candidates. To assess the experiences of URM Ph.D.s, Smith surveyed nearly 300 doctoral-level minority and non-minority scholars, 93 percent of whom held doctorates from research institutions, who had been recipients of prestigious Ford, Mellon, and Spencer Founda-

---

[2]"Active" learning techniques include the use of cooperative learning, student presentations, group projects, student-designed learning activities, class discussion, and other activities that "enable students to exercise initiative and assume responsibility for their own learning" (Milem, 2001, p. 235). Research indicates that active learning techniques enhance student learning and development (Astin, 1993) and facilitate student interaction across racial, ethnic, and socioeconomic groups. Active learning is therefore one of several important benefits of classroom diversity (Hurtado et al., 1999).

tion Fellowships. These fellowships are designed to support the careers of scientists and academicians in a range of fields.

Perhaps one of the most pervasive myths, Smith found, is that qualified URM candidates are few and far between and, therefore, are often the subject of "bidding wars" as institutions compete among each other to recruit candidates. While it is true that URM Ph.D.s are less numerous relative to non-URM scholars, only a small fraction of the URM Ph.D.s in Smith's sample (11 percent) reported that they were recruited and encouraged to apply for a faculty position. This percentage was even smaller among Puerto Rican Ph.D.s, as only 3 percent of this group reported being encouraged to apply for a job. When job candidates had a choice of offers, respondents reported that these institutions were typically limited to two or three institutions, and these usually were not their top choices.

Another myth is that faculty of color who are recruited to nonelite campuses are often lured away by more prestigious institutions, or that URM faculty are leaving academia for better-paying government or industry jobs. The majority of respondents in Smith's sample, however, reported that they were unwilling to change jobs primarily for salary or prestige. Those who did change jobs were as likely to report that they moved because of "dual-career choices, questions of fit, or unresolved problems with their institutions, such as having to deal with multiple demands as a result of being one of just a few faculty of color in a department or an institution" (Smith, 2000, p. 50).

In light of the experiences reported by these highly qualified minority scholars, Smith recommends several steps for institutions to improve their efforts at recruiting minority faculty. To begin, institutions should carefully examine their mission statement and assess how faculty diversity assists the institution to meet its goals. Such an analysis "positions diversity at the center of what is taught, how it is taught, and to whom students are exposed" (Smith, 2000, p. 51). These institutions should examine how faculty diversity can influence teaching and scholarship; many universities, for example, are instituting new diversity requirements in the curriculum and are exploring ways to improve the classroom environment and pedagogy for an increasingly diverse student body. URM faculty can assist in these efforts.

Identifying and recruiting qualified URM candidates for faculty positions can be improved by utilizing active search processes, Smith argues, that go beyond simply posting positions and recruiting though networks that are familiar to the faculty. Active searches require developing personal connections with individuals who have expertise in needed areas of scholarship and demonstrating flexibility regarding candidates' specialties. Similarly, search committees should be diverse, to help in assessing and evaluating candidates of different backgrounds, and should have a close working relationship with the university administration to ensure the success of the search process (Smith, 2000). Identifying potential URM faculty candidates should not be limited to external searches; in many instances, potential faculty can be found among an institution's URM graduate and postdoctoral health professions students (see example provided by Formicola et al. [2003] in section titled, "A Comprehensive Strategy to Increase URM Applications, Admission, and Success—One Dental School's Example").

Once qualified candidates are identified, personal support in the form of a "champion," someone willing to facilitate communication, advise the candidate, and advocate for him or her during the search process, can ensure that the search committee has "the opportunity to fully assess the candidate's talent" (Smith, 2000, p. 52). Finally, Smith notes, posthiring support is critical for many URM faculty. Institutional politics, the challenges of earning tenure, balancing teaching and research, and other faculty concerns may be exacerbated for faculty of color, who are often expected to assume a larger role than non-URM faculty in mentoring students, serving on committees, and other tasks (Smith, 2000).

Recruitment of Underrepresented Minority Students

As noted earlier in this chapter, increasing the proportions of underrepresented minority students in health professions training settings is an important *initial* step toward transforming the institutional climate. Health professions training institutions have experimented with a wide range of strategies to recruit URM students, with varying degrees of success. Recruitment efforts are affected by a number of factors, such as the quality of primary and secondary education for URM students, changes among students in career interests, competition from other nonhealth fields for talented students (e.g., almost all health professions schools have seen modest declines in the overall number of applicants since the late 1990s; Grumbach et al., 2001), and competition among health professions disciplines for students from the same applicant pool. Such competition poses particular problems for some disciplines, such as nursing, which has declined in popularity as a health professions career choice as opportunities for women and minorities in other fields have increased and as wages and working conditions for nurses have failed to improve substantially (Buerhaus and Auerbach, 1999).

Strategies for recruitment of URM students generally fall into several categories, including, but not limited to:

- The use of targeted marketing materials, outreach, and information campaigns to interest high school and college students in health professions careers;

• Efforts to inform pre-health-career advisors of opportunities in health professions and entrance and admissions requirements;
• Educational enrichment programs aimed at URM and educationally disadvantaged students, which typically expose high school and college-level students to health professions education curriculums and to the programs and services of health professions schools; and
• Partnerships between majority- and historically minority-serving institutions, to foster student exchanges and encourage URM students to pursue further study in health professions.

Several examples of these recruitment efforts are highlighted in published literature (see Boxes 5-3 and 5-4). Few of these programs, however, have been evaluated to determine their effectiveness and/or which components of recruitment efforts are most useful.

Retention of URM Students

Recruitment, admission, and matriculation of URM students represent only the first steps for health professions training programs to ensure successful educational experiences for URM students. While data are not uniformly available for all health professions, URM medical students experience higher rates of academic failure, withdrawal, and lower graduation rates than non-URM medical students (Rainey, 2001), trends that are also likely to occur in dentistry, nursing, and psychology training programs.

This pattern of poorer success in health professions training settings is likely the result of many factors. As noted earlier in this report, because of inequitable educational opportunities, URM students often receive an inferior academic preparation in K-12 and college relative to non-URM students. URM students also face greater financial challenges than non-URM students, particularly in the face of rising tuition costs at almost all public and private universities. The dearth of URM faculty results in fewer opportunities for URM students to obtain mentoring from individuals who are most familiar with the cultural and economic background of these students (Rainey, 2001). Incidents of racial discrimination and unfair treatment on the basis of race and ethnicity are, unfortunately, not rare events for health professions students (e.g., more than one in seven medical students who reported being mistreated also reported being subjected to racially or ethically offensive remarks; AAMC, 2000). Furthermore, URM students typically report higher levels of alienation from the campus environment and may not find appropriate social supports to counter these feelings.

A growing number of HPEIs are developing comprehensive strategies to improve retention among URM students, with a range of programs that may include intervention efforts to increase academic preparation,

---

BOX 5-3
Recruiting a Diverse Nursing Student Workforce—
Two Universities' Experiences

Nursing is facing workforce shortages that threaten to short-circuit efforts to increase the safety and efficiency of American health care. Recognizing that the fastest-growing share of the potential nurses of the future are students of color, nursing programs are expanding efforts to attract these students.

Washington State University's Intercollegiate College of Nursing was recently highlighted for its efforts to increase the pool of future URM nursing students through targeted efforts to recruit from some of the state's most medically underserved communities (Rosseter, 2002). The college has:

• Received funding to initiate the Aid Latino Community to Attain Nursing Career Employment (ALCANCE) project, which targets recruitment of Latino and American Indian nursing students. The program provides culturally congruent community mentors for high school and prenursing students, culturally congruent advanced nursing student mentors, and mentors from the National Association of Hispanic Nurses for beginning nursing students, and stipends for Latino and American Indian students who pursue nursing education. In addition, the project offers an entry-level position to nursing through the Hispanic Health Care Broker Class, where bilingual high school students study medical terminology, basic anatomy, confidentiality, and ethics and serve as interpreters for monolingual Spanish-speaking clients at Yakima Valley Farmworkers Clinic.
• Launched a statewide recruitment campaign with a consortium of area universities and hired a member of the Nez Perce tribe to serve as a recruitment coordinator. A summer camp for students interested in health care and ongoing contact with the coordinator provide support and encouragement to pursue a career in nursing.

The College of Nursing at the University of Nebraska Medical Center uses a combination of recruitment efforts to attract men and minority students. In 2000–2001, the number of minority applicants increased 84 percent, and the school's minority enrollment increased 43 percent. Some of the school's specific steps have been to:

• develop outreach materials in Spanish and target information to URM students' parents regarding the shortage of American Indian, Hispanic, and African American nurses;
• develop a system to attract URM potential recruits and follow-up with personal contact;
• recruit in minority communities and encourage families to attend an "exploratorium for kids," with current nursing students on hand to teach children about nursing (Rosseter, 2002).

BOX 5-4
Institutional Partnerships to Increase URM Students' Preparation and Interest in Health Professions Careers

In recent years, several institutions have developed partnerships to increase URM students' exposure to, interest in, and preparation for heath professions careers. These can include partnerships between majority- and historically minority-serving institutions, as the following examples illustrate:

A Partnership Between St. Louis University and the Atlanta University Center

The four historically black colleges that constitute the Atlanta University Center (AUC), including Clark-Atlanta University, Morehouse College, Morris Brown College, and Spelman College, are collaborating with Saint Louis University (SLU) to promote interest among African American students in careers in research psychology. Undergraduate students from AUC colleges are selected to participate in the program, which provides mentoring and exposes students to psychological research. Students join a research team in the fall of their sophomore year and are asked to develop during the academic year a research proposal, complete with literature search and institutional review board approval. The following summer, these students attend an 8-week summer session at SLU, during which they live on campus and complete their research, while taking a course in research ethics. In addition, the students participate in a graduate admissions workshop, in which they will request and complete actual applications for graduate admission. The summer session concludes with a formal research conference at which students present their research findings. Students are provided with faculty follow-up and mentoring as they return to their home institutions.

This program, which is supported by a grant from the National Science Foundation, was honored with the 1999 Richard Suinn Award by the American Psychological Association for its innovative efforts to increase diversity in the field of psychology (APA, 2000).

The Fisk University-Vanderbilt University School of Nursing Joint BSN Program

Fisk University, a historically black college, and the Vanderbilt University School of Nursing (VUSN) have entered into a unique agreement for a collaborative degree program that allows Fisk to award a Bachelor of Science in Nursing (BSN) to its students by completing core liberal arts coursework at Fisk and BSN equivalent curriculum at VUSN. VUSN, which offers only master's and doctoral nursing degree programs, will commit resources toward the Fisk BSN program, saving the latter institution the expense of creating an undergraduate nursing program from scratch, including developing specialized classrooms and skill labs and employing nursing faculty. After completing the Fisk BSN degree, students will have the foundation for graduate study in nursing and therefore may consider continuing their graduate education at VUSN. VUMC has agreed to provide support funding to the new program for Fisk BSN graduates, who agree to work at VUMC at full salary for a specific period of time. The graduates can then enroll in the MSN program at VUSN and take advantage of the VUMC tuition support benefit.

The program is being hailed as an innovative means of both increasing the numbers of URM nurses and addressing Tennessee's nursing shortage, which is expected to exceed 9,000 nursing positions by the year 2020 (Hurst, 2003).

mentoring, financial support, academic support, psychosocial support, and professional opportunities (Grumbach et al., 2002; Rainey, 2001). Rainey (2001), noting that many such efforts are splintered and unsystematic, calls for coordinated efforts to address such factors as:

- HPEI curriculum and pedagogy (e.g., switching emphasis from lecture-based teaching to more active learning approaches, such as small-group problem-based learning, and reducing the "boot camp mentality" operative during the first few months of a student's medical school career);
- Student orientation (e.g., by giving greater attention to helping students manage the fast-paced, content-rich curriculum through the teaching of specific study skills and learning strategies);
- Financial aid (e.g., by providing consistency in financial aid, even if a student is required to repeat a year, to avoid placing greater pressures on students facing academic difficulty); and
- Remedial strategies (e.g., by providing remedial services that are coordinated between student and academic affairs offices and keep the student in the academic environment, so that the student maintains contact with on-campus resources and faculty).

Observing that few institutions have adopted such a coordinated approach, Rainey notes:

> Once a student experiences an academic failure that results in a projected delayed graduation date, there appears to be a cumulative effect that significantly increases the chances the student will never graduate. The student no longer has the support of friends and classmates. She has increased financial pressures. She believes that her failures are common knowledge. . . . Early identification of academic failure, swift and intense efforts to provide assistance by faculty and administration, making every effort to keep the student on schedule, and providing continuing and adequate financial aid are essential elements of a successful remediation strategy, especially for first- and second-year academic problems (Rainey, 2001, p. 352).

In developing and implementing student academic and social support programs, many HPEI administrators are often faced with the question of whether to target programs to URM and other students at risk for academic difficulties, or to provide remedial and support services to all students, regardless of background and prior levels of preparation. Rainey (2001) argues against the former approach, noting that "these strategies run the risk of stigmatizing the student doing poorly and of increasing his or her already high level of anxiety" (Rainey, 2001, p. 350). Instead, Rainey argues, HPEIs should provide comprehensive learning assistance support, make students and faculty aware of differences in learning styles, and find alternative remedial strategies that do not segregate students experiencing academic difficulty.

Establishing an Informal, Confidential Mechanism for Mediation: The Role of the Ombuds Office

HPEI students, faculty, staff, and administrators occasionally experience barriers to achieving institutional diversity goals, such as behaviors, attitudes, or speech that are racially or ethnically offensive and are counter to goals of inclusiveness. The creation of an institutional ombuds office may be useful in addressing these concerns, thereby assisting broader efforts to improve the institutional climate for diversity. An ombudsperson is a formally designated, neutral, trained practitioner whose major function is to provide confidential and informal assistance to all constituents of the university community. The ombuds may serve as a fact-finder, counselor, or mediator between two or more parties but operates outside of the typical management structure and is an independent agent (UCOA, 2003). The ombuds does not, however, participate in formal grievance processes, testify in lawsuits, make administrative decisions, determine the "guilt" or "innocence" or those accused of wrong-doing, or assign sanctions. The informal, internal nature of the ombuds' operation is therefore often an effective supplement to more formal institutional conflict resolution, compliance, and equal employment/equal opportunity policies and procedures (Steinhardt and Connell, 2002).

Central to the operation of the ombuds office are the characteristics of neutrality, independence, informality, and confidentiality. Ombuds must remain neutral within the organization, both in perception and practice, and independent of the traditional lines of authority. In addition, ombuds must ensure absolute confidentiality of operations, in order to provide a safe environment for individuals registering complaints and for dispute mediation. The characteristics of ombuds offices allow the ombuds to serve effectively as a "fact-finder" to gather information about complaints, advise individuals about how to resolve disputes informally, mediate disputes and seek "win–win" resolution of problems, and advise individuals about more formal grievance procedures should informal efforts fail (Steinhardt and Connell, 2002).

Transforming the Health Professions Education Curriculum

In many health professions training settings, the curriculum is perhaps the most resistant to change (Rainey, 2001). Training institutions face growing demands to provide students with new skills and knowledge, and faculty find it increasingly difficult to adopt new curriculum and pedagogy

within limited classroom time. Yet curricular change can serve as an important component of an overall strategy to support and harness the benefits of
classroom diversity. Such changes are consistent with the growing need to
produce new health professionals who possess cross-cultural skills and can
meet the demands of an increasingly diverse patient population (Betancourt
et al., 2002; Brach and Fraser, 2000; Tedesco, 2001).

Cross-cultural education strategies—defined as programs to help trainees to understand the sociocultural dimensions underlying a patient's health
values, beliefs, and behavior, with the goal of preparing trainees to care for
patients from diverse social and cultural backgrounds and to recognize and
address racial, cultural, and gender biases in health-care delivery—are increasingly being developed and implemented in medical, dental, nursing,
and professional psychology training settings (Brach and Fraser, 2000).
These strategies have been developed to meet at least three demands. First,
cross-cultural education is expected to provide students with the skills and
knowledge that they will need as future health professionals working with
diverse patient populations. Second, cross-cultural education can be expected to help improve patient outcomes and narrow the racial–ethnic gap
in health-care quality observed in many studies. Third, such training is
increasingly being required by accreditation and licensure bodies
(Betancourt, 2003).

Three conceptual approaches are predominant in cross-cultural education models. The first, which emphasizes teaching cultural sensitivity and
awareness, is "based on the attitudes central to professionalism—humility,
empathy, curiosity, respect, sensitivity, and awareness of all outside influences on the patient" (Betancourt, 2003, p. 561). The primary focus of this
approach is to expand trainees' awareness of the impact of sociocultural
factors, such as culture, racism, social class, and the social construction of
gender roles, on patients' health attitudes and behaviors (Brach and Fraser,
2000). Furthermore, this model of training explores how sociocultural factors influence the provision and quality of health care and health-care
outcomes (Betancourt et al., 2002). As noted above, such training can be
enhanced by the diverse backgrounds and experiences of a multiracial,
multiethnic student and faculty body and by the sharing of diverse experiences and perspectives in the classroom.

A second cross-cultural education model, focused on multicultural or
categorical approaches, emphasizes the acquisition of knowledge about the
attitudes, values, beliefs, and behaviors of cultural groups. Such training,
however, risks promoting stereotypes through the use of broad-based gen-
eralizations that fail to account for the heterogeneity within cultural groups.
Effective forms of this approach train students to develop methods of community assessment and evidence-based facts regarding cultural groups, such

as disease incidence and prevalence, historical factors that might shape health behaviors, and ethnopharmacology (Betancourt, 2003).

A third conceptual model, the cross-cultural approach, focuses on developing communication skills and tools for providers to "be aware of certain cross-cutting cultural issues, social issues, and health beliefs while providing methods to deal with information clinically once it is obtained" (Betancourt, 2003, p. 562). These include tools to help providers to better understand patients' conceptions of health and illness, methods to assess patients' social contexts, and strategies to facilitate patient–provider negotiation and participatory decision making (Brach and Fraser, 2000; Betancourt, 2003).

A limited number of studies have evaluated the impact of cross-cultural education strategies on trainees, in part because of methodological limitations. For example, investigators are often limited in their ability to accurately assess students' cross-cultural attitudes following training, and "fact-based evaluation" in some cases runs counter to the goal of cross-cultural education (i.e., cross-cultural education strategies often attempt to assist trainees in managing complex information about culture and language, rather than imparting "facts" about racial and ethnic groups, which may inadvertently promote stereotyping of different racial, cultural, or linguistic groups). Several studies, however, have demonstrated gains in trainees' cross-cultural knowledge and skills following training (Brach and Fraser, 2000; Betancourt, 2003). It is reasonable to assume that racial and ethnic diversity among faculty and students in HPEIs may enhance the quality of cross-cultural education, as such diversity can provide a rich exchange of ideas and opportunities to challenge assumptions. In addition, cross-cultural education programs may assist in efforts to attract URM students to health professions education (e.g., URM students may have greater interest in HPEI programs that include significant cross-cultural education components), and to develop a supportive institutional climate for diversity.

The importance of cross-cultural training is increasingly reflected in the ethical and professional principles and guidelines of many health professions disciplines. The American Psychological Association, for example, has published guidelines for multicultural education, training, research, practice, and organizational change for psychologists that "reflect knowledge and skills needed for the profession in the midst of dramatic historic sociopolitical changes in U.S. society, as well as needs of new constituencies, markets, and clients" (APA, 2003, p. 377). The guidelines (summarized in Box 5-5) are designed to provide psychologists with a rationale for addressing multicultural concerns in their professional work, relevant research and information that support the guidelines, and paradigms that broaden the purview of psychology as a profession. Moreover, the guidelines are founded on the following principles:

• "Ethical conduct of psychologists is enhanced by knowledge of differences in beliefs and practices that emerge from socialization through racial and ethnic group affiliation" (APA, 2003, p. 382);
• The quality of education, training, and research in psychology can be enhanced by understanding the interface between racial and ethnic group affiliation and socialization experiences;
• The understanding and treatment of all people can be enhanced by understanding how race and ethnicity intersect with other dimensions of identity, such as gender, age, sexual orientation, disability, and other factors;

BOX 5-5
Guidelines on Multicultural Education, Training, Research, Practice, and Organizational Change for Psychologists

Commitment to Cultural Awareness and Knowledge of Self and Others
Guideline 1: Psychologists are encouraged to recognize that, as cultural beings, they may hold attitudes and beliefs that can detrimentally influence their perceptions of and interactions with individuals who are ethnically and racially different from themselves.

Guideline 2: Psychologists are encouraged to recognize the importance of multicultural sensitivity/responsiveness to, knowledge of, and understanding about ethnically and racially different individuals.

Education
Guideline 3: As educators, psychologists are encouraged to employ the constructs of multiculturalism and diversity in psychological education.

Research
Guideline 4: Culturally sensitive psychological researchers are encouraged to recognize the importance of conducting culture-centered and ethical psychological research among persons from ethnic, linguistic, and racial minority backgrounds.

Practice
Guideline 5: Psychologists are encouraged to apply culturally appropriate skills in clinical and other applied psychological practices.

Organizational Change and Policy Development
Guideline 6: Psychologists are encouraged to use organizational change processes to support culturally informed organizational (policy) development and practices.

SOURCE: APA, 2003.

• Understanding of the underrepresentation of some racial and ethnic minority groups in the discipline is explained, in part, by psychology's history of viewing cultural differences as "deficits" and underappreciation of the role of race and ethnicity in the development of personal and social identity;

• Psychologists' ability to promote racial and ethnic equity and social justice is enhanced by an understanding of race, ethnicity, and culture; and

• "Psychologists' knowledge about the roles of organizations, including employers and professional psychological associations, is a potential source of behavioral practices that encourage discourse, education and training, institutional change, and research and policy development that reflect, rather than neglect, cultural differences" (APA, 2003, p. 382).

A Comprehensive Strategy to Increase URM Applications, Admission, and Success—One Dental School's Example

Throughout this discussion, the committee has emphasized the importance of comprehensive, multipronged strategies to create and support diversity in health professions training programs. Some common elements of successful strategies include efforts to:

• conduct a self-assessment, identify areas where support for diversity efforts must be improved, and develop a strategic plan for improvement;
• recruit URM applicants;
• reduce barriers to the admission of URM students, while maintaining the academic quality of admits;
• reduce financial barriers to URM student participation; and
• recruit URM faculty.

Columbia University's School of Dental and Oral Surgery (SDOS) has undertaken such a comprehensive approach, with the result that the school has dramatically increased the racial and ethnic diversity of its students, faculty, and staff and is much better positioned to address the oral health care needs of the region and nation. This change process began with a reassessment of past institutional efforts, which had been less than successful. Until the early 1980s, SDOS enrolled few African American, American Indian, or Hispanic students, and the full-time D.D.S. faculty was almost entirely composed of white males. Recognizing that the school's reputation as a local and national leader in dental education and ability to serve an increasingly diverse population would suffer without improved diversity efforts, SDOS developed a number of initiatives to transform the school's climate for diversity (Formicola et al., 2003).

SDOS began in the early 1980s by rethinking its admissions processes, which were heavily dependent upon applicants' college grade point average, Dental Aptitude Test scores, letters of recommendation, and a personal interview. These policies were typical of other dental schools, but "[led] to considering a narrow range of students for admission and did not permit adequate consideration of a student's full range of intellectual, social, and personal traits" (Formicola et al., 2003, p. 492). In response, the admissions committee broadened its criteria to include a greater emphasis on applicants' personal attributes and background, extracurricular activities, difficulties overcome, and other qualitative factors. To facilitate this change of emphasis, admissions committee members were provided with training in interview skills and understanding qualitative attributes that might be beneficial to the school and to the profession. In addition, a new survey instrument was developed to help guide the interviews and ensure that applicants' qualitative attributes were assessed. Finally, a subcommittee on minority enrollment was appointed to assist the admissions committee in interviewing and assessing applicants with diverse educational and professional backgrounds. As a result, more minority students were admitted; in the 59-year period between 1923 and 1982, SDOS graduated 16 African American and Latino students, while in the period from 1984 to 2001, the school admitted 57 African American and Latino students, graduating 51 of them (Formicola et al., 2003).

With the admission of greater numbers of diverse students, SDOS realized that variation in students' educational background required that the institution provide academic support services. As a result, the school developed tutorial services for first-year students and a summer preenrollment academic enrichment program. These services were offered initially to all students whose records indicated that their preparation could be improved. Gradually, the first-year tutorial program expanded and improved its ability to serve all students, and the summer enrichment program was suspended (Formicola et al., 2003).

During this same period, SDOS also sought opportunities to expand its postdoctoral training, while at the same time improving its service to the local community and increasing the numbers of URM faculty. These goals were met with a unique collaboration between SDOS and the Harlem Hospital Medical Center. At the time, Harlem Hospital had expanded its dental service from mainly emergency and oral surgical care to comprehensive care, and expanded its dental clinic facility. This created an opportunity for SDOS and the dental department at Harlem Hospital to collaborate to develop a postdoctoral specialty training program for dentists completing their residency at Harlem Hospital. The residents, who were mainly African American and Hispanic, were required to commit to service in the community as members of the hospital staff, or as faculty in the dental school and/ or in practice in the Harlem community. In return, Harlem Hospital paid the salary for residents admitted to the postdoctoral program, and tuition was waived by the SDOS. SDOS also realized that the program provided an opportunity to recruit URM graduates into full- and part-time faculty positions at Columbia. These goals have been met: from 1988 to 2000, the program provided postdoctoral training to 21 African American and Latino graduates of the Harlem Hospital Dental Department residency program, 15 of these graduates practice in the Harlem community on the hospital staff, and 12 have faculty appointments at Columbia SDOS. In addition, Harlem Hospital now has a full range of dental specialists available to provide comprehensive care to the community and provide training to general practice residents (Formicola et al., 2003).

Following the development of these programs, SDOS also took several other steps to assess and improve the institutional climate for diversity. By the mid-1990s, the school established a faculty Search Committee that included members external to the department and whose recommendations were reviewed by Columbia University's Health Sciences Affirmative Action Committee. This committee ensured that all faculty search committees conducted a thorough review and considered racial and ethnic minority candidates. In addition, SDOS conducted a climate study, using focus groups composed of randomly selected groups of faculty, staff, and students. The purpose of the climate study was to determine how students from diverse background perceived the dental school environment and to identify areas for improvement. The climate study resulted in several recommendations, ranging from student training and faculty/staff development programs designed to increase awareness of cultural pluralism and diversity, to efforts to ensure that all students were provided equal access to information and opportunities for research activities, internships, and other activities (Formicola et al., 2003).

SUMMARY AND RECOMMENDATIONS

The institutional climate for diversity—defined as the perceptions, attitudes, and expectations that define the institution, particularly as seen from the perspectives of individuals of different racial or ethnic backgrounds—can exert a profound influence on diversity efforts. Diversity is most often viewed as the proportion and number of individuals from groups underrepresented among students, faculty, administrators, and staff (i.e., structural diversity). Diversity, however, can also be conceptualized as the *diversity of interactions* that take place on campus (e.g., the quality and quantity of interactions across diverse groups and the exchange of diverse ideas), as well as *campus diversity-related initiatives and pedagogy* (e.g., the range and quality of curricula and programming pertaining to diversity, such as cultural activities and cultural awareness workshops; Milem, Dey, and White, this volume). Each of these elements of diversity must be carefully considered as institutions assess their diversity goals.

The institutional climate for diversity is influenced by several elements of the institutional context, including the degree of structural diversity, the historical legacy of inclusion or exclusion of students and faculty of color, the psychological climate (i.e., perceptions of the degree of racial tension and discrimination on campus), and the behavioral dimension (i.e., the quality and quantity of interactions across diverse groups and diversity-related pedagogy; Hurtado et al., 1999). Each of the dimensions of the institutional climate may influence diversity efforts, in both positive and negative ways. More importantly, the institutional climate is malleable and can be altered through systemic intervention efforts aimed at each of the elements of the institutional context.

Research on Diversity and Learning

A growing body of research demonstrates that college students, of all racial and ethnic backgrounds, benefit from interaction with a diverse group of college student peers (see also discussion in Chapter 1). Gurin and colleagues (2002), for example, found that college students' informal and classroom interactions with students from diverse racial and ethnic groups were associated with students' subsequent learning outcomes (defined as the use of active thinking, intellectual engagement and motivation, and academic skills) and democracy outcomes (i.e., citizenship engagement, belief in the compatibility of group differences and democracy, the ability to take the perspective of others, and cultural awareness and engagement). While the majority of this research has been conducted with undergraduate students, recent research has extended these findings to medical students (Whitla et al., 2002), and many of the principles regarding diversity's benefits extend to health professions training settings (Tedesco, 2001).

How Can Health Professions Educational Institutions Ensure the Success of Diversity Efforts?

Building on this research and theory, Hurtado et al. (1999) outline 12 strategies to achieve an improved climate for diversity. More importantly, these strategies can help institutions to maximize the benefits of diversity. The first four principles (i.e., affirm the value of diversity, systematically assess the climate, develop a plan of action, and institute ongoing evaluation of the plan) are "core" to any institutional efforts for change, while the remaining eight offer guidance for the development of new programmatic initiatives and policies. Hurtado and colleagues stress that these principles represent a comprehensive, "holistic" approach to institutional change and require that institutions possess strong leadership, adequate resources to support change efforts, strong planning and evaluation, and a long-term commitment.

Recruitment, Hiring, and Retention of Underrepresented Minority Faculty

Enhancing the racial and ethnic diversity of health professions education faculty can provide support for URM students in the form of role models and mentors, lead to important pedagogical changes, and "bring new kinds of scholarship to an institution, educate students on issues of growing importance to society, and offer links to communities not often connected to our campuses" (Smith, 2000, p. 51). Many health professions training programs have struggled, however, to increase the proportion of URM faculty members. To a degree, these failures are the result of common myths regarding URM faculty recruitment (e.g., that qualified URM faculty candidates are few, too highly sought-after to invest significant efforts into recruiting, and apt to leave following offers from more prestigious institutions; Smith, 2000).

Health professions training institutions can take several steps to improve their efforts at recruiting minority faculty. To begin, institutions should carefully examine their mission statement and assess how faculty diversity assists the institution to meet its goals. Identifying and recruiting qualified URM faculty candidates can be improved by utilizing active search processes that go beyond simply posting positions and recruiting though networks that are familiar to the faculty. Search committees should be diverse, to help in assessing and evaluating candidates of different backgrounds, and should have a close working relationship with the university administration to ensure the success of the search process. Once qualified candidates are identified, personal support in the form of a "champion"— someone willing to facilitate communication, advise the candidate, and advocate for the candidate during the search process—can ensure that the search committee has the opportunity to fully assess the candidate. Finally, posthiring support is critical for many URM faculty to address the challenges of earning tenure, balancing teaching and research, and other faculty concerns (Smith, 2000).

Minority Student Recruitment and Retention

Several health professions training programs have implemented successful URM student recruitment and retention programs. Some elements of successful recruitment efforts include developing academic and educational partnerships with minority-serving institutions, addressing financial barriers, targeting outreach to URM students, and engaging prehealth advisors. Just as importantly, institutions should develop comprehensive strategies to retain URM students, by providing a range of academic and social supports, including faculty and peer mentoring, tutoring, academic skills assessment, and instruction in study skills. Institutions may increase opportunities for URM students to integrate themselves into the campus community (and take advantage of support programs) through both ethnic- and racial-group interest organizations, as well as general campus programs, such as orientation programs that clearly outline the institutions' expectations regarding diversity-related policies and goals, and sensitivity training programs that increase awareness and understanding of diversity in the campus context.

> Recommendation 5-1: HPEIs should develop and regularly evaluate comprehensive strategies to improve the institutional climate for diversity. These strategies should attend not only to the structural dimensions of diversity, but also to the range of other dimensions (e.g., psychological and behavioral) that affect the success of institutional diversity efforts. These strategies include, but are not limited to efforts to:
>
> • recruit and retain URM students and faculty through a range of academic and social supports, including but not limited to mentoring programs, academic supports, and other strategies integrated into ongoing programs;
> • educate faculty and students regarding the benefits of diversity to the institutional mission; and
> • encourage participation by diverse faculty on core institutional committees, including but not limited to admissions, faculty search, internal review, and promotions and tenure.

Education is a critically important initial step toward increasing diversity at many HPEIs. HPEIs must provide all members of the campus community with an explicit rationale for diversity efforts and communicate the principles that underlie such efforts. Educational programs should be ongoing, integrated into regular programming, and regularly evaluated to assess their effectiveness. As with other institutional goals, faculty should be evaluated, as part of ongoing merit and promotion review, on their progress toward achieving the institution's diversity-related objectives.

> Recommendation 5-2: HPEIs should proactively and regularly engage and train students, house staff, and faculty, via orientation programs and ongoing training, regarding institutional diversity-related policies and expectations, the principles that underlie these policies, and the importance of diversity to the long-term institutional mission. Faculty

should be able to demonstrate specific progress toward achieving these goals as part of the promotion and merit process.

Because of the often difficult nature of racial/ethnic dialogue and potential for conflict, HPEIs should consider developing appropriate conflict mediation and dispute resolution services that may serve to increase understanding and cooperation. An ombuds program may assist efforts to improve the campus climate for diversity by providing an informal, confidential process to assess and resolve disputes.

Recommendation 5-3: HPEIs should establish an informal, confidential mediation process for students and faculty who experience barriers to institutional diversity goals (e.g., experiences of discrimination, harassment). Such a process can be established by appointment of an ombudsman who can serve as an arbitrator with the power to investigate complaints and mediate disputes.

Innovative institutional diversity models also take into consideration the quality of diversity training experiences that students receive. Well-supported training experiences that expose all students to diverse patient populations increase students' knowledge and skills in working with underserved groups. Moreover, as the experiences of Formicola et al. (2003) illustrate, training affiliations with community-based health-care facilities can increase access to health care among diverse patient populations and attract more URM students and faculty to training settings.

Recommendation 5-4: HPEIs should be encouraged to affiliate with community-based health-care facilities in order to attract and train a more diverse and culturally competent workforce and to increase access to health care.

REFERENCES

American Psychological Association (APA). 2000. *Model Strategies for Ethnic Minority Recruitment, Retention, and Training in Higher Education.* Compiled by the Office of Ethnic Minority Affairs, American Psychological Association, May 2000. Washington, DC: American Psychological Association.

American Psychological Association (APA). 2003. Guidelines on multicultural education, training, research, practice, and organizational change for psychologists. *American Psychologist* 58:377–402.

Association of American Medical Colleges (AAMC). 2000. *LCME Graduation Questionnaire.* Washington, DC: Association of American Medical Colleges.

Astin AW. 1993. *What Matters in College: Four Critical Years Revisited.* San Francisco: Jossey-Bass.

Betancourt JR. 2003. Cross-cultural medical education: Conceptual approaches and frameworks for evaluation. *Academic Medicine* 78(6):560–569.

Betancourt JR, Green AR, Carrillo JE. 2002. *Cultural Competence in Health Care: Emerging Frameworks and Practical Approaches.* New York: The Commonwealth Fund.

Brach C, Fraser I. 2000. Can cultural competency reduce racial and ethnic health disparities? A review and conceptual model. *Medical Care Research and Review* 57:181–217.

Buerhaus PI, Auerbach D. 1999. Slow growth in the United States of the number of minorities in RN workforce. *Image: Journal of Nursing Scholarship* 31(2):179–183.

Chang MJ. 2001. The positive educational effects of racial diversity. In: Orfield G, Kurlaender M, eds. *Diversity Challenged: Evidence on the Impact of Affirmative Action.* Cambridge, MA: The Civil Rights Project, Harvard University and Harvard Education Publishing Group. Pp. 175–186.

Davis SP, David M. 1998. Experiences of ethnic minority faculty employed in predominantly white schools of nursing. *Journal of Cultural Diversity* 5(2):68–76.

Formicola AJ, Klyvert M, McIntosh J, Thompson A, Davis M, Cangialosi T. 2003. Creating an environment for diversity in dental schools: One school's approach. *Journal of Dental Education* 67(5):491–499.

Frankenberg E, Lee C. 2002. *Race in American Public Schools: Rapidly Resegregating School Districts.* Cambridge, MA: The Civil Rights Project, Harvard University.

Grumbach K, Coffman J, Rosenoff E, Muñoz C. 2001. Trends in underrepresented minority participation in health professions schools. In: Smedley BD, Stith AY, Colburn L, Evans CH, eds. *The Right Thing to Do, The Smart Thing to Do: Enhancing Diversity in the Health Professions.* Washington, DC: National Academy Press. Pp. 185–207.

Grumbach K, Coffman J, Muñoz C, Rosenoff E, Gándara P, Sepulveda E. 2002. *Strategies for Improving the Diversity of the Health Professions.* University of California, San Francisco: Center for California Health Workforce Studies.

Gurin P, Dey EL, Hurtado S, Gurin G. 2002. Diversity and higher education: Theory and impact on educational outcomes. *Harvard Education Review* 72(3):330–366.

Hurst J. 2003. Fisk, VU Team to Offer Rx for Shortage of Nurses. *The Tennessean,* June 16, 2003.

Hurtado S. 2001. Linking diversity and educational purpose: How diversity affects the classroom environment and student development. In: Orfield G, Kurlaender M, eds. *Diversity Challenged: Evidence on the Impact of Affirmative Action.* Cambridge, MA: Harvard Education Publishing Group.

Hurtado S, Milem JF, Clayton-Peterson A, Allen WA. 1998. Enhancing campus climates for racial/ethnic diversity: Educational policy and practice. *Review of Higher Education* 21(3):279–302.

Hurtado S, Milem J, Clayton-Peterson A, Allen W. 1999. *Enacting Diverse Learning Environments: Improving the Climate for Racial/Ethnic Diversity in Higher Education.* ASHE-ERIC Higher Education Report Volume 26, No. 8. Washington, DC: George Washington University, Graduate School of Education and Human Development.

Inglehart M, Quiney C, Kotowicz W, Tedesco L, Getchell K, Jordan J, Kanar H, Kozin W, Perkins KG, Rehemtulla S, Robinson E, Ueda N, Voss C, Chesler M, Reed B. 1997. Cultural audits: Introduction, process, and results. *Journal of Dental Education* 61(3):283–288.

Kalkwarf KL. 1995. Creating multicultural dental schools and the responsibility of leadership. *Journal of Dental Education* 59(12):1107–1110.

Krislov M, Alger J, Caminker E, Kessle PJ, Niehoff LM, Long B, Mahoney M, Ballenger JS, Pickering JH, Payton J, Benitez BA, Delery S, Goldblatt C. 2003. *Brief for Respondents, Barbara Grutter, Petitioner, vs. Lee Bollinger, Dennis Shields, and the Board of Regents of the University of Michigan, Respondents.* No. 02-241 in the Supreme Court of the United States.

Milem JF. 2001. Increasing diversity benefits: How campus climate and teaching methods affect students outcomes. In: Orfield G, Kurlaender M, eds. *Diversity Challenged: Evidence on the Impact of Affirmative Action.* Cambridge, MA: Harvard Education Publishing Group. Pp. 233–249.

Milem JF, Dey EL, White CB. This volume. Diversity considerations in health professions education. In Smedley BD, Stith-Butler A, Bristow LR, eds. *In the Nation's Compelling Interest: Ensuring Diversity in the Health-Care Workforce.* Washington, DC: The National Academies Press.

Monts LP. 1995. Diversity and multiculturalism: Institutional leadership at the University of Michigan. *Journal of Dental Education* 59(12):1113–1118.

Myers HF, Echemendia RJ, Trimble JE. 1991. The need for training ethnicity minority psychologists. In: Myers HF, Wohlford P, Guzman LP, Echemendia RJ, eds. *Ethnic Minority Perspectives on Clinical Training and Services in Psychology* Washington, DC: American Psychological Association. Pp. 3–11.

Rainey ML. 2001. How do we retain minority health professions students? In: Smedley BD, Stith AY, Colburn L, Evans CH, eds. *The Right Thing to Do, The Smart Thing to Do: Enhancing Diversity in the Health Professions.* Washington, DC: National Academy Press. Pp. 328–357.

Rosseter R. 2002. Reshaping recruiting strategies for increasing diversity in academic nursing programs. *Association of Women's Health, Obstetric and Neonatal Nurses (AWHONN)* 6(3):196–200.

Smith D. 2000. How to diversify the faculty. *Academe* 86(5):48–52.

Steinhardt R, Connell M. 2002. Reporting of wrongdoing and resolving disputes: The value of ombudsmen and hotlines in the corporation. In: Banks TL, Banks FZ, eds. *Corporate Legal Compliance Handbook.* New York: Aspen Publishers. Pp. 6-1–6-34.

Tedesco L. 2001. The role of diversity in the training of health professionals. In: Smedley BD, Stith AY, Colburn L, Evans CH, eds. *The Right Thing to Do, The Smart Thing to Do: Enhancing Diversity in the Health Professions.* Washington, DC: National Academy Press. Pp. 36–56.

University and College Ombuds Association (UCOA). 2003. *The Role of a University or College Ombuds Office.* [Online]. Available: http://www.ucoa.org/the_ombuds.html.

University of Michigan. 2000. *The Compelling Need for Diversity in Higher Education.* [Online]. Available: http://www.umich.edu/~urel/admissions/legal/expert/index.html [accessed April 10, 2000].

Whitla DK, Orfield G, Silen W, Teperow C, Howard C, Reede J. 2003. Educational benefits of diversity in medical school: A survey of students. *Academic Medicine* 78(5):460–466.

6

Community Benefit as a Tool for Institutional Reform

The preceding chapters provide the evidence and justification for definitive action by health professions education and training institutions to
increase the diversity of the health-care workforce. A key question is
whether community benefit can be used as a tool to frame the responsibility
of these institutions to play a role in responding to major societal imperatives. This chapter reviews the historical and legal origins of community
benefit, the evolution of policies and practices, and the potential application to health professions education and training institutions.

HISTORICAL ORIGINS AND LEGAL ANTECEDENTS

Community benefit is a legal term that applies to charitable activities
that benefit the community as a whole. The term grows out of an English
common law concept, articulated in a 1891 legal decision that defined four
types of charitable organizations: trusts for the relief of poverty; trusts for
the advancement of education; trusts for the advancement of religion; and
trusts for other purposes beneficial to the community.[1] The outlines of this
framework were adopted into U.S. law with the passage of the first federal
taxation act in 1894.[2] Although this law was ruled unconstitutional[3] with
the ratification of the 16th Amendment[4] and passage of Congressional

---

[1]*Commissioners for Special Purposes of Income Tax v. Pemsel*, A.C. 531-592 (1891).
[2]U.S. Congress, Act of August 1894, chap. 349, 28 Stat. 553.
[3]*Pollock v. Farmers' Loan & Trust Co.*, 158 U.S. 601 (1895).
[4]16th Amendment to the U.S. Constitution (1913).

legislation in 1913[5] allowing for federal personal and corporate income taxation, the charitable trust framework providing for income tax exemption for qualifying eleemosynary organizations (nonprofits that served "religious, charitable, scientific, literary, or educational purposes")[6] was adopted and maintained in every update of the tax code since the original ruling.

In this era of the advent of corporate income taxation and accompanying tax exemption in the United States, there also arose an accompanying effort to establish a more uniform regulatory structure for the formation of nonprofit organizations. While the size of the nonprofit sector was relatively small at this point in U.S. history, legislators also recognized a need for a more uniform process to determine which organizations qualified for tax exemption and the extent of their tax preferred status. This became increasingly important in the twentieth century, as the nonprofit sector entered a period of dramatic growth.

A major factor in this trend was the emergence of nonprofits that derived the majority of their income from the sale of personal services. Chief among these types of organizations were voluntary hospitals. By 1910, there were approximately 4,000 such institutions in the United States (Stevens, 1982). Rapid advances in medical technology during the 1930s and 1940s transformed the hospital into a provider of highly sophisticated services. The modern hospital bore little resemblance to the almshouses of the eighteenth and nineteenth centuries, which had a limited role to provide free custodial care to poor people. The hospital now operated fully in the marketplace, charging fees for an increasing array of costly services. Services for the poor were limited to what could be covered by a combination of donations, public sector contracts, and surplus revenue from fees charged to insured populations (Stevens, 1982).

By 1956, concern about medical care for the poor contributed to the issuance of IRS Revenue Ruling 56-185, which established explicit "relief of poverty" criteria for hospitals to qualify for tax exemption as 501(c)(3) nonprofit organizations.[7] While the ruling included language that acknowledged the practical limits to the volume of charitable services that could be provided by nonprofit hospitals,[8] only services to the poor would qualify the organization for tax exemption.

The relief of poverty interpretation of charity remained the standard for nonprofit hospitals until the issuance of IRS Revenue Ruling 69-545 in

---

[5]Revenue Act of 1913.
[6]*Pollock v. Farmers' Loan & Trust Co.*, 158 U.S. 601 (1895).
[7]Rev. Rul. 56-185, 1956-1 C.B. 202.
[8]Rev. Rul. 56-185, 1956-1 C.B. 202; section 2.

1969.[9] This ruling modified the criteria of 56-185 to remove the requirement to provide services for the poor, and identified the promotion of health (i.e., community benefit) as a charitable purpose. In promulgating this alternative standard for granting tax exemption to hospitals, the IRS created a controversy that has now lasted over 30 years over the issue of what exactly is expected of a nonprofit hospital to meet the "community benefit standard."

It is important to note that this ruling was issued 4 years after the passage of the Medicare/Medicaid Act of 1965. Some have suggested that these events contributed to an impression among government officials that problems of access for the medically indigent would be solved in the near future, and hence it would be appropriate to broaden the criteria for charitable purposes (Fox and Schaffer, 1991).

In the 1970s, major changes in health-care financing and ownership contributed to increased scrutiny and the withdrawal of some privileges for nonprofit hospitals. Rising costs, application of federal cost-containment measures, expansion in the number of investor-owned hospitals, growing numbers of medically indigent, and two economic recessions contributed to an amplification of competitive behavior among hospitals. In the public sector, local governments were faced with a reduction in federal and state support at the same time they were confronted with significant increases in social safety net costs. In some cases, these pressures led to legal actions that challenged the tax exemption of individual institutions. The most notable of these occurred in 1985 with *Utah County v. Intermountain Health Care*.[10]

At the federal level, a series of regulatory actions were taken in the 1970s and 1980s to withdraw privileges from nonprofit organizations. Notable examples include the elimination of exemption from federal labor law,[11] elimination of the exemption to pay Social Security taxes (with the exception of employees of schools, colleges, and universities),[12] and clarification that there was no nonprofit health-care exception under the antitrust laws.[13] Federal action was also taken against specific classes of nonprofit

---

[9]Rev. Rul. 69-545, 1969-2 C.B. 117.

[10]*Utah County v. Intermountain Health Care*, 709 P.2d 265 (Utah 1985).

[11]Cornell University, 183, N.L.R.B. 329 (1970) and St. Aloysius Home, 224 N.L.R.B. 1344 (1976).

[12]Social Security Amendments of 1983, Pub. I., No. 98-21, § 102, 97 Stat. 65, 70-71 (codified as amended in scattered sections of 26 & 42 U.S.C.); 42 U.S.C. § 410(a)(10)(A) & (B) (1986).

[13]See, e.g., *Marjorie Webster Junior College v. Middle States Association of Colleges and Secondary Schools*, 432 F.2d 650, 654055 (C.C. Dir.) cert. Denied, 400 U.S. 965 (1970), and *National Collegiate Athletic Association v. Board of Regents*, 468 U.S. 85, 98-120 (1984).

organizations. The 1986 Tax Reform Act eliminated tax exemption for life and health insurance companies.[14] It has been suggested that these actions were driven by substantial growth in the number of commercial nonprofits and observations of their operations in the marketplace (Hansmann, 1989).

The community benefit standard articulated in IRS Revenue Ruling 69-545 was reaffirmed with the issuance of IRS Revenue Ruling 83-157 in 1983. Revenue Ruling 83-157 provided some clarification of the "promotion of health" language in 69-545, indicating that the class of beneficiaries "must be sufficiently large . . . so that the community as a whole benefits."[15] The only significant amendment to 69-545 was an easing of the emergency room requirement. Ruling 83-157 indicated "nonprofit hospitals are not required to operate an emergency room where a state or local health planning agency has found that this would unnecessarily duplicate emergency services and facilities that are adequately provided by another medical institution in the community."[16]

The community benefit standard for nonprofit organizations, established with 69-545 and reaffirmed with 83-157, provided an important backdrop for the U.S. Supreme Court's 1983 decision in *Bob Jones University v. the United States*.[17] In that case, the Court was asked to rule on a challenge to the tax-exempt status of Bob Jones University because of its racially discriminatory policies. The university denied admission to applicants who were in an interracial marriage or known to advocate interracial dating. While the IRS Revenue Rulings were intended to address the specific obligations of nonprofit hospitals, the Court determined that the obligation to confer a public benefit by not being in violation of public policy was applicable to an educational organization as well—and for that matter to all 501(c)(3) organizations. Accordingly, the Court found that that the policy of overt racial discrimination at Bob Jones University vitiated its eligibility for income tax exemption. The importance of the ruling is that it at least suggests that all tax-exempt organizations have certain public policy responsibilities that, if left unfulfilled, can place them at risk of losing some important privileges that government can confer.

Debate over the charitable obligations of nonprofit hospitals entered the federal policy arena in 1991 with the introduction of two bills in the House of Representatives. Rep. Edward Roybal (CA) introduced HR 790,

---

[14]Tax Reform Act of 1986, Pub. I. No. 99-514. § 1012, 1986 U.S. Code Cong & Admin. News (100 Stat.) 2085, 2390 (codified at I.R.C. § 501(m) (1986)).

[15]Rev. Rul. 83-157, 1983-2 C.B. 94; Restatement (Second) Trusts, § 368, comment (b) and § 372, comment (b) and (c); IV Scott on Trusts §§ 368, 372.2 (3d ed. 1967).

[16]Ibid.

[17]*Bob Jones v. United States*, 461 U.S. 474 (1983).

and Rep. Brian Donnelly (MA) introduced HR 1372.[18] Both bills sought to establish minimal financial thresholds for a combination of charity care and "qualified" community benefit activities, and both included substantial penalties for noncompliance. While neither bill made it to the floor of the House for a vote, the scope of issues raised in public hearings conveyed a strong sense of concern among policy makers about the market behavior of nonprofit hospitals. Both bills faced strong opposition from congressional opponents, industry representatives, and the George H.W. Bush administration.

By the time Roybal and Donnelly introduced their bills at the federal level, two states had already taken action. Section 2803-1 of the New York Public Health Law was adopted as part of legislation passed in 1990 and requires the development and implementation of "community service plans" by nonprofit hospitals. Requirements include an annual review of the hospital mission statement, publication of hospital assets and liabilities, an assessment of community needs and hospital strategies to address them, and the solicitation of input from community stakeholders.[19]

In the same year, the Utah State Tax Commission issued a set of formal guidelines for nonprofit hospitals and nursing homes that included a requirement for a minimum financial threshold of contributions that exceed the annual property tax liability of each facility.[20] Categories of sanctioned contributions included care to the medically indigent, community education and service, medical discounts, and donations of time and money. These legal requirements were a direct outgrowth of the 1985 challenge to the tax exemption of Intermountain Healthcare.

The initial ruling by the Utah Supreme Court was notable in that in interpreting its State Constitution, it rejected the community benefit standard in favor of the more narrow "relief of poverty" interpretation of charity, viewing community benefit activities as "any of countless private enterprises might provide"[21] (p. 265). The rejection of the community benefit standard was also based on the contention that it "entangles the state in the impossible task of valuing the relative contributions of organi-

[18]U.S. Congress, House of Representatives, Committee on Ways and Means. 1991. *Tax-exempt status of hospitals, and establishment of charity care standards. 102nd Congress, 1st Sess. July 10, 1991* (includes selected excerpts from presentations by the Department of the Treasury, the American Hospital Association, the Catholic Health Association, and texts of H.R. 790-Roybal bill, H.R. 1374-Donnelly bill, and Texas S.B. 557).
[19]Section 2803-1 of the New York Public Health Law; Chapter 922 (1990).
[20]Nonprofit Hospital and Nursing Home Charitable Property Tax Standards, Utah State Tax Commission (1990).
[21]Rev. Rul. 69-545, 1969-2 C.B. 117.

zations in the community.[22] The court enacted a set of strict standards consistent with the more narrow interpretation, which were reversed less than a year later, and the community benefit standard was codified in the 1990 State Tax Commission guidelines.

The New York and Utah legal requirements placed upon nonprofit health-care providers reflect two alternative approaches that have marked subsequent state actions in this arena: a general reporting requirement (NY) and the establishment of a minimum financial threshold (UT). Between 1990 and 2001, a total of 11 states implemented some form of legal mechanism to increase the accountability of nonprofit health care providers. Eight of the eleven (CA–1994,[23] ID–1999,[24] IN–1994,[25] MD–2001,[26] MA– 1994 [Harshbarger and MA Attorney General's Office, 1994], NH–2000,[27] NY–1990, WV–1990 [28]) took the general reporting requirement approach; three (PA–1997,[29] TX–1993,[30] UT–1990) took the minimum financial threshold approach.

Eight of the eleven states also require community assessments to identify local unmet needs; three do not (NY [limited to consultation with community members], PA, WV). Six of the eleven states require solicitation of community input in the development of community benefit plans; one state suggests it as an option (MD) and four do not address the issue (ID, PA, UT, WV). Five of the eleven states call for a review of organizational mission statements to reflect a commitment to address community health needs (CA, IN, MA, NY, TX); two require submittal of existing mission statements (MD, NH); and four do not address the issue (ID, PA, UT, WV). Finally, eight of the eleven states specifically identify unreimbursed costs of health professional training and research as reportable community benefit activities; three do not (ID, MD, WV).

Among the 11 states, there are a few unique characteristics worth noting. In Massachusetts, the state mechanism is a set of voluntary guidelines promulgated by the Office of the Attorney General, rather than a statute. In addition, a parallel set of voluntary guidelines was developed for

---

[22]Rev. Rul. 69-545, 1969-2 C.B. 117, p. 343.

[23]S.B. 697, enacted January 1, 1995, Cal. Health and Safety Code Ann. §§ 127340-127365.

[24]H.B. 154, 55th Leg., 1st Reg. Sess. Idaho 1999).

[25]House Enrolled Act No. 1023, 108th Leg., 2d Reg. Sess. (Ind. 1994).

[26]HB 15, Ch. 178, 11r1292, 2001 Reg. Sess.

[27]SB 69-Local, LSR 924, Chap. 0312, enacted January 2000.

[28]W. VA. Code State R. Tit. 110 § 24.1 (1990).

[29]Institutions of Purely Public Charity Act, November 26, 1997, 10 PA. Cons. Stat. Ann. §§ 371-55.

[30]SB 427, Tex. Health and Safety Code Ann. §§ 311.031-.048; enacted September 1, 1993.

health maintenance organizations (HMOs) (Harshbarger and Massachusetts Attorney General's Office, 1996). These guidelines are particularly notable in that they apply to all HMOs, both nonprofit and investor-owned. The basic reasoning provided by the Attorney General is that "all HMOs share responsibility for the health care needs of medically-underserved Massachusetts residents" (Harshbarger and Massachusetts Attorney General's Office, 1998).

In three states, the statutes apply to other nonprofit organizations in addition to hospitals. As noted previously, Utah's guidelines also apply to nursing homes, and New Hampshire's law applies to all health-care charitable trusts. Pennsylvania's statute applies to "institutions of purely public charity," which is general language drawn from their state constitution. While this term has contributed to uncertainty about the scope of application, key elements in the statute suggest that major providers of health-care services (i.e., hospitals) are the central focus of attention. Perhaps the most unusual element of Pennsylvania's statute is an option for applicable institutions to fulfill their charitable obligations by making payments in lieu of taxes (PILOTs) to government agencies, in essence, to pay property tax revenues that had been exempted. To encourage this practice, the state offers up to 350 percent credit for such payments, depending upon the size of the contribution in relation to annual revenues.

The most recent federal regulatory action in the community benefit arena came in March 2001 with the issuance of an IRS Field Service Advice Memorandum.[31] The advisory reviews case law in the period since IRS Revenue Ruling 69-545 and offers two significant conclusions. First, it indicates that charity care is an important part of a hospital's community benefit contributions, beyond simply the operation of an emergency room. Second, it indicates that it is insufficient simply to state that hospitals have established policies that ensure access for the medically indigent; that a hospital "must show that it actually provided significant health services to the indigent."[32] This action provided validation of recent efforts by consumer advocates to increase the volume of charity care provided by nonprofit hospitals, particularly in states with high numbers of medically indigent.

The actions taken by legislators, regulators, and the courts over the course of the last half-century reflect a clear inclination to respond to changing societal imperatives and emerging trends in organizational behavior. The most significant societal imperative driving actions related to hos-

---

[31]IRS Field Advisory, Subject: Exempt Hospitals' Compliance with Treas. Reg. Section 1.501(c)(3)-1(c).
[32]Ibid.

pitals is the persistent and system-wide problem of access to care for the uninsured. This problem is exacerbated by growing fiscal constraints on safety net funding in the public sector, downward pressures on reimbursement among health-care providers in the private sector, and rapid increases in the cost of care.

At different points in time, promising efforts to improve access for the medically indigent have led to an emphasis on a broader role for hospitals to promote health in local communities. Rising costs have also led some hospitals to focus on strategies to address the causes of persistent health problems in an effort to reduce demand for high-cost medical care among medically indigent populations. While this reflects an appropriate interest in a more cost-effective and sustainable approach to health improvement, near-term pressure to increase the volume of charity care has made it difficult for hospitals to expand investment in this arena.

Two major trends in organizational behavior have served as drivers for regulatory activism: nonprofit hospital closures and/or conversions to investor-owned facilities, and periodic reports of institutional practices that are inconsistent with public expectations. With conversions, concerns about the loss of public assets, reduced access for the medically indigent, and a decline in support for community health initiatives have led some states (e.g., CA Assembly Bill 3101,[33] RI Hospital Conversion Act of 1997[34]) to pass conversion statutes that use community benefit principles to determine what responsibilities should be maintained by an investor-owned purchaser of a nonprofit provider or HMO. Similar concerns are raised in transactions among nonprofit hospitals. In one case, a proposed merger between two nonprofit hospitals in New Hampshire was challenged over concerns about the loss of essential services (New Hampshire Attorney General's Office, 1998). In Michigan, the FTC imposed a Consent Decree in 1996 as a condition for a merger of two nonprofit hospitals that limited price increases and established an annual minimum financial threshold for community benefit contributions.[35]

Examples of institutional practices that have provided the impetus for regulatory activism range from aggressive bill collections among medically indigent populations to the use of surplus revenues for purposes other than improving the quality of services and facilities. In most cases, however, the core issue is the net volume of quantifiable charitable contributions pro-

---

[33]CA Assembly Bill No. 3101, Chapter 1105, Section 5913, Division 2 of Title 1 of the Corporations Code, February 23, 1996.

[34]Hospital Conversions Act, Chapter 23-17.14, State of Rhode Island, March 12, 1997.

[35]*Federal Trade Commission v. Butterworth Health Corporation and Blodgett Memorial Medical Center*, Civil Action No. 1:96CV49, October 25, 1996.

vided by an organization. In a number of states, concerns about the behavior of one organization can provide the impetus for regulatory actions that impact the entire field. The community benefit statutes in Idaho, Texas, and Utah were all outgrowths of challenges to the tax-exemption of individual nonprofit providers.

The next section provides an overview of the implementation of public and private sector community benefit initiatives and explores the evolution nonprofit health care organization practices during the last decade.

EVOLUTION OF POLICIES AND PRACTICES

The implementation of state community benefit initiatives provides important lessons for the potential application of community benefit principles to institutions engaged in health professions education and training. Insights can also be gleaned from the implementation of private sector initiatives that have sought to enhance the community benefit practices of nonprofit hospitals. This section highlights key lessons from experience to date and explores the evolution in the practices of nonprofit health-care organizations during the last decade.

Implementation of State Initiatives

As indicated in the preceding section, states have taken two basic approaches in the design of community benefit initiatives: the establishment of a general reporting requirement that outlines steps to plan, implement, and document community benefit contributions; or the establishment of specific minimum financial thresholds. The following discussion will explore common and distinctive characteristics in the implementation of both approaches.

Perhaps the most common characteristic among all state initiatives is a failure to allocate sufficient resources to the state agency responsible for monitoring compliance. The net effect is that for states with general reporting requirements, initial concerns among nonprofit health-care providers about the quality and veracity of documentation are gradually eroded by knowledge that reports are filed with minimal review. Moreover, any effort to conduct a systematic review is confounded by a lack of uniformity in documentation. A review of reports from multiple states confirms that there is profound variation in the quality and specificity of reporting. This variation makes it impossible to conduct a comparative analysis of performance. The only alternative would be a detailed audit of individual reports, an approach that would be highly resource-intensive and infeasible, given the paucity of resources.

Some state agencies have managed to secure additional resources on a temporary basis to enhance monitoring capability and to facilitate increased awareness among nonprofit health-care providers. California's Office of Statewide Health Planning and Development (OSHPD) conducted a series of workshops and site visits in the first few years following the passage of Senate Bill 697 and produced a report that summarized findings from a general review of reports.[36] A state advisory committee was also formed to support the implementation of the statute. The state legislature provided a small pool of funds in 1999 to support the enhancement of OSHPD's monitoring capacity but withdrew those funds the following year as part of a general cost-saving measure in state government. In a recent survey of nonprofit hospital community benefit practices in California, respondents identified a lack of clarity in the current legislation on the reporting process as a significant challenge (Barnett, 2002). To date, OSHPD staff are limited in their ability to provide specific guidance beyond the current language in the statute, since the law prohibits the promulgation of specific standards without direct action by the California legislature.[37]

In Massachusetts, the Office of the Attorney General recently completed a multiyear process to develop uniform reporting guidelines and establish a searchable website for posting of community benefit reports. This was made possible by a combination of proceeds from class action insurance settlements and private foundation support.[38] While the guidelines lack the specificity needed for a reliable comparative analysis of performance in quantitative terms, the searchable function provides a rich opportunity for qualitative analysis. As public competence in the use of Internet technology increases, access to detailed information by a full spectrum of stakeholders offers significant potential to increase local accountability.

In New Hampshire, the enactment of SB 69 in January 2000 was accompanied by the parallel funding of a statewide health planning process by the state legislature.[39] The health planning process focused primarily on the assessment of health-care needs and the development of strategies to increase access to health care, but it also included funding for a series of

---

[36]"Not-for-Profit Hospital Community Benefit Legislation (SB 697) Report to the Legislature," January 1998, Office of Statewide Health Planning and Development, California Health and Welfare Agency.

[37]SB 697, section 449.30 states that "nothing in this part shall be construed to authorize or require specific formats for hospital needs assessments, community benefit plans, or reports until recommendations pursuant to Section 449.35 (requiring a report from OSHPD to the Legislature by October 1, 1997) are considered and enacted by the Legislature."

[38]A grant from the W.K. Kellogg Foundation.

[39]New Hampshire State Health Plan, a series of reports on the health care environment in NH, implemented by the Office of Planning and Research, New Hampshire Department of Health and Human Services.

workshops to increase understanding of community benefit requirements associated with New Hampshire's statute. In addition, the state Department of Health and Human Services and the Office of the New Hampshire Attorney General secured funding from a private foundation[40] to conduct an evaluation of first-year report filings and to hold a state conference to highlight exemplary practices. Findings from the evaluation are consistent with experience in other states; there are numerous examples of promising programs, but substantial variability in the quality and specificity of reporting make it impossible to conduct a reliable comparative analysis of performance. As is the case with California's community benefit statute, further action is required by the state legislature in order to promulgate uniform guidelines for reporting.[41]

In states with minimum financial thresholds (PA, TX, UT), monitoring is a less challenging prospect, but experience to date suggests that compliance with requirements has not yielded the intended outcome, that is, improved access for medically indigent populations. Two predictable trends have emerged. First, hospitals have devoted increased attention to the development of sophisticated accounting methods to maximize the compilation of contributions. Second, there has been a de-emphasis on more proactive approaches to address persistent health problems in partnership with local community stakeholders. The first trend presents a challenge for state agencies in determining whether specific elements of reported contributions are consistent with the letter and intent of the statute. The second trend raises concerns that community hospitals may be moving toward a more inward focus, limiting the allocation of charitable resources to the provision of costly emergency and inpatient care for what are often preventable illnesses among the medically indigent populations.

Until recently, the implementation of community benefit statutes at the state level has been a relatively benign process with submissions of annual reports and a cursory review by state monitoring agencies. Federal funding of state programs to increase coverage for children and families in the 1990s produced measurable gains[42] and may have reduced pressure for

---

[40]Grant from the NH Endowment for Health to the Community Health Institute, in partnership with the Office of Planning and Research, NH Department of Health and Human Services to conduct a statewide study of community benefit reports submitted in compliance with Senate Bill 69.

[41]Section 312:3 of Senate Bill 69 indicates that "the provisions of this act shall be subject to further legislative review and amendment based upon the results of the statewide health planning process to be implemented during the fiscal year ending June 30, 2000 and the initial reports by the health care charitable trusts in compliance with this act."

[42]Title XXI of the Social Security Act, the State Children's Health Insurance Program (SCHIP), Centers for Medicare and Medicaid Services (CMS).

further action in the state policy arena. In the last three years, however, rising costs, job losses, and the general economic downturn have contributed to a steady increase in the number of uninsured and underinsured people. Attention is once again turning to nonprofit hospitals as a resource to fill the growing gaps in the social safety net. Consumer advocates are applying pressure on state policy makers to act, and some have acquired new tools to conduct independent analyses of nonprofit hospital charitable contributions and overall expenditures.

Given the current fiscal crisis in many states, passage of a community benefit statute with minimum financial thresholds may be viewed by some policy makers as a low-risk alternative to taking on the problem of access to health care in a more systematic manner. A coalition of consumer advocates and organized labor groups recently collaborated with policy makers in California to propose minimum financial thresholds of charity care for nonprofit hospitals. While the initial effort was unsuccessful, a similar proposal is expected in the next legislative session.

There is also evidence that state legislators may be moving in the direction of prescribing the specific content focus of charitable contributions. A bill passed in New Hampshire in 2002 established a study committee that explores strategies to increase the number of physician residents in medically underserved areas (MUAs) in the northern part of the state and includes the consideration of securing funding from health-care charitable trusts as a component of their community benefit responsibility.[43] Continued fiscal pressure and growing numbers of medically indigent persons suggest that other states will consider more prescriptive approaches to community benefit in the foreseeable future.

Private Sector Initiatives

Two national demonstrations funded by the W.K. Kellogg Foundation in the last 15 years focused on increasing the accountability of nonprofit hospitals and encouraging the engagement of community stakeholders to address local unmet health needs. The Hospital Community Benefit Standards Program (HCBSP) ran from 1989 to 1992 and was administered by the Robert F. Wagner Graduate School of Public Services at New York University. The primary goal of the initiative was to recognize hospitals committed to improve community health, and to support the enhancement of their efforts. Forty-nine hospitals were selected from a pool of 331

---

[43]House Bill 1131, (Chapter 37:2, Laws of 2002), increasing the number of physicians who are New Hampshire residents and making a technical change Study Committee.

190   IN THE NATION'S COMPELLING INTEREST

applicants. Participants were challenged to meet a set of specific standards
that demonstrated their commitment to play an ongoing role in addressing
health problems in local communities and participated in a survey at the
end of the demonstration to assess their performance.

The second national demonstration was the Community Care Network
Demonstration (CCN), which ran from 1996 to 2000, and was administered by the Health Research and Educational Trust of the American Hospital Association. Twenty-five local partnerships of hospitals and local community partners were selected from a pool of over 300 applicants to develop
and implement a series of community projects and institutional reforms.
Both HCBSP and CCN provided valuable insights into alternative approaches to address persistent health problems in local communities. They
also provided insights into the challenges associated with aligning institutional governance, management, and operations to ensure long-term commitment and to facilitate the optimal use of charitable resources. The Catholic Health Association of the United States (CHA) and VHA (formerly
Voluntary Hospitals of America) have provided ongoing leadership by
authoring publications and sponsoring conferences and workshops over the
last two decades. Among the most notable publications was the Social
Accountability Budget (SAB) (Trocchio et al., 1989), a comprehensive
manual for planning and implementing community benefit programs activities in local communities. CHA and VHA collaborated to develop an elec-
tronic software package[44] based on SAB for the documentation of program
activities that is currently used by over 800 hospitals nationwide.

A study published by the Public Health Institute in 1997 outlined a
strategy for planning, implementing, and evaluating community benefit
program activities and offered a conceptual framework for community
benefit that provides insights into public expectations associated with the
exemption of local, state, and federal taxes for nonprofit institutions
(Barnett, 1997). The Public Trust Model outlines six public expectations
associated with tax exemption, including:

1. **Redistributive intent**—nonprofit health-care organizations are exempted from tax liabilities with the expectation that they will focus a
substantial portion of their charitable contributions in proximal communities where there is a disproportionate volume of unmet health-related needs.

2. **Assumption of Special Skills**—nonprofit health-care organizations
are expected to bring special skills and capacity to address health-related
problems in their immediate geographic locale.

---

[44]Lyon Software, Lyon and Associates, Sylvania, OH.

3. **Protection from Political Influence**—exemption from taxation reflects a desire to shield those revenues from the exigencies of the political process and ensure that they are carefully allocated to address unmet health needs.

4. **Collaborative governance**—decision making regarding the use of charitable resources should reflect the scope of interests, knowledge, and priorities of local communities.

5. **Cost-effectiveness**—the loss of tax revenues associated with exemption should be substantially offset by surplus value generated by private sector fulfillment of a public responsibility.

6. **Pluralism**—tax exemption encourages a more pluralistic expression of charity than would be accomplished by an expansion of the public sector.

A study by Schlesinger and colleagues (1998) offers a typology of community benefit that applies more broadly to all types of health-care institutions (including health plans) and highlights four different, but overlapping, perspectives that inform the debate regarding the roles and obligations of nonprofit health-care institutions. The *Legal/Historical* perspective focuses on the historical responsibilities of nonprofit hospitals, which provides the basis for current law (with exceptions cited previously in UT, NH, and MA). The *Market-Failures* perspective focuses on the costs and benefits of medical care experienced by communities and society at large. The *Community Health* perspective focuses on strategies to develop evidence-based linkages between medical services and efforts to address the causes of health problems. The *Healthy Community* perspective focuses on strategies to strengthen the social institutions that influence health and quality of life in local communities.

The Legal/Historical perspective draws it strength from the public expectations as outlined in the Public Trust Model and is reinforced by observations associated with the Market-Failures perspective (i.e., that market failures in American health-care financing result in negative externalities). While these expectations and the negative externalities associated with a market-based system of health-care financing have been applied primarily to nonprofit hospitals, there is at least the basis in principle for a broader application of similar societal expectations to other institutions that receive any form of public funding.

The Community Health perspective draws its strength from the proposition that the demand for high-cost medical care can be substantially reduced by targeted provision of preventive services and the promotion of health in local communities. For nonprofit hospitals, this approach often represents an effort to reduce hospitalizations and emergency room utilization for preventable illnesses.

Finally, the Healthy Communities perspective envisions diverse stake-holders (including nonprofit, public, and investor-owned organizations) as ongoing partners in efforts to create a local environment that will support and sustain optimal health and quality of life. Healthy Communities is an outgrowth of the Healthy Cities concept developed by Hancock and Duhl (1988) and has been implemented in cities throughout the world by the World Health Organization since 1988. This perspective significantly broadens the scope of contributions that may be viewed as community benefits to encompass activities such as economic development, neighborhood revitalization, and building social capital. While nonprofit institutions may be viewed as having special responsibilities, accountability for improved health and quality of life is shared among all local stakeholders.

As noted previously, there have been a variety of studies examining the community benefit obligations of nonprofit hospitals, ranging from quantitative comparisons of the volume of charity medical care provided by nonprofit and investor-owned hospitals (Kane, 1994; Sofaer et al., 1990; Herzlinger and Krasker, 1987; Norton and Staiger, 1994; Pattison and Katz, 1990; Nicholson et al., 2000) to more qualitative analyses of exemplary practices (Schlesinger et al., 1996; Shortell et al., 1995; Rundall, 1994). In the aggregate, these studies highlight the fact that there is significant variation in the charitable behavior of nonprofit hospitals that is driven by a range of factors, including, but not limited, to the following:

- Local demographics and level and form of health-care coverage
- Level of competition with other providers
- Local/regional market penetration
- Availability of public sector safety net services
- Reimbursement rates from public and private sector payers
- Links, leverage, and support from other facilities
- Brand-name status
- Endowments

These and other factors play a major role in determining the relative ability of nonprofit hospitals to generate surplus revenues that can be directed toward charitable purposes. For this reason, it is difficult, if not inappropriate, to judge the charitable intent of nonprofit hospitals (and other institutions that receive public funding) based upon a single standard such as the volume of free medical care provided to medically indigent populations. This understanding is crucial in the evolution of state community benefit statutes that permit the documentation of a broad spectrum of activities viewed as addressing priority concerns in local communities, as well as societal imperatives.

Organizational Practices

As noted previously, the charitable behavior of nonprofit health-care institutions is significantly influenced by historical and situational factors at the local level, as well as by major trends at the societal level (e.g., number of uninsured people, changes in reimbursement structures), and actions in the regulatory arena. While variations in both requirements and documentation have made it impossible to evaluate the impact of state community benefit statutes in any systematic manner, observation suggests the emergence of some common strengths and areas for improvement in organizational practices.

Strengths

In the eight states that require nonprofit hospitals to conduct periodic needs assessments, anecdotal information suggests that hospitals and local partners acquire increased knowledge of the scope of local unmet needs and an increased understanding of linkages between health problems and a range of causal factors. This knowledge provides the basis for the design of more comprehensive approaches to health improvement that may yield sustainable impacts in the aggregate. Anecdotal information also suggests that there has been an increase in the engagement of diverse community stakeholders, in the best situations resulting in the leveraging of scarce local resources. A recent study of hospital community benefit practices in California (Rundall, 1994) identified four common elements among exemplary programs:

- Clear targeting of community benefit activities to serve communities with disproportionate unmet health-related needs
- Meaningful engagement of diverse community stakeholders
- Strategic allocation of charitable resources to build on existing community assets
- Alignment of organizational governance, management, and operational functions with the charitable mission of the organization

In the best cases, nonprofit hospitals have increased the diversity of their governance structures to reflect more clearly the diversity of local communities, established interdepartmental performance measures to increase the accountability of leadership and staff, hired dedicated staff with appropriate competencies to support an ongoing process of quality improvement, and shielded community benefit decision-making processes from marketing and business development imperatives.

Areas for Improvement

There are a plethora of examples across the nation where nonprofit hospitals have demonstrated a strong commitment to fulfill their charitable obligations. At the same time, there are a number of areas where greater attention and improvement are needed. Many nonprofit hospitals lack the internal infrastructure and competencies to design, implement, and monitor community benefit activities. Unfortunately, increasing financial pressures have led many hospitals to reduce dedicated staff support, undermining their ability to produce high-quality results. In addition, community benefit management in many hospitals is an isolated and marginal functional unit, lacking connections to senior leadership and/or organizational strategic planning processes. In this situation, staff turnover is high, program quality is compromised, and measurable impacts are absent.

The ability to demonstrate value and accountability in local communities is impeded by a lack of data at the subcounty level. Many hospitals are faced with the option of allocating substantial charitable resources to collect primary data in local communities or limiting their monitoring process to documenting the volume of inputs. Increased engagement of local public health agencies, colleges and universities, and other local stakeholders with special competencies is needed.

In summary, the charitable behavior of the best organizations provides valuable insights into potential contributions and roles that nonprofit hospitals, as well as other institutions, can play to address unmet needs at the local and societal level. Increasing public understanding of these potential benefits, roles, and expectations may yield substantial impact upon charitable practices and organizational behavior in general.

RELEVANCE TO HEALTH DISPARITIES AND HEALTH WORKFORCE DIVERSITY

Are there applicable laws or regulations—based on community benefit principles—that could function as "carrots" or "sticks" to better ensure that organizations such as teaching hospitals and colleges and universities would feel more obligated to advance key public policy goals tied to workforce diversity? More particularly, because the origins of the community benefit principles flow from the arena of income tax exemption, it is logical to first ask: Is there a legal obligation tied to the grant of tax-exempt status that obligates nonprofit hospitals, colleges, and universities to advance workforce diversity goals? The simple answer is probably not. Nevertheless, it is worthwhile to explore this question further and see where the legal precedents have taken us to date.

Applicability to Nonprofit Hospitals

In the hospital context, as noted previously, there is certainly a rich history supporting the notion that nonprofit hospitals are expected to meet community benefit standards as a quid pro quo for tax exemption. It is notable that teaching hospitals (hospitals that are centers of learning for physicians, nurses, and other allied health professionals) are expected to meet the same operational standard for tax exemption as those that are only involved in patient care. With the focus of this report on issues related to workforce diversity, an interesting issue arises regarding whether or not the formal educational activities of a teaching hospital are subject to scrutiny under a set of community benefit principles.

A review of Revenue Rulings 69-545 and 83-157 indicates no references to the educational mission or function of hospitals; their focus is on the operational characteristics of hospitals tied to patient care.[45] Certainly, under the Internal Revenue Code, hospitals could not remain tax exempt while practicing overt racial discrimination tied to patient care or employment.[46] However, absent such overt discrimination, even in the patient care context, there do not appear to be affirmative expectations that hospitals make their patient care environments more welcoming to persons of color in order to remain tax exempt. Even in the face of growing concern over health disparities confronting our nation, or in dealing with the reality of a more diverse patient populations, to date there has not been any hint that the grant of tax exemption will be tied to hospital efforts to address language barriers for non-English speaking patients,[47] provide needed cultural competency training of staff, and/or recruit and retain a more diverse cadre of provider staff. While these efforts individually or collectively may be part of a hospital's community benefits plan, from the operative Revenue Rulings as well as the limited case law in this area, it appears that no one factor is determinative of a hospital's eligibility for tax exemption.[48]

If one wanted to find an opportunity to push the limits of the community benefit standard as applied to hospitals, one possibility would be to build on the initial step taken by the IRS in its 2001 IRS Field Service

---

[45]Revenue Ruling 69-545, 1969 –2 C.B. 117 and Revenue Ruling 83-157, 1983 2- C.B. 94.

[46]*Bob Jones v. United States*, 461 U.S. 474 (1983).

[47]There has been a growing legal effort tied to care of patients who are not English-language-proficient. On August 11, 2000, President Clinton issued Executive Order (EO) 13166, entitled *Improving Access to Services for Persons with Limited English Proficiency*, 65 Fed. Reg. 50121 (Aug. 16, 2000). It requires all organizations that receive federal assistance, such as Medicare or Medicaid, to provide translation services for their non-English-speaking patients.

[48]See for example, *Redlands Surgical Services v. Commissioner*, 113 T.C. 47, 73 (1999), appeal docketed, No. 99-71253 (9th Cir., Sept. 17, 1999).

Advisory Memorandum #200110030 (referenced previously) which arguably represents a first tentative step in the direction of revisiting the specificity of what hospitals must do to meet the expectations of the community benefit standard. While the IRS memorandum seems to do that with respect to charity care and related policies, it also suggests that the IRS could further try to add some specificity to a hospital's "promotion of health" obligations by requiring it to address issues such as workforce diversity and racial and/or ethnic health disparities as a key factor to maintain tax-exempt status. Establishing such explicit requirements, however, would represent a radical departure from the historical practices of the IRS in this arena.

Applicability to Colleges and Universities

Colleges and universities derive their tax-exempt status by qualifying under the category of "educational" as delineated in Section 501(c)(3) of the Internal Revenue Code. While the IRS has never established a general community benefit requirement tied to the operational test for qualifying educational organizations in determining eligibility for tax-exempt status, the ruling of the U.S. Supreme Court in its 1983 decision, *Bob Jones*,[49] adopted a "public policy" test that applies to all 501(c)(3) organizations, including those that qualify under the category of "educational."

Tying this to the health professions workforce diversity issue, it is possible to argue that if such diversity goals are found to be part of established public policy, then the failure of colleges and universities to make sufficient efforts in this regard through their admissions, retention, and related policies should jeopardize their tax-exempt status for being in violation of established "national public policy." Admittedly, reading the Supreme Court's decision in this way might be considered a significant reach from the original decision. As the Court itself noted in the decision, ". . . a declaration that a given institution is not 'charitable' should be made only where there can be no doubt that the activity involved is contrary to fundamental public policy."

Accordingly, the question here centers on the issue of whether the overt failure of health professional schools in recent decades to enroll and graduate sufficient numbers of underrepresented minorities (URMs) represents an action (or omission) that is contrary to established or fundamental public policy. If so, then *Bob Jones* tells us that such organizations may be in jeopardy of losing their tax-exempt status and hence, more likely to be actually engaged in efforts to address health-care workforce diversity issues.

---

[49]*Bob Jones v. United States*, 461 U.S. 474 (1983).

Another application of community benefit principles to colleges and universities, beyond the tax exemption context for nonprofits, is the issue of what expectations should be placed on governmentally sponsored institutions. These institutions receive the bulk of their revenues from state appropriations (U.S. Department of Education, 2002). Health professionals training schools based at these public institutions often receive significant appropriations from state governments. It would certainly seem to make sense to ask if these public institutions of higher education are meeting their "community benefit" expectations in advancing societal goals tied to health-care workforce diversity. Such an expectation surely could be part of a state legislature's quid pro quo for sending over significant taxpayer dollars to these public institutions.

PUBLIC POLICY OPTIONS: PRECEDENTS, OPPORTUNITIES, AND PITFALLS

From a public policy perspective, it is clear that health professionals training schools and hospital based training programs have made only limited progress in advancing workforce racial and ethnic diversity goals in the United States. Though community benefit principles offer an attractive framework for holding health professionals training programs and their institutional sponsors accountable for advancing goals tied to racial and ethnic diversity of their students and trainees, from a legal perspective, it is important that the principles be applied in the most effective venue. In that regard, while community benefit laws and associated public expectations have evolved out of a tax exemption context, it is reasonable to suggest that the most practical application of concepts for increased institutional accountability are outside of the tax exemption arena. Specifically, they are best applied in the accreditation world affecting health professionals training programs. Furthermore, for publicly sponsored colleges and universities, community benefit concepts might also be part of a scheme that in some way ties governmental subsidies for these public institutions of higher education to performance measures related to student and trainee diversity goals. These concepts apply for a number of reasons:

1. Legally, based on the relevant IRS Revenue Rulings, there is no current tax exempt status requirement that would necessitate either charitable teaching hospitals or private, nonprofit colleges and universities to make affirmative workforce diversity efforts in order to maintain tax-exempt status. It would likely be too much of a stretch for the IRS (even if motivated to do so) to make such a regulatory change absent new Congressional legislation that modifies the language of 501(c)(3) of the IR Code. This is especially true with respect to colleges and universities, which, at present, have only the *Bob Jones* "public policy" test (as described above)

for their community benefit expectations attendant to their tax-exempt status.

2. Tax exemption is only a factor of importance to nonprofit organizations. For public teaching hospitals, colleges, and universities, a community benefit standard aimed at advancing racial and ethnic diversity tied to tax exemption would have no impact on such governmental organizations, as they derive their exempt status as being units of government. In fact, reliance upon tax exemption as a framework for accountability could have the consequence of placing more legal expectations for advancing diversity goals on private, nonprofit institutions than on institutions that receive direct governmental subsidies as public entities.

3. If tied to tax exemption, the failure of a program to advance diversity goals would lead to the entire organization losing its tax-exempt status. How should one handle a university where diversity goals were being achieved in a variety of schools but failed in the ones that are part of health professionals training? Under the tax code, while there are intermediate sanctions for certain prohibited transactions, failure to meet the overall operational test for community benefit would result in revocation of the entire organization's tax-exempt status.

4. Accreditation is an oversight scheme that is attendant to all of the education programs that educate independently licensed health professionals. For some health professions (physician training, for example), there are distinct educational programs for different stages of professional training, each with its own separate accreditation program under a distinct sponsorship. Given the breadth and reach of the various accreditation programs and their ability to independently set standards based on high professional norms, it is a logical place to enforce a set of expectations tied to advancing diversity goals. In addition, the accreditation process often allows institutional individuality in how standards are met, thus encouraging creative approaches to meeting the underlying goals of the accreditation process. Such flexibility has some important advantages when approaching issues like racial and ethnic diversity.

5. While the issues are complex, it is the case that health professions schools and hospitals of all forms (i.e., nonprofit, investor-owned, and public) receive varying amounts of public resources, whether through tax deferrals, public third-party payments, or direct subsidies. This is especially true in health professions education, which is quite expensive and heavily subsidized for participating students and trainees (Chhabra, 1996). As discussed in Chapter 3, Medicare Graduate Medical Education (GME) provides a significant source of funding for the costs of educating health professionals, particularly physicians. Indirect funding, covering additional teaching costs associated with caring for Medicare patients, is also provided to academic health centers. In 1998, Medicare paid approximately $2 bil-

lion in direct payments and approximately $5 billion in indirect payments (COGME, 2000). In 2000, $260 million were provided for nursing and allied health programs (Medicare Payment Advisory Commission, 2001 as cited in IOM, 2003). In addition to Medicare funding, support for training is provided by the Health Resources and Services Administration (HRSA) and the National Institutes of Health (NIH). In 2002, approximately $400 million was provided by HRSA and about $650 million was provided by NIH to individuals (IOM, 2003; NIH, 2003). These public resources should come with an expectation that the institutions are responsible to societal imperatives. Community benefit offers insights into how these responsibilities can be framed and the scope of potential contributions. State legislatures or other bodies granting state taxpayer monies to these schools of higher learning rarely set policy quid pro quos related to the mission and activities of these higher education programs. There is certainly an opportunity for state government officials to be more explicit about their goals and expectations for higher education in the diversity arena. Such a mandate has periodically led to some focused and successful programs over the years. A very good example is the University of Illinois College of Medicine (Girotti, 1999).

SUMMARY AND RECOMMENDATIONS

This chapter of the report seeks to educate the public on an issue that has received limited attention outside of the nonprofit health-care arena. In the most basic sense, community benefit principles provide insights for the public expectations of both nonprofit health-care providers and institutions that train these providers. Just as nonprofit hospitals are expected to play a role in addressing priority unmet needs in local communities, health professions schools can appropriately be expected to play a direct role in responding to priority unmet health needs at the local and/or societal level. Specifically, we suggest that community benefit principles form a conceptual cornerstone by which accreditation organizations for health professional training programs and state governments can set expectations for the advancement of societal goals tied to racial and ethnic diversity of the health-care workforce. The historical and legal antecedents outlined in the first section of this chapter validate the concept of a social contract. Moreover, they demonstrate that changes in social priorities justify periodic adjustments in public expectations and requirements. The Supreme Court in its recent decision in *Grutter v. Bollinger et al.*[50] sent the message that, if

---

[50]*Barbara Grutter, Petitioner v. Lee Bollinger et al.*, no 02-241, (June 23, 2003).

accomplished without fixed numerical quotas, such affirmative diversity efforts are permissible under the U.S. Constitution. We think that it is time for those entities that maintain significant leverage over health professionals schools and training programs to exercise those incentives.

The committee offers three core recommendations to encourage definitive action by academic medical centers and health professions education institutions in support of the societal imperative to increase the diversity of the health-care workforce. They include:

> **Recommendation 6-1:** HPEI governing bodies should develop institutional objectives consistent with community benefit principles that support the goal of increasing health-care workforce diversity including, but not limited to (1) ease financial and non-financial obstacles to URM participation (redistributive intent), (2) increase involvement of diverse local stakeholders in key decision-making processes (collaborative governance), and (3) undertake initiatives that are responsive to local, regional, and societal imperatives (response to local needs) (see Recommendation 5-4).

> **Recommendation 6-2:** Health professions accreditation institutions should explore the development of new standards that acknowledge and reinforce efforts by HPEIs to implement community benefit principles as they relate to increasing health-care workforce diversity.

> **Recommendation 6-3:** HPEIs should develop a mechanism to inform the public of progress toward and outcomes of efforts to provide equal health care to minorities, reduce health disparities, and increase the diversity of the health-care workforce.

> **Recommendation 6-4:** Private and public entities (e.g., federal, state, and local governments) should convene major community benefit stakeholders (e.g., community advocates, academic institutions, health-care providers), to inform them about community benefit standards and to build awareness that placing a priority on diversity and cultural competency programs is a societal expectation of all institutions that receive any form of public funding.

REFERENCES

Barnett K. 1997. *The Future of Community Benefit: An Expanded Model for Planning and Assessing the Participation of Health Care Organizations in Community Health Improvement Activities*. Berkeley, CA: Public Health Institute and the Western Consortium for Public Health. Published jointly with the AHA/HRET.

Barnett K. 2002. *The Status of Community Benefit in California: A Statewide Review of Exemplary Practices and Key Challenges.* Commissioned by The California Endowment. Berkeley, CA: Public Health Institute.

Chhabra A. 1996. Medical school tuition and the cost of medical education. *Journal of the American Medical Association* 275(17):1372–1373.

Council on Graduate Medical Education (COGME). 2000. *Fifteenth Report: Financing Graduate Medical Education in a Changing Health Care Environment.* [Online]. Available: http://www.cogme.gov/15.pdf [accessed October 10, 2003].

Fox DM, Schaffer DC. 1991. Tax administration as health policy: Hospitals, the Internal Revenue Service, and the courts. *Journal of Health Politics, Policy, and Law* 16(2):251–279.

Girotti JA. 1999. The Urban Health Program to encourage minority enrollment at the University of Illinois at Chicago College of Medicine. *Academic Medicine* 74(4):370–372.

Hancock T, Duhl L. 1988. Promoting health in the urban context. *WHO Healthy Cities Papers Series* 1:24.

Hansmann H. 1989. The evolving law of nonprofit organizations: Do current trends make good policy? *Case Western Reserve Law Review* 39:807–827.

Harshbarger LS, Massachusetts Attorney General's Office. 1994. *Community Benefits Guidelines for Nonprofit Acute Care Hospitals.* Boston: Attorney General Commonwealth of Massachusetts.

Harshbarger LS, Massachusetts Attorney General's Office. 1996. *Community Benefits Guidelines for Health Maintenance Organizations.* Boston: Attorney General Commonwealth of Massachusetts.

Harshbarger LS, Massachusetts Attorney General's Office. 1998. *The Attorney General's Report on Community Benefits by Health Maintenance Organizations* (excerpt from paragraph one of cover letter). Boston: Attorney General Commonwealth of Massachusetts.

Herzlinger RE, Krasker WS. 1987. Who profits from non-profits? *Harvard Business Review* 65(1):93–106.

Institute of Medicine (IOM). 2004. *Academic Health Centers: Leading Change in the 21st Century.* Washington, DC: The National Academies Press.

Kane NM. 1994. *Nonprofit Hospital Status: What Is It Worth?* Boston: Harvard School of Public Health.

National Institutes of Health (NIH). 2003. *NIH Awards by Fiscal Year and Mechanism.* [Online]. Available: http://grants1.nih.gov/grants/award/trends/budg9202.htm [accessed October 10, 2003].

New Hampshire Attorney General's Office. 1998. *New Hampshire Attorney General's Report on Optima Health.* March 10, Concord: Office of the Attorney General.

Nicholson S, Pauly MV, Burns LR, Baumritter A, Asch DA. 2000. Measuring community benefits provided by for-profit and nonprofit hospitals. *Health Affairs* 19(6):168–177.

Norton EC, Staiger DO. 1994. How hospital ownership affects access to care for the uninsured. *Rand Journal of Economics* 25(1):171–185.

Pattison RV, Katz HM. 1990. Investor-owned and not-for-profit hospitals: A comparison based upon California hospitals. *New England Journal of Medicine* 309:347–353.

Rundall TG. 1994. The integration of public health medicine. *Frontiers of Health Service Management* 10(4):3–24.

Schlesinger M, Gray B, Bradley E. 1996. Charity and community: The role of nonprofit ownership in a managed health care system. *Journal of Health Politics, Policy and Law* 21(4):697–752.

Schlesinger M, Bradford G, Carrino G, Duncan M, Gusmano M, Antonelli V, Stuber J. 1998. A broader vision for managed care. 2. A typology of community benefits. *Health Affairs* 17(5):26–49.

Shortell SM, Gillies RR, Devers KJ. 1995. Reinventing the American hospital. *Milbank Quarterly* 73(2):131–160.

Sofaer S, Rundall TG, Zellers WL. 1990. Restrictive reimbursement policies and uncompensated care in California hospitals, 1981–1986. *Hospital and Health Services Administration* 35:189–206.

Stevens R. 1982. A poor sort of memory: Voluntary hospitals and government before the depression. *Millbank Memorial Fund Quarterly/Health and Society* 60(4):551–586.

Trocchio J, Eckels T, Hearle K. 1989. *Social Accountability Budget for Not-for-Profit Healthcare Organizations*. St. Louis: The Catholic Health Association of the United States; Washington, DC: Lewin/ICF.

U.S. Department of Education, National Center for Education Statistics. 2002. *Digest of Education Statistics, 2001*. Washington, DC: U.S. Department of Education. Pp. 390–392.

7

Mechanisms to Garner Support for Institutional and Policy-Level Diversity Initiatives

The committee's analysis in the preceding chapters of this report documents that several barriers exist at the institutional (e.g., health professions educational institutions [HPEIs]) and policy level (e.g., federal and state policies and resources regarding financing of health professions education) that may contribute to the underrepresentation of many racial and ethnic minority groups in health professions careers. These barriers are largely unintentional policies, practices, and attitudes that have been understudied in relation to the problem of increasing the supply of well-prepared underrepresented minority (URM) students who are highly motivated to enter heath professions careers. Greater study of and attention to these barriers may therefore assist efforts to create greater opportunities for URM students to participate in health professions training and enter health professions careers. Institutional and policy-level barriers include:

- Among health professions educators, governance bodies, administrators, students, and the general public, a lack of understanding of and commitment to the important role of diversity in strengthening the health professions workforce and in improving the educational experiences and training of *all* health professions students;
- The lack, in many HPEIs, of statements in the institutional mission addressing the role of diversity in the institutional mission and its educational goals;
- Admissions policies and practices that disproportionately emphasize applicants' quantitative data, such as performance on standardized tests,

and fail to place appropriate emphasis on qualitative attributes of applicants that may more accurately predict success in health professions careers (e.g., empathy, leadership, commitment to service, cross-cultural experience, linguistic ability, and interpersonal skills);

• The absence, in many HPEIs, of appropriate training for admissions committee members regarding diversity issues, of inclusion of representatives of relevant stakeholder groups that are affected by admissions decisions on admissions committees, and of rewards and incentives for faculty for committee service and other efforts to enhance diversity in the institution;

• Unmet financial need that may disproportionately limit URM participation in health professions education programs and inconsistent federal and state support for health professions education programs that encourage minority participation in health professions careers and provide services to medically underserved communities;

• The failure of some health professions accreditation bodies to establish, monitor, and enforce strong diversity-related program standards, and the failure of the U.S. Department of Education to encourage the development of such standards;

• The failure of HPEIs to recognize the need to develop and regularly evaluate comprehensive strategies to improve the institutional climate for diversity; and

• The lack of information for key constituency groups—such as health-care consumer groups, leaders of communities served by academic health centers, and others—regarding diversity among the health professionals that serve them and the potential benefits of diversity for health-care consumers.

These institutional and policy-level barriers to greater URM participation in health professions can be reduced through a series of interventions aimed at a range of stakeholders. Health professions education leaders, their institutions, and the organizations that govern their operation (e.g., governance bodies, accrediting organizations) figure prominently in this effort. The hallmark of any profession is the obligation to set standards to serve the needs of the public. Accordingly, these groups must provide leadership by educating their constituencies about the benefits of diversity and establishing policies and standards that promote greater diversity among health professionals. These efforts should be directed toward HPEIs; their students, faculty, and others involved in health professions education; health professions education accrediting organizations; public and private sources of financial aid for health professions students; and all institutions that directly or indirectly serve the public and are accountable for the use of public resources to improve the public's health.

Mechanisms to Encourage Support for Diversity Initiatives

Through the recommendations that it has generated, the study committee has identified several mechanisms to encourage the development and implementation of institutional and policy-level strategies. These mechanisms include major "fulcrum" points, such as program accreditation and sources of student financial aid, that offer incentives, as well as reprimands, to encourage diversity efforts. For example, accreditation bodies can encourage member institutions to address diversity issues in student and faculty recruitment, curriculum, and training arrangements. And federal and state health agencies must evaluate and provide greater support for programs found to be effective in increasing URM participation in health careers, and innovative partnerships with private organizations that share workforce goals should be established.

Needed Data and Research Efforts

Implementation of these strategies should begin with efforts to collect data and conduct additional research to assess diversity among health professionals and in health professions education and to further identify the benefits of diversity for health-care service delivery. As noted earlier in this report, the availability of data regarding the representation of racial and ethnic minority groups in health professions varies considerably, as data on URM participation in medical education are generally more systematic and widely available than in other health professions disciplines. Data are needed to identify trends in the number of URM applicants to HPEIs; their rates of acceptance, matriculation, enrollment, and degree completion; the number of URM administrators, staff, and faculty in HPEIs, including full- and part-time faculty at all levels; and the participation of URM professionals in the health professions workforce. In addition, data are needed on the total cost of health professions education, including tuition, books and equipment, living expenses, average URM student educational debt (both prior to and after completion of training), the availability and receipt of both need- and merit-based student financial aid, and the impact of debt and financial aid on URM student participation in health professions training. Health professions institutions, as well as their governing bodies and professional associations, should increase efforts to collect and report such data to key stakeholders, including health policy makers, educators, health-care consumers, and the general public.

Similarly, additional research is needed to further assess and describe the benefits of diversity in health professions education and health-care delivery. As noted in Chapter 1, these benefits are considerable, with evidence to date demonstrating that diversity is associated with benefits for student learning, increasing access to care among minority and medically underserved populations, and improving patient choice and satisfaction, among other benefits. Additional research is needed to quantify the benefits of diversity in health-care delivery. Such research should assess, for example, whether there are economic benefits associated with greater diversity among health professionals. Evidence summarized in Chapter 1 suggests that diversity among health professionals—associated with improved access to and satisfaction with care among racial and ethnic minority patients—can lead to better patient understanding of and compliance with treatment regimens, higher rates of follow-up and adherence, and fewer patient misunderstandings of treatment recommendations, all of which may influence patients' health-care outcomes. The implications of this research are that better health-care outcomes among racial and ethnic minority patients—many of whom suffer from disproportionately high rates of illness, disability, and premature death—offer broad economic benefits for individuals, families, employers, and the nation as a whole, in the form of improved health status, fewer preventable illnesses, lower health-care costs, reduced workplace absenteeism, and greater productivity. These relationships should be assessed to contribute to the evidence base regarding the benefits of diversity among health professionals, and the results of such research should be widely communicated.

> Recommendation 7-1: Additional data collection and research are needed to more thoroughly characterize URM participation in the health professions and in health professions education and to further assess the benefits of diversity among health professionals, particularly with regard to the potential economic benefits of diversity.

Educational Strategies

Increasing support for diversity efforts also requires strategies to educate health professions leaders, faculty, administrators, students, and others in the HPEI community regarding the benefits of greater diversity among health professionals. HPEIs should proactively and regularly engage and train students, house staff, and faculty regarding institutional diversity-related policies and expectations and the importance and benefits of diversity to the long-term institutional mission. Similarly, health policy makers, health systems administrators, and health professionals should understand how diversity improves their ability to serve the community. To achieve this goal, HPEIs can benefit from model curricula for training, including course material, workshops, and other educational strategies. Professional associations can assist in the development and dissemination of model curricula components and can serve as clearinghouses for this information. The most powerful mechanism to encourage such educational efforts is program accreditation. HPEIs, academic health centers, and teaching hospitals should strive to meet high accreditation standards that articulate the value of diversity in the health professions and that require specific steps toward achieving diversity goals.

Educational strategies must not be limited to health professionals and health system administrators. Health-care consumers and the general public are among the most important stakeholders in the effort to increase diversity among health professionals. Public and private groups who share the goal of increasing diversity in health professions should engage in coordinated efforts to inform the public of the importance of diversity in health professions. These efforts should be directed to a range of individuals and groups that are affected by insufficient attention to diversity among health professionals, including grassroots advocacy and health-care consumer groups; businesses and corporations, particularly those that employ a racially and ethnically diverse workforce; educators, including primary and secondary school teachers and others involved in "pipeline" efforts; students; organized labor; elected officials at all levels of government; state and local health departments; religious groups, including churches, synagogues, temples, and others concerned with community health; health and education philanthropic organizations; as well as many other public and private groups. These educational strategies should emphasize the potential benefits of diversity for all Americans who are consumers of health care.

Several recent initiatives offer examples of innovative efforts to increase awareness of diversity issues and involve diverse, powerful constituents in the effort to increase diversity in health professions. The Sullivan Commission on Diversity in the Healthcare Workforce, funded by the W.K. Kellogg Foundation, has attempted to increase public awareness regarding the problem of insufficient health workforce diversity and generate broad support among the public and policy makers for diversity efforts. The commission, named for former U.S. Secretary of Health and Human Services Louis Sullivan, M.D., includes 15 health, business, and legal professionals and other leaders. Former U.S. Senate Majority Leader Robert Dole and former U.S. Representative and Congressional Health Subcommittee Chairman Paul Rogers are honorary co-chairs. The Sullivan Commission has held field hearings in six cities across the country, providing an opportunity for commissioners to gather data and hear testimony from health experts, community advocates, business leaders, local governmental officials, and consumers. In the process, the commission has increased public awareness of the problem of minority underrepresentation in health professions and of the need for broad and effective strategies to address the problem. A final report of the commission will be released in Spring 2004.

The Washington Business Group on Health (WBGH) has led efforts to increase business leaders' awareness of racial and ethnic disparities in health and access to health care and the implications of these disparities for employee productivity and well-being. WBGH is exploring ways in which businesses can become involved in solutions to improve the health and productivity of all its employees, serving as an information source to employers on health disparities and providing the tools and resources necessary to address the health needs of their diverse employees. For example, WBGH recently introduced a computer-based evaluation tool to assist health plan purchasers in assessing efforts by health plans to reduce racial and ethnic disparities in care, including tools to assess the diversity of health plan providers.

These local and national efforts share a common goal: to increase understanding of the imperative to enhance diversity among health professionals and to build consensus among a range of stakeholders regarding steps that should be taken toward this goal.

> **Recommendation 7-2: Local and national efforts must be undertaken— through community dialogues, forums, and other educational initiatives—to increase understanding of the imperative to enhance diversity among health professionals and to build consensus among a range of stakeholders regarding steps that should be taken to achieve this goal.**

Building Coalitions to Support Diversity Efforts

Educational efforts, as well as institutional and policy-level interventions to increase diversity, represent only the first steps toward action in support of institutional and policy-level strategies to increase diversity. Just as important are efforts to build coalitions of broad stakeholder groups— including, as identified above, health professions leaders, health-care consumer groups, grassroots and community organizations, business leaders, educators, and others—that can provide effective advocacy for change. Such coalition-building and advocacy can be viewed within the framework of community benefit principles discussed in the previous chapter. Community benefit principles provide insights for the public expectations of both nonprofit health-care providers and institutions that train these providers. Just as nonprofit hospitals are expected to play a role in addressing priority unmet needs in local communities, HPEIs can appropriately be expected to play a direct role in responding to priority unmet health needs at the local and/or societal level. Community benefit principles should therefore form a conceptual cornerstone by which health professions education accreditation organizations and state governments can set expectations for the advancement of societal goals tied to racial and ethnic diversity of the health-care workforce.

Efforts to build coalitions can benefit from strategies to increase the involvement of diverse stakeholders in key decision-making processes and to inform the public of progress toward efforts to increase the diversity of the health-care workforce. In addition, private and public (e.g., federal, state and local governments) entities should convene community stakeholders to inform them about community benefit standards and to build awareness that placing a priority on diversity and cultural competency programs is a societal expectation of all institutions that receive any form of public funding.

Several examples exist of initiatives that seek to build coalitions and utilize community benefit principles to increase support for health workforce diversity. As an example, Community Catalyst, with support from the W.K. Kellogg Foundation, has initiated the Physician Diversity Project in two sites (Boston and New York) to identify community-based strategies to increase medical workforce diversity. The overarching goals of the Physician Diversity Project are:

- to increase key stakeholders and other community leaders' awareness of the problems associated with the lack of physician diversity in the workplace,
- to gain the commitment of key stakeholders and other community leaders to make efforts to increase physician diversity a key policy priority, and
- to develop models from the existing sites that can be replicated in other locations.

To achieve these goals, Community Catalyst has organized and supported efforts to address public and private policies and increase community involvement in health-care priority-setting as part of a larger health-care reform effort. The Boston site will develop a highly visible campaign that will include activities such as campaign strategy development and implementation, leadership recruitment and mobilization, constituency and coalition building, and legislative and policy research and analysis. The New York City site is attempting, through the reauthorization of the Health Care Reform Act (HCRA), which governs Medicaid reimbursement rates for hospitals, hospital uncompensated care pool financing, and state allocations for the cost of training medical residents, to gain stakeholder support for public policy designed to promote diversity in medical education and the physician workforce. Activities at the New York City site include coalition building, setting and promoting the coalition's policy agenda, and other activities.

The W.K. Kellogg Foundation also supports the Community Voices Program, which is designed to strengthen community support services and strengthen the health-care safety net for vulnerable and medically under-served populations. Thirteen communities across the nation are participating in this 5-year initiative; each community is piloting different approaches and strategies tailored to the specific needs of the populations served. Among the initiative's goals are to increase access to health services for the vulnerable (with a focus on primary care and prevention) and to develop models of best practice for communities to adapt to their unique circumstances. As part of this effort, each project develops plans to help communities become informed about and empowered to improve the health-care infrastructure in their communities. This is accomplished by the development of:

- a plan and capacity for informing the public and marketplace policy;
- community involvement in strategic planning and activities that includes all the key members of the community;
- efforts to link the provider and community network together through infrastructure that includes management of information systems, legal agreements and initiatives to establish and expand provider–community relationships;
- explicit responsiveness to the community's culture and environment for creating health and wellness; and
- other efforts to help community members to assume leadership roles in shaping community-based health-care delivery.

These and other efforts to stimulate coalition building at the grassroots and national levels should be supported to pursue a coordinated agenda aimed at encouraging policy changes among HPEIs, their accrediting bodies, health-care providers (e.g., health professionals, hospitals, health plans), and others.

> Recommendation 7-3: Broad coalitions of stakeholder organizations—including health professions leaders, health-care consumer groups, grassroots and community organizations, business leaders, and others—should vigorously encourage HPEIs, their accreditation bodies, and federal and state sources of health professions student financial aid to adopt policies to enhance diversity among health professionals.

SUMMARY

Several mechanisms offer promise to garner support among a diverse array of stakeholder groups to increase diversity among health professions. Broad support is needed among many groups—including health professionals, the HPEI community, health policy makers, affected communities, educators, corporate and business leaders, organized labor, and the general public—in order to create the necessary "push" to support institutional and policy-level strategies to increase diversity among health professionals. As a start, health professions organizations should assess and disseminate information about HPEI applicants, matriculants, and graduates from URM groups, as well as the participation of URMs among HPEI faculty, staff, and professionals in the workforce. Educational efforts are also an important step to raise awareness of the problem among these stakeholders. Local and national efforts must be undertaken to increase understanding of the imperative to enhance diversity among health professionals and to build consensus among a range of stakeholders regarding steps that should be taken to achieve this goal. In addition, efforts to develop coalitions of stakeholder groups can help to create a political impetus for federal, state, and local strategies to increase diversity. Broad coalitions of stakeholder organizations—including health professions leaders, health-care consumer groups, grassroots and community organizations, business leaders, and others—should encourage HPEIs, their accreditation bodies, and federal and state sources of health professions student financial aid to adopt policies to enhance diversity among health professionals. Finally, federal and state government health agencies should increase support for policies that increase diversity among health professionals and should explore new initiatives to create incentives for HPEIs to adopt diversity efforts.

A

Data Sources and Methods

In order to respond to the study charge, several steps were undertaken to assess data regarding strategies for increasing diversity in the health professions. Sources of data and information included the assembly of a committee with appropriate knowledge and expertise; review of literature regarding admissions practices, accreditation policies, financing arrangements, community benefit principles, and the institutional climate; commissioned papers; and public workshops.

STUDY COMMITTEE

A 15-member study committee was convened to assess available data and respond to the study charge. The committee comprised members with expertise in areas such as health professions education, minority health, health-care service delivery, economics, law, statistics, and health policy. The committee convened for five 2-day meetings between November 2002 and September 2003.

LITERATURE REVIEW

The committee's review of the literature included, but was not limited to, articles published in peer-reviewed journals. The review focused on data regarding trends in minority health; underrepresented minority (URM) representation in the targeted health professions fields; admissions and accreditation policies for psychology, nursing, medicine, and dentistry; federal and private sources of funding for health professions students, including a review of evidence of their efficacy; and the role of institutional climate and community benefit standards in supporting and increasing diversity.

COMMISSIONED PAPERS

The study committee commissioned several papers, which were intended to provide in-depth information on the benefits of diversity, accreditation standards, admissions policies, financing of health professions, and institutional climate. Some of these papers are published with this report volume. These topics and the paper authors were determined by the study committee. The commissioned papers were not intended to serve as a substitute for the committee's own review and analysis of the literature. The committee independently deliberated on data regarding these topics, prior to receiving the draft commissioned papers.

PUBLIC WORKSHOPS

The study committee hosted six one-day public workshops in conjunction with its February, April, and June 2003 meetings in order to gain additional information from the public on key aspects of the study charge. Two workshops were conducted at each of these three meetings. The topics and nature of the workshops were determined by the study committee.

The first workshop was intended to allow the committee to hear the perspectives of racial and ethnic minority and nonminority health professions organizations on the importance of diversity. Subsequent workshops were focused on admissions policies and practices; the role of accreditation standards in increasing diversity; the potential application of community benefits standards; ways in which the climate of institutions can support diversity; and the financing of health professions education, including federal and nonfederal sources of support. The agendas, with lists of participants, are presented in Boxes A-1 through A-3.

BOX A-1

Public Workshop
IOM Committee on Institutional and Policy-Level Strategies for Increasing the Diversity of the U.S. Health Care Workforce

Wednesday, February 5, 2003
The National Academies, 500 Fifth Street, NW, Room 109

AGENDA

10:00 a.m. **WELCOME AND INTRODUCTIONS**

Lonnie R. Bristow, M.D.
Chair, IOM Committee on Institutional and Policy-Level
Strategies for Increasing the Diversity of the U.S. Health Care
Workforce

10:15 a.m. **PRESENTATIONS FROM INTEREST GROUPS AND STAKEHOLDERS**

L. Natalie Carroll, M.D.
President, National Medical Association

David Johnsen, D.D.S.
President, American Dental Education Association

Hilda Richards, Ed.D., R.N.
President, National Black Nurses Assocation, Inc.

Charles Terrell, Ed.D.
Vice President, Division of Community Minority Programs
Association of American Medical Colleges

Barbara Blakeney, M.S., A.P.R.N., B.C., A.N.P.
President, American Nurses Association

Phyllis Kopriva
Director, Women and Minority Services
and
Kevin McKinney, M.D.
Chair, Minority Affairs Consortium
American Medical Association

Geraldine Bednash, Ph.D., R.N., F.A.A.N.
Executive Director, American Association of Colleges of Nursing

Elena Rios, M.D.
National Hispanic Medical Association

Ben Muneta, M.D.
President, Association of American Indian Physicians

Continued

BOX A-1 Continued

11:00 a.m.	**QUESTION AND ANSWER PERIOD**
12:00 p.m.	**LUNCH SERVED IN MEETING ROOM**
1:00 p.m.	**ADMISSIONS POLICIES AND PRACTICES**

Speakers will present for 30 minutes. Committee members will participate in a 15-minute question and answer period following each presentation.

1:00 p.m.	*Dean Whitla, Ph.D.* Director, National Campus Diversity Project Harvard Graduate School of Education
1:45 p.m.	*Ella Cleveland, Ph.D.* Association of American Medical Colleges
2:30 p.m.	**BREAK**
2:45 p.m.	*Gabriel Garcia, M.D.* Associate Dean of Medical School Admissions Stanford University
3:30 p.m.	*Joshua Aronson, Ph.D.* Assistant Professor, Department of Applied Psychology New York University
4:15 p.m.	**ADJOURN**

BOX A-2

Public Workshop
IOM Committee on Institutional and Policy-Level Strategies for Increasing the Diversity of the U.S. Health Care Workforce

Wednesday, April 9, 2003
The National Academies, 500 Fifth Street, NW, Room 109

AGENDA

8:30 a.m.	**WELCOME AND INTRODUCTIONS**

Lonnie R. Bristow, M.D.
Chair, Committee on Institutional and Policy-Level Strategies for Increasing the Diversity of the Health Care Workforce

BOX A-2 Continued

8:45 a.m.	**WORKSHOP—WHAT IS THE ROLE OF ACCREDITATION STANDARDS IN PROMOTING RACIAL AND ETHNIC DIVERSITY IN HEALTH PROFESSIONS TRAINING PROGRAMS?**
8:45 a.m.	*Barbara Grumet* National League for Nursing Accrediting Commission
9:30 a.m.	*Dr. Charlotte Beason* Commission on Collegiate Nursing Education
10:15 a.m.	*Karen Hart* Commission on Dental Accreditation
11:00 a.m.	**BREAK**
11:15 a.m.	*Dr. David Stevens* Liaison Committee on Medical Education
12:00 p.m.	*Dr. Susan Zlotlow* American Psychological Association Committee on Accreditation
12:45 p.m.	**LUNCH SERVED IN MEETING ROOM**
1:15 p.m.	**WORKSHOP—WHAT IS THE ROLE OF COMMUNITY BENEFIT STANDARDS IN PROMOTING RACIAL AND ETHNIC DIVERSITY IN HEALTH PROFESSIONS TRAINING PROGRAMS?**
	Presentation—Community Benefit: Policies, Practices, and Potential Application to Health Professions Education
	Dr. Kevin Barnett Public Health Institute *Dr. Paul Hattis* Tufts University
	Panel Discussion
	Dr. JudyAnn Bigby Brigham and Women's Hospital and Harvard Medical School *Dr. Bradford Gray* New York Academy of Medicine *Dr. William Vega* UMDNJ–Robert Wood Johnson Medical School
4:15 p.m.	**ADJOURN**

BOX A-3

Public Workshop
IOM Committee on Institutional and Policy-Level Strategies for
Increasing the Diversity of the U.S. Health Care Workforce

Monday, June 30, 2003
The National Academies, 2101 Constitution Avenue, NW,
Room 150

AGENDA

9:00 a.m.   **WELCOME AND INTRODUCTIONS**

Lonnie R. Bristow, M.D.
Chair, Committee on Institutional and Policy-Level Strategies for
Increasing the Diversity of the Health Care Workforce

9:15 a.m.   **WORKSHOP—WHAT IS THE ROLE OF INSTITUTIONAL**
CLIMATE IN PROMOTING RACIAL AND ETHNIC DIVERSITY
IN HEALTH PROFESSIONS TRAINING PROGRAMS?

Enacting Diversity on Campus: A Framework for
Conceptualizing and Assessing the Campus Racial Climate
Jeffery F. Milem, Ph.D.
Associate Professor
Department of Education Policy and Leadership
University of Maryland
and
Eric L. Dey, Ph.D.
Associate Professor
Center for the Study of Higher and Postsecondary Education
University of Michigan School of Education

Efforts to Retain Ethnic Minority Health Professions
Students
Michael Rainey, Ph.D.
Associate Dean for Academic Advisement
Stony Brook University School of Medicine

Efforts to Recruit and Retain Ethnic Minority Faculty
Daryl G. Smith, Ph.D.
Professor of Education and Psychology
School of Educational Studies
Claremont Graduate University

Efforts to Recruit and Retain Ethnic Minority Faculty—
ACE Perspective
William B. Harvey, Ed.D.
Vice President and Director
Office of Minorities in Higher Education
American Council on Education

BOX A-3 Continued

12:00 p.m. **LUNCH SERVED IN MEETING ROOM**

1:00 p.m. **WORKSHOP—WHAT IS THE ROLE OF FINANCING OF HEALTH PROFESSIONS TRAINING IN PROMOTING RACIAL AND ETHNIC DIVERSITY IN HEALTH PROFESSIONS TRAINING PROGRAMS?**

Federal and Nonfederal Sources of Financial Assistance for Health Professions Students
Karen Matherlee
Consultant to the Study Committee
President, KRM Policy

Bureau of Health Professions Programs That Address Financial Barriers
Henry Lopez, Jr.
Director, Division of Health Careers Diversity and Development
Bureau of Health Professions, Health Resources and Services Administration

Potential of Two Colorado Programs to Increase Access to and Interest in Dental Careers Among Underrepresented Students
Howard Landesman, D.D.S., M.Ed.
Dean, School of Dentistry
University of Colorado Health Science Center

3:30 p.m. **ADJOURN**

B

Committee and Staff Biographies

COMMITTEE BIOGRAPHIES

Lonnie R. Bristow, M.D., *Chair,* (New York University College of Medicine) is a former president of the American Medical Association, after earlier serving as vice chair and chair of the AMA's Board of Trustees. Dr. Bristow has written and lectured extensively on medical science as well as socioeconomic and ethical issues related to medicine. He is a board-certified internist and has practiced medicine for more than 30 years. He is a member of the Institute of Medicine and was appointed to its Quality of Health Care in America committee, which in 1999 and 2001 respectively, authored the widely read reports *To Err Is Human* and *Crossing the Quality Chasm.* Dr. Bristow's research interests and expertise are eclectic and, over the decades, his writings have included papers on medical ethics, socialized medicine as practiced in Great Britain and Canada, health-care financing in America, professional liability insurance problems, sickle cell anemia, and coronary care unit utilization. Dr. Bristow has recently served as vice chair for the Physician Leadership for a New Drug Policy and also, by Presidential appointment, he served for 6 years as chair of the board of regents of the Uniformed Services University of Health Sciences (Bethesda, MD). He continues as an active member of both groups. In addition he is a reviewer for the *Journal of the American Medical Association.* Dr. Bristow recently retired from private practice but continues his other activities as a professional consultant.

Colleen Conway-Welch, Ph.D., R.N., CNM, FAAN, *Vice-Chair*, has been dean and professor at Vanderbilt University School of Nursing since 1984. She has served on the Tennessee Board of Nursing, the National Bipartisan Commission on the Future of Medicare, the Advisory Council of the NIH National Center for Nursing Research, and the Advisory Board of the Agency for Health Care Policy and Research (AHCPR), now the Agency for Health Care Research and Quality (AHRQ). Dr. Conway-Welch is also a member of the Secretary's Council on Public Health Preparedness, Office of the Assistant Secretary for Public Health Emergency preparedness, DHHS, appointed by Secretary Tommy Thompson. Among her many honors, in 2000 Dr. Conway-Welch was awarded the Nancy and Hilliard Travis Endowed Chair in Nursing and in 2001 received the National Association of Childbearing Centers Public Advocate Award. She is a member of the Institute of Medicine, a Fellow of the American Academy of Nursing, a charter Fellow of the American College of Nurse-Midwives, and a member of Sigma Theta Tau, among other distinctions. Dr. Conway-Welch received her B.S.N. degree from Georgetown University School of Nursing, an M.S.N. degree from Catholic University, and her Ph.D. degree in nursing from New York University.

Brenda E. Armstrong, M.D., associate dean and director of Medical School Admissions, associate professor of pediatrics in the Division of Pediatric Cardiology, and associate vice provost at Duke University. She is also program director of the Duke University Summer Biomedical Science Institute, funded by the Robert Wood Johnson Foundation, and director of the Fellowship Training Division of Pediatric Cardiology at Duke University Medical Center. Previously, she was medical director of the Raleigh Multi-Specialty Pediatric Clinic and has served as a consultant to the U.S. Army and U.S. Air Force. She is a Fellow of the American Academy of Pediatrics and is board certified in pediatrics and pediatric cardiology. Among her many professional activities, Dr. Armstrong serves on the Accreditation Council for Graduate Medical Education Appeals Committee, specialty in pediatric cardiology, and serves as a consultant to the Durham County General Hospital. Among her many awards and honors are the Distinguished Faculty Award, Duke University School of Medicine, 2001, and the Association of Black Cardiologists "Hero" Award, 2002. Dr. Armstrong received a B.A. degree from Duke University in 1970 and an M.D. degree from St. Louis University School of Medicine in 1974.

Kevin Barnett, Dr.PH, M.C.P., is a senior investigator for the Public Health Institute (PHI) in Oakland, California. His work with the PHI focuses on applied research and technical assistance in population health planning, policy analysis, health system reform, and community problem solving. Dr.

Barnett received his doctorate in public health and master's in city planning from the University of California at Berkeley. He has devoted much of the last 15 years to the facilitation and evaluation of broad-based, inter-sectoral partnerships between organizations and community resident groups to address persistent health-related problems ranging from access to health care to violence, housing, and economic development. A major focus during the last decade has been research into the role of not-for-profit health care organizations in community health improvement. He currently leads a multistate community benefit demonstration program to develop uniform standards for documenting, quantifying, and evaluating institutional performance.

Joseph Betancourt, M.D., M.P.H., is senior scientist at the Institute for Health Policy, director for Multicultural Education, Multicultural Affairs Office at Massachusetts General Hospital, and assistant professor of medicine at Harvard Medical School. Previously, he served as the assistant professor of medicine and public health and the associate director for multinational and minority health at New York Presbyterian Hospital–Weill Medical College of Cornell University. Dr. Betancourt's research has focused on several areas relevant to the study charge, including: cross-cultural communication and its relationship to adherence, utilization, and health outcomes; cultural competence in health policy; determinants of racial/ethnic disparities; and the impact of disease management programs in Medicaid managed care. His most current work has involved examining Hispanic health services utilization, cultural competence in health care, and racial differences in lung cancer treatment. Dr. Betancourt was a member of the IOM Committee on Understanding and Eliminating Racial and Ethnic Disparities in Health Care which produced the 2003 report, *Unequal Treatment: Confronting Racial and Ethnic Disparities in Health Care.*

Michael V. Drake, M.D., is vice president for health affairs of the University of California (UC) system. He oversees education and research activities at UC's 15 health sciences schools located on 7 University of California campuses. Previously, he served as vice chair, Department of Ophthalmology; senior associate dean for Admissions and Extramural Academic Programs; interim associate dean for student affairs; professor of ophthalmology; associate dean for admissions and student programs; and chief, Vision Care and Research Unit, Beckman Vision Center, all at the UCSF School of Medicine. He maintains his position as Stephen P. Shearing Professor of Opthalmology and is engaged in teaching, research, and patient care on a limited basis. He received his A.B. degree from Stanford University in 1974 and his M.D. degree from UCSF in 1975. Dr. Drake has served in many roles within the UC system, including service on the UC Medical School

Admissions/Diversity Task Force, and has testified before the California State Senate and Assembly on diversity issues. Among his numerous awards and distinctions, he is president of the Alpha Omega Alpha Honor Medical Society. Dr. Drake is a member of the Institute of Medicine

Jay Alan Gershen, D.D.S., Ph.D., is executive vice chancellor and professor in the School of Dentistry at the University of Colorado Health Sciences Center. In addition to assisting the chancellor in administering the campus, Dr. Gershen has had responsibility for resource development, external and community affairs, technology transfer, information systems, diversity, ombuds, and telehealth programs. Concurrently, from 2000 to 2002, Dr. Gershen served as interim vice president for academic affairs and research, University of Colorado. Dr. Gershen holds a B.A. in psychology from the State University of New York at Buffalo (1968) and a D.D.S. from the University of Maryland (1972). After a one year general dentistry internship at Eastman Dental Center, Rochester, New York, he completed both a clinical specialty in pediatric dentistry and a Ph.D. in education at the University of California, Los Angeles, in 1976. Concurrently, he served as a postdoctoral scholar in child psychiatry at UCLA's Neuropsychiatric Institute. Dr. Gershen joined the faculty of the School of Dentistry at UCLA in 1976. For 6 years (1976–1982) he directed the UCLA Mobile Dental Clinic, serving children of migrant workers in rural California. Dr. Gershen was awarded a Robert Wood Johnson Health Policy Fellowship (1982–1983), sponsored by the Institute of Medicine. In this capacity he worked on health policy issues and legislation in the Committee on Energy and Commerce in the U.S. House of Representatives. Dr. Gershen served as associate dean for policy and program development from 1983 to 1984, and professor and chair in the Section of Public Health Dentistry from 1988 to 1995. As acting dean of the School of Dentistry (1995–1996), he was the first dental dean in the nation to gain Graduate Medical Education (GME) support funds for all of the School of Dentistry's postdoctoral programs.

Lazar J. Greenfield, M.D., is on sabbatical with the Center for Medical Devices, FDA. He is emeritus executive vice president for Medical Affairs at the University of Michigan (U-M) and interim chief executive officer of the U-M Health System. Dr. Greenfield attended Rice University before graduating with honors from Baylor University College of Medicine in 1958. He trained in general and thoracic surgery at the Johns Hopkins Hospital from 1958 to 1966. Dr. Greenfield began his academic surgical career as assistant professor of surgery and chief of surgical services at the Veteran's Administration Hospital, University of Oklahoma Medical Center in 1966. He was named a Markle Scholar and became professor of surgery in 1971. In 1974, Dr. Greenfield was appointed the Stuart McGuire Professor and chairman of the Department of Surgery at the Medical College of Virginia, Virginia Commonwealth University. He remained in that position until 1987, when he was appointed the F.A. Coller Distinguished Professor of Surgery and chairman of the Department of Surgery at the University of Michigan School of Medicine. Dr. Greenfield is a Fellow of the American College of Surgeons and has served on the board of governors. He served on the board of the national honor society, Alpha Omega Alpha, and has been elected president of the American Surgical Association, the American Venous Forum, American Association of Vascular Surgery, and the Halsted Society. He has been a director of the American Board of Surgery and past Chairman of the national ACGME-Residency Review Committee for Surgery. In 1995, Dr. Greenfield was elected to the Institute of Medicine. In 1996, he was designated a Johns Hopkins Society Scholar and in 1999 he received the Rice University Distinguished Alumnus Award.

Robert L. Johnson, M.D., is professor and chair of pediatrics, professor of psychiatry and director of the Division of Adolescent and Young Adult Medicine at the New Jersey Medical School of the University of Medicine and Dentistry of New Jersey. His research focuses on adolescent physical and prevention/reduction programs, with specific emphasis on substance and alcohol abuse, sexuality and sexual dysfunction, male sexual abuse, suicide, and AIDS. He currently serves on the U.S. Department of Health and Human Services Council on Graduate Medical Education, the Board of Health Care Services of the National Academy of Sciences, and chairs the Newark Ryan White Planning Council. Dr. Johnson is a Fellow of the American Academy of Pediatrics. He has previously been a member of the National Council of the National Institute of Mental Health, member of the NIH AIDS Research Council, member of the Institute of Medicine Committee on Unintended Pregnancy, chair of the National Commission on Adolescent Sexuality, president of the New Jersey State Board of Medical Examiners and chair of the Board of Advocates for Youth. Dr. Johnson has published widely, and he conducts an active schedule of teaching, research, and clinical practice at the New Jersey Medical School.

Ciro V. Sumaya, M.D., M.P.H.T.M., is a native of Brownsville, Texas, dean of the School of Rural Public Health (SRPH), and holder of the Cox Endowed Chair in Medicine at Texas A&M University Health Science Center in College Station. Before coming to the SRPH, Dr. Sumaya served as a presidential appointee for 4 years at the U.S. Department of Health and Human Services. He first served as administrator of Health Resources and Services Administration, a federal focal point for innovation in health-care delivery and health professions education, and subsequently served as deputy assistant secretary for Health, spearheading the federal initiative on the Future of Academic Health Centers. Before federal service, Dr. Sumaya was associate medical dean at the University of Texas Health Science Center at San Antonio. As associate dean he established the South Texas Health Research Center, Area Health Education Center of South Texas, and a Medical Treatment Effectiveness Research Center. He has also held academic positions at the UCLA School of Medicine. Dr. Sumaya was one of the six Founding Scholars in Academic Administration and Health Policy of the Association of Academic Health Centers and executive committee member of the Surgeon General's National Hispanic Health Initiative. In 1993 he was selected as a group leader of the Health Care Workforce workgroup of the Presidential Task Force on Health Care Reform. He received a B.A. degree (1963) with high honors from the University of Texas at Austin, where he was also elected to Phi Beta Kappa. His M.D. degree (1966) was obtained from the University of Texas Medical Branch in Galveston, where he was inducted into the Alpha Omega Alpha Honor Medical Society.

Lisa Tedesco, Ph.D., is vice president and secretary of the university and professor of dentistry, at the University of Michigan and during 2001 served as interim provost. As vice president and secretary, she is the liaison officer for the board of regents; responsible for facilitation, coordination, and management of policy matters and communications pertaining to the board, the president, and executive officers of the university. Throughout her academic and administrative career, Dr. Tedesco has been involved with programs to increase student and faculty diversity on campus. She was coprincipal investigator of the University of Michigan Health Occupations Partners in Education (HOPE) project funded through the American Association of Medical Colleges Health Professions Partnership Initiative to provide academic preparation and social support to disadvantaged and minority youth for careers in the health professions. In October 1995 she was inducted as an honorary member of the American Dental Association, in recognition for her contributions to academic dentistry, and in May 1998 she received the Distinguished Alumni Award from the State University of New York at Buffalo, Graduate School of Education. Dr. Tedesco earned her master's degree in education in 1975 and her doctorate in educational psychology in 1981, both from the State University of New York at Buffalo.

Ena Vazquez-Nuttall, Ed.D., is associate dean and director of the graduate school of Bouve College of Health Sciences at Northeastern University in Boston. This graduate school contains programs in counseling and school psychology, pharmaceutical sciences, nursing, and allied health. She started at Northeastern in 1989 as a professor in the Department of Counseling Psychology, Rehabilitation and Special Education. From 1975 to 1988,

Vazquez-Nuttall was a professor in the Counseling and School Psychology Program at the University of Massachusetts, Amherst. She has served in many state and national professional committees and boards. She was chair of the Training and Education Group of the Commission on Ethnic Minority Recruitment, Retention, and Training in Psychology (CEMRRAT) of the American Psychological Association (APA) from 1994 to1996. For 5 years, Dr. Vazquez-Nuttall was a member of the Committee on Accreditation of APA (1998–2002). She is a fellow of Division 16 (school psychology) of APA, and member of Division 17 (counseling psychology) and 35 (women's division). She served on the Massachusetts Board of Registration from 1988 to 1993. She has been a member of several editorial boards, including *School Psychology Quarterly, School Psychology Review, American Journal of Counseling and Development,* and the *Journal of Counselor Education and Supervision.* At present she is on the editorial board of *Applied School Psychology.* Dr. Vazquez-Nuttall has written two books with collaborators *Assessing and Screening Preschoolers* (1999, Allyn & Bacon, with Romero & Kalesnik) and *Multicultural Counseling Competencies: Individual and Organization Development* (1998, Sage, with Sue, Carter, Casas, Fouad, Ivey et al). She has received several NIMH research awards and OSEP personnel preparation grants. She has extensive program evaluation experience, including of bilingual education programs and a National Science Foundation-funded parent involvement grant. She obtained a bachelor's degree from the University of Puerto Rico, master's degree in social psychology from Radcliffe, and Ed.D. from Boston University.

Judith A. Winston, J.D., is the former under secretary and general counsel of the U.S. Department of Education and former executive director of the President's Initiative on Race. Ms. Winston is currently a lawyer in private practice and a principal and cofounder of the legal consulting firm Winston Withers & Associates, LLC, in Washington, DC. She assists businesses, schools, colleges, universities and nonprofit entities in understanding and developing effective equity, diversity, and equal opportunity management and organizational strategies consistent with legal requirements and best practices. Prior to her most recent government service, Winston served as research professor of law at the Washington College of Law at American University. Her research and teaching responsibilities included constitutional law, education law and policy, civil rights, and civil procedure. Ms. Winston has received a number of honors and citations, including the prestigious Thurgood Marshall Award, from the District of Columbia Bar Association, recognizing her lifetime commitment to the cause of civil rights, and the Margaret Brent Women Lawyers of Achievement Award from the American Bar Association's Commission on Women in the Profession. She has served on numerous boards and committees including the board of directors of National Public Radio, Partners for Democratic Change, and the Southern Education Foundation, and the National Law Center on Poverty and Homelessness. She is the author of many articles on civil rights, employment discrimination, women of color in the workplace, and education. Ms. Winston is a graduate of the Georgetown University Law Center and Howard University.

Vickie Ybarra, R.N., M.P.H., is director of planning and development for the Yakima Valley Farm Workers Clinic, one of the largest community/ migrant health care systems in the country, with clinics in Washington and Oregon. She has extensive experience in development, oversight, and evaluation of community programs targeting Hispanic and Spanish-speaking populations. She earned her undergraduate degree in nursing from the University of Washington School of Nursing and in 1996 completed her master's in public health at the University of Washington. In her role as a member of the Washington State Board of Health she has provided leadership for the board's health disparities efforts and in May 2001 coauthored the board's report on health disparities, focusing on diversifying the state health-care workforce. Ms. Ybarra has been active in efforts to connect local communities to institutions of higher education. She has conducted research related to the presence and service needs of local undocumented women and children. She also served as a member of the Community-Campus Partnerships for Health board of directors from 1995 to 2000. Ms. Ybarra is active in her community in Hispanic academic achievement. She works with a local group to distribute scholarship dollars and provide community-wide recognition for academic success of local outstanding Hispanic high school graduates. She has conducted research with the local school district demonstrating the wide gap in college preparedness between Hispanic and non-Hispanic students. Ms. Ybarra is also a recently appointed member of the local school board, with a particular focus on closing the achievement gap between Hispanic and non-Hispanic students.

IOM STAFF BIOGRAPHIES

Andrew Pope, Ph.D., is director of the Board on Health Sciences Policy at the Institute of Medicine. With expertise in physiology and biochemistry, his primary interests focus on environmental and occupational influences on human health. Dr. Pope's previous research activities focused on the neuroendocrine and reproductive effects of various environmental substances on food-producing animals. During his tenure at the National Academy of Sciences and, since 1989, at the Institute of Medicine, Dr. Pope has directed numerous reports; topics include injury control, disability prevention, biologic markers, neurotoxicology, indoor allergens, and the enhancement of environmental and occupational health content in medical and nursing school curricula. Most recently, Dr. Pope directed studies on NIH priority-setting processes, fluid resuscitation practices in combat casualties, and organ procurement and transplantation.

Brian D. Smedley, Ph.D., is a senior program officer in the Division of Health Sciences Policy of the Institute of Medicine (IOM), where he most recently served as study director for the IOM report, *Unequal Treatment: Confronting Racial and Ethnic Disparities in Health Care.* Previously, Smedley served as study director for the IOM reports, *Promoting Health: Intervention Strategies from Social and Behavioral Research; The Right Thing to Do, The Smart Thing to Do: Enhancing Diversity in the Health Professions;* and *The Unequal Burden of Cancer: An Assessment of NIH Research and Programs for Ethnic Minorities and the Medically Underserved.* Smedley came to the IOM from the American Psychological Association, where he worked on a wide range of social, health, and education policy topics in his capacity as director for public interest policy. Prior to working at the APA, Smedley served as a congressional science fellow in the office of Rep. Robert C. Scott (D-VA), sponsored by the American Association for the Advancement of Science, and as a postdoctoral research fellow in the Education Policy Division of the Educational Testing Service in Princeton, NJ. Among his awards and distinctions, in 2000 and 2003 Smedley was awarded the National Academy of Sciences' Individual Staff Award for Distinguished Service, in April 2002 he was awarded the Congressional Black Caucus "Healthcare Hero" award, and in August 2002 he was awarded the Early Career Award for Distinguished Contributions to Psychology in the Public Interest by the American Psychological Association.

Adrienne Stith Butler, Ph.D., is a program officer with the Board on Health Sciences Policy at the Institute of Medicine (IOM). She is currently a staff officer for the IOM Committee on Institutional and Policy-Level Strategies for Increasing the Diversity of the U.S. Health Care Workforce. She recently served as study director for the IOM report *Preparing for the Psychological Consequences of Terrorism: A Public Health Strategy,* conducted within the Board on Neuroscience and Behavioral Health. Previously she served as staff officer for the IOM report *Unequal Treatment: Confronting Racial and Ethnic Disparities in Health Care,* conducted within the Board on Health Sciences Policy. Prior to working at the IOM, Dr. Butler served as the James Marshall Public Policy Scholar, a fellowship cosponsored by the Society for the Psychological Study of Social Issues and the American Psychological Association (APA). In this position, based at the APA in Washington, DC, she engaged in policy analysis and monitored legislative issues related to ethnic disparities in health care and health research, racial profiling, and mental health counseling provisions in the reauthorization of the Elementary and Secondary Education Act. Dr. Butler, a clinical psychologist, received her doctorate in 1997 from the University of Vermont. She completed a postdoctoral fellowship in adolescent medicine and pediatric psychology at the University of Rochester Medical Center in Rochester, New York.

Thelma Cox is a senior project assistant in the Board on Health Sciences Policy. During her years at the Institute of Medicine (IOM), she has also provided assistance to the Division of Health Care Services and the Division of Biobehavioral Sciences and Mental Disorders. Ms. Cox has worked on several IOM reports, including *Unequal Treatment: Confronting Racial and Ethnic Disparities in Health Care; Designing a Strategy for Quality Review and Assurance in Medicare; Evaluating the Artificial Heart Program of the National Heart, Lung, and Blood Institute; Federal Regulation of Methadone Treatment; Legal and Ethical Issues Relating to the Inclusion of Women in Clinical Studies;* and *Review of the Fialuridine (FIAU/FIAC) Clinical Trials.* She has received the National Research Council Recognition Award and the IOM Staff Achievement Award.

Commissioned Papers

Editors' Note:

The following papers were commissioned by the study committee to provide additional analysis and information regarding several key areas of the study charge. For each paper, nationally known experts were asked to review available literature and draw upon their professional expertise to provide an in-depth analysis of institutional and policy-level strategies to increase diversity in the health professions workforce.

The papers were prepared independently of the IOM study committee's deliberations and analysis, although some of the commissioned paper authors were asked to present their findings before the study committee in public meetings. The opinions expressed in the papers are solely those of the authors. Several of the papers include findings and recommendations; these should not be confused with the findings and recommendations of the study committee, as indicated in the preceding committee report.

Paper Contribution A
Increasing Diversity in the Health Professions: A Look at Best Practices in Admissions

Gabriel Garcia, Cathryn L. Nation, and Neil H. Parker

In fiscal year 2001–2002, Americans spent more than $1.4 trillion on the cost of health care (CMS, 2003). Despite this staggering investment, an estimated 41.2 million individuals were uninsured and another 92 million lacked adequate access to care (Mills, 2002; KFF, 2002). Not surprisingly, a disproportionate number of these more than 133 million people live in inner cities, rural areas, low-income neighborhoods, and communities with large numbers of minority residents. The diversity of the U.S. population continues to grow, yet the lack of diversity among its health providers is striking by any measure. Recent bans on affirmative action, together with persistent inequities in educational opportunity for many poor and minority students, pose major challenges for schools seeking to diversify their classes. In the face of these realities, a growing sense of urgency has emerged. Evidence regarding race- and ethnicity-based disparities in health status is mounting, and the need to increase diversity in the health workforce as a strategy for improving the nation's health is both logical and clear.

This paper builds on previous work undertaken by the authors as part of the Medical Student Diversity Task Force appointed by University of California President Richard C. Atkinson in October 1999 (UCOP, 2000). The paper uses medicine as a model and starting point for examining admissions practices and institutional strategies for increasing the diversity of health professions classes. It begins with a review of the increasing diversity of the population and the profound disparities in health status among racial and ethnic groups as an imperative for change. A commentary about the responsibilities of U.S. medical schools for training clinicians, researchers, and leaders who will collectively meet the needs of the public follows. The paper briefly reviews the history of affirmative action and recent challenges that affect admissions. The medical school admissions process is described in detail, with a focus on strategies and best practices essential to recruiting and enrolling diverse classes of students. Special commentaries for clinical psychology, nursing, and dentistry are also provided. Across the health professions, however, the authors concur that institutional commitment, strong leadership, support for comprehensive strategies, and thinking "outside the box" have never been needed more urgently.

DIVERSITY IN THE HEALTH PROFESSIONS

The Demographic Imperative

Major advances in science and technology have enabled the quality of medical care to improve for many individuals. Notwithstanding these achievements, significant disparities in health status continue to exist between white people and other racial and ethnic minority groups. In a landmark report issued in 1985 by the U.S. Department of Health and Human Services (DHHS), these disparities were described in terms of excess deaths for six health conditions: cancer, cardiovascular disease and stroke, chemical dependency, diabetes, unintentional injuries, and infant mortality (DHHS, 1985). Fifteen years later in 2000, the Surgeon General reported that minority groups continue to have substantially higher morbidity and mortality associated with the same and other health conditions as their white counterparts. These gaps were so great that a national *Race and Health* initiative was launched by DHHS in 1998. The project was recently expanded and incorporated as part of *Healthy People 2010*, a national public health initiative calling for the elimination of these disparities by 2010.

For many individuals, race- and ethnicity-based disparities in health status are compounded by reduced access to services, lack of adequate insurance, and inadequate availability of physicians and other health-care professionals. Among the nation's more than 284 million people (U.S. Census Bureau, 2003), an estimated 133 million lack adequate access to care (Mills, 2002; KFF, 2002). In California alone, more than 4 million residents live in 165 areas designated by the state and federal governments as medically underserved or as health professions shortage areas (Grumbach et al., 1999). Nationally, this number jumps to a stunning 56 million (BHPR, 2003). Although differences exist in the criteria used by state and federal agencies to make such designations, health professions shortage areas, overwhelmingly, are home to poor and minority communities that lack access to health services and to adequate numbers and types of health-care personnel.

The ramifications of these findings for the health of the nation are substantial. By the year 2020, the U.S. population is projected to reach nearly 325 million. Of these, an estimated 117 million will be nonwhite (U.S. Census Bureau, 1999). Research relevant to these changes shows that physicians from groups traditionally underrepresented in medicine are more likely than others to serve those from minority and economically disadvantaged backgrounds, to practice in physician shortage areas, and to serve patients with chronic illness and multiple diagnoses (UCOP, 2000).

The Educational Mission of U.S. Medical Schools

The mission of U.S. medical schools is to meet the needs of the citizenry by training competent and compassionate physicians.

Meeting Public Health Needs

Public support and investment in medical education totals more than $10 billion annually through federal Medicare and Medicaid payments alone (MedPAC, 1998). This investment stems from the view that medical schools and teaching hospitals are a "public good" that benefit society by training tomorrow's practitioners, providing state-of-the-art patient care, and offering promise of new treatments for alleviating human illness and suffering. In fulfilling this trust, medical schools have an obligation to recruit, admit, and train graduates who will collectively meet the health needs of the public. As the public becomes increasingly diverse, the need for medical schools nationwide, and particularly those in racially and ethnically diverse states such as California, Texas, and New York, to diversify student enrollments is clearly evident from the standpoint of educational opportunity, public health, and workforce need.

Despite the select successes of some medical schools, diversity efforts on a national scale have had limited overall success. Medical student education in the United States is conducted in 126 allopathic and 19 osteopathic medical schools. Together, these schools admit approximately 20,000 new students each year. Yet among students who started medical school in fall 2002, fewer than 1,970 (or less than 10 percent) are from groups traditionally underrepresented in medicine (AAMC, 2003; AACOM, 2003).

Preparing Clinicians, Scientists, and Leaders

Although the lack of diversity in medicine is long-standing, U.S. medical schools and teaching hospitals have been subject to increasing awareness and criticism by the public, managed care organizations, and policy makers, who argue that medical education is not adapting to meet changing societal needs. In response to this claim, the Hastings Center brought together representatives from 14 countries to develop a consensus view of what society expected of its doctors (Callahan, 1996). The American Association of Medical Colleges (AAMC) began to address the need for changes in medical education and developed several white papers through its Medical School Objectives Projects I–IV (MSOP). The first such report in this series, entitled "Learning Objectives for Medical Education," focused on "expressed concerns that new doctors were not as well prepared as they should be to meet society's expectation of them" (AAMC, 1998, p. 1).

Four areas were identified in the report as essential characteristics of practicing physicians; these are that doctors be altruistic, knowledgeable, skillful, and dutiful. The AAMC (1998, p. 4) report stated that, "physicians must be compassionate and empathetic in caring for patients and must be trustworthy and truthful in all of their professional dealings. . . . They must understand the history of medicine, the nature of medicine's social compact, the ethical precepts of the medical profession, and their obligations under law. . . . They must seek to understand the meaning of the patients' stories in the context of the patients' beliefs and their family and cultural value. . . . As members of a team addressing individual or population-based health care issues, they must be willing both to provide leadership when appropriate and to defer to the leadership of others when indicated."

At the turn of the past century, doctors tended to the ill in their homes or in public hospitals. Advances in technology and the development of the modern hospital required that students become clinical scientists prepared to care for the sick in hospital settings. Students were selected for their abilities to master a curriculum heavily weighted to the basic and clinical sciences. They were rewarded for being science majors and for achieving high grade point averages (GPAs) and Medical College Admissions Test (MCAT) scores. Although Americans have always had high expectations about the knowledge and skill of their doctors, the growing diversity of the population has created new expectations. Patients today speak many languages and virtually all want doctors who are able to communicate with them in languages and ways they understand.

Increasing attention by accreditation bodies and state and national policy makers has similarly focused on the need for medical schools to better address changing societal needs. The Liaison Committee for Medical Education, which accredits allopathic schools, recently added a requirement that medical schools produce graduates who are culturally competent. Discussions at various state and national levels have also begun to consider the value of adding a language requirement as a prerequisite for admission to medical school. These and other initiatives addressing both undergraduate and graduate medical education are driven by growing recognition of the need to improve access to care, reduce disparities in health status, and respond more effectively to the changing needs of the public.

The need for diversity in the scientific and research community is equally compelling. Graduates of medical schools frequently do more than just practice medicine. Many are directly and indirectly involved in research at the basic science and clinical levels. All medical students and physicians should be trained to understand research design and its applications and limitations to various patient populations. Research and provider communities should understand that the number of research and clinical trials involving individuals from all races and ethnicities is inadequate, and that this insufficiency limits the application of some research findings.

To improve health outcomes, clinicians and researchers will require increased understanding of the disparities in health status that exist between racial and ethnic groups. Improving health outcomes will also require that health-care providers make efforts to improve their own cultural competency and to enhance their awareness of the diversity of belief systems and behavioral determinants that are characteristic of the patient populations they serve.

PAST AND PRESENT CHALLENGES TO DIVERSITY

Public health needs in America have changed, but efforts to diversify the health professions workforce are by no means new concepts or goals. Just as the achievements of individual schools have varied over time, so have the obstacles to their progress been influenced by changing law, public policy, and societal values. Past challenges remain and new ones have emerged. Critical to the success of some institutions is the use of affirmative action policies that encourage and allow consideration of race/ethnicity as one among many factors considered in the admissions process. Recent bans on affirmative action, however, have created new obstacles for a number of public institutions seeking to diversify their student bodies. A brief review of the history of affirmative action and recent major state initiatives and legal challenges in this area provides useful context for those charged with developing effective institutional policies in the future.

Historical Ramifications of Segregation

For the first two-thirds of the twentieth century, U.S. medical schools were de facto segregated. The Flexner Report of 1910, which shaped medical education in the subsequent century, encouraged the support of medical education at the historically black colleges and universities to provide a physician workforce that would serve black Americans, yet its recommendations resulted in the closure of five of the seven majority medical schools that trained African American physicians (Shea and Fullilove, 1985). As recently as 1964, 93 percent of all medical students in the United States were men and 97 percent were non-Hispanic whites. Of the remaining 3 percent, all but a few were enrolled in the nation's (then) two predominantly black medical schools, Howard University in Washington, DC, and Meharry Medical College in Nashville, Tennessee. At that time, less than 0.2 percent of all medical students were Mexican American, Puerto Rican, American Indian, or Alaskan Native. Prevailing societal values and practices within the profession were reflected in restricted opportunities for minority medical school graduates to participate in specialty training, medical society membership, hospital staff membership, and other professional activities.

Affirmative Action as a Remedy

Beginning in the late 1960s, a handful of other medical schools changed their admissions policies and favored a more integrated student body through affirmative action. An example at the time was the University of California Davis campus, where the medical school guaranteed 16 percent of the seats in each incoming class to African American and Mexican American applicants. By 1970, the AAMC adopted a recommendation to medical schools that strongly encouraged vigorous expansion of efforts to recruit and enroll minority students. The AAMC's stated goal was "to achieve equality of opportunity by relieving or eliminating inequitable barriers and constraints to access to the medical profession" (AAMC, 1970).

The widely recognized underrepresentation of minorities in medicine during the middle of this century was one of the driving forces behind the passage of the Federal Comprehensive Health Manpower Training Act of 1971 and its articulation of a new national policy intended to produce a physician workforce that would draw on the knowledge and skills of people from all segments of society. These efforts yielded promising early results. In the 6-year period between 1968 and 1974, enrollment of minority students increased from 3 percent of all entering students to approximately 8 percent nationwide (AAMC, 2000).

No significant changes in minority enrollment in medical schools occurred until 1990, when the AAMC established *Project 3000 by 2000*. This initiative called on U.S. medical schools to increase the number of minority students to 3,000 entering students by the year 2000. It recognized that medical schools have the means and the responsibility to improve educational opportunities for young people and their communities, but that they cannot solve the problem of minority underrepresentation alone. The initiative established both enrichment programs for college students and educational exercises for medical school admissions committee members, which led to a slow but steady rise in minority enrollment until peak levels of 2,014 students (12.4 percent) were reached in 1994.

The Bakke Decision

In the mid-1970s, and the years that followed, previous gains leveled off. Among the prime causes was a 1974 reverse discrimination lawsuit heard by the U.S. Supreme Court and brought by Allan Bakke against the University of California (UC). Bakke was a 33-year-old white man who applied to the UC-Davis School of Medicine during the time when positions in the entering class were "reserved" for qualified minority students. When Bakke was denied admission, he argued that the admissions process at UC-Davis was discriminatory because only minority students could compete for those seats.

The complexity of the Supreme Court's 1978 decision was reflected in the more than 150 pages and nine opinions necessary to express its result. Six justices wrote separate opinions, with no more than four agreeing fully in their reasoning. Justice Powell cast the deciding vote. In his written opinion, Powell stated, "the State has a substantial interest that legitimately may be served by a properly devised admissions program involving the competitive consideration of race and ethnic origin." He also quoted the president of Princeton University regarding the benefits of diversity on the learning process, stating that, "it occurs through interactions among students of both sexes; of different races, religions and backgrounds . . . who are able, directly or indirectly, to learn from their differences and to stimulate one another to examine even their most deeply held assumptions about themselves and their world" (Powell, 1978).

As a result of the Court's decision, Bakke was admitted to medical school at UC-Davis and the school's special admissions program was invalidated insofar as it reserved seats for minority applicants. More significantly, however, the Court's decision affirmed the use of race as one among many factors that could be considered as part of the medical school admissions process. Throughout the 1980s and early 1990s, the Supreme Court's decision set the standard for U.S. medical schools—and for many higher educational institutions nationwide—that sought to increase the diversity of their student bodies.

Recent Anti-Affirmative Action Initiatives

In the mid-1990s, several high-profile changes in public higher education challenged the use of affirmative action in admissions. The first occurred in July 1995, when the University of California Board of Regents approved a new policy prohibiting the use of "race, religion, sex, color, ethnicity, or national origin as criteria for either admission to the University or to any program of study." Within 18 months of the regents' action, two other challenges to affirmative action occurred. In March 1996, the U.S. Supreme Court refused to review the Fifth District Court of Appeals decision in *Hopwood v. Texas*, which found that the civil rights of four white applicants had been violated by the minority admissions process of the University of Texas School of Law. The Court ruled that the school could not use race as a factor in its admissions process. Although not binding for the rest of the nation, this ruling prohibits the consideration of race in the admissions process among all public higher educational institutions in Texas, Louisiana, and Mississippi.

In the November 1996 state general election, California voters passed Proposition 209, thereby adding state constitutional backing to the anti-affirmative action effect of the (then) new regents policy. Proposition 209 provided that the state, including the University of California, "shall not discriminate against, or grant preferential treatment to, any individual or group on the basis of race, sex, color, ethnicity, or national origin in the operation of public employment, public education, or public contracting." Although the regents rescinded the policy in May 2001, the effects of Proposition 209 nevertheless prohibit the consideration of race in the admissions process. The state of Washington subsequently passed a similar initiative and other states have considered measures intended to achieve the same goal. These state mandates have had significant effects on the rates of admission of underrepresented minority students to medical schools in these states. In fact, reductions in minority student enrollments in these states have been a major cause of the nearly 12 percent decline in the matriculation of underrepresented students at U.S. medical schools between 1995 and 2001 (Cohen, 2003) (Table PCA-1).

The Supreme Court Ruling in the University of Michigan Lawsuits

The U.S. Supreme Court recently heard two admissions cases, *Grutter v. Bollinger* and *Gratz v. Bollinger,* involving the University of Michigan and the constitutionality of using race-conscious decisions as part of its admissions process. Although neither case directly involved medical school or other health profession admissions, the Court's ruling was widely recognized as one that would have profound bearing on the future of affirmative action in public higher education nationwide.

In June 2003, the Court ruled on these separate but parallel cases. In *Grutter v. Bollinger,* the justices voted 5-4 to uphold the University of Michigan's law school affirmative action policy. Writing the majority opinion, Justice O'Connor wrote that diversity served a compelling interest in

TABLE PCA-1 Underrepresented Minority Matriculants to U.S. Medical Schools, 1995–2001

State	1995	2001	Change	% Change
California	179	126	−53	−29.6
Louisiana	46	35	−11	−23.9
Mississippi	14	5	−9	−64.3
Texas	218	181	−37	−17.0
Washington	14	6	−8	−57.1
All other states	1,554	1,433	−121	−7.8
Total	2,025	1,786	−239	−11.8

SOURCE: Cohen, 2003.

higher education, thereby enabling the school to continue taking race and ethnicity into account. Avoiding the use of quotas, the Court ruled that the school may take steps to "narrowly tailor" its admissions program. In *Gratz v. Bollinger,* the Court's 6-3 vote struck down the affirmative action policy for undergraduate admissions, which awarded points related to ethnic background on an admissions rating scale. With these rulings, the Supreme Court recognized the value of diversity in higher education and preserved the ability to consider race as a factor in admissions decisions.

Although the Supreme Court's ruling is a victory for those committed to success in this area, it does not change the fact that affirmative action is now prohibited in some of the most populous states in the nation. It also does not change the fact that bans already in effect for several large and prominent public higher education systems have contributed substantially to the decline in the enrollment of minority students in U.S. medical schools. Further challenges to affirmative action appear likely; if enacted, these can be expected to have similar effects.

Ramifications and Implications of Affirmative Action Bans

It has been estimated that if affirmative action is prohibited nationally, the number of minority medical students will decrease from 10 percent to fewer than 3 percent (Cohen, 2003). Should this occur, the effect would be less diverse student populations and diminished ability for students to learn in an environment that increases cultural competence and promotes understanding and tolerance of individuals with different backgrounds and opinions. This change would decrease the diversity of future faculty, thereby decreasing the minority representation among those involved in research, teaching, and future leadership of health sciences schools, physician groups, and clinics and medical centers. The applicant pools for these professions will again shrink as prohibitions against race-conscious admissions impact access to undergraduate higher education. Outreach programs and efforts targeted at segments of the population historically underrepresented in the sciences and health professions will be jeopardized, and highly successful programs such as the Robert Wood Johnson Medical Minority Education Program would likely decrease or cease to exist. Scholarship programs to address the financial needs of minority students also could be ruled illegal.

The Small Size of the Applicant Pool

Although affirmative action policies have provided a mechanism by which higher educational institutions can—or could—pursue diversity initiatives, the small size of the minority applicant pool in the health professions is a persistent challenge. By its nature, medical education in the United States is a graduate educational program. A requirement for all applicants is completion of the necessary premedical requirements, which for most prospective applicants means earning an undergraduate college degree. A review of the output of all U.S. undergraduate institutions shows that the likelihood that a person 18 years or older will obtain a college degree is 82 percent for whites, yet only 6.9 percent for African Americans and 4.5 percent for Hispanics (U.S. Department of Education, 2000). The admissions process at the nation's most selective colleges and universities yields a class composed of 69.8 percent white students but only 6.3 percent African Americans and 5.5 percent Hispanics (IPEDS, 1999). These long-standing disparities in educational opportunity and achievement ensure that many of the nation's poor and minority students will disproportionately fail to achieve entrance to medical school in proportion to their representation in society.

The term "underrepresented minority" (URM) has been used by the AAMC since the early 1970s to define minority groups excluded from participation in the medical profession through societal discriminatory practices. To date, the four groups recognized as URMs include African Americans or blacks, Mexican Americans, Native Americans (American Indians, Alaskan Natives, and native Hawaiians), and mainland Puerto Ricans. Changes in the racial and ethnic demography of the United States over the past three decades have motivated the AAMC to look again at this definition. Because eligibility for participation in minority enrichment programs sponsored by the AAMC is tied to this definition, alternative guidelines have been established by the federal government that define how race and ethnicity information is collected. Concern about the admissions practices of medical schools created by recent attacks on affirmative action increases the urgency for a new definition.

DHHS recognizes underrepresented minorities as "racial and ethnic populations that are underrepresented in the health profession relative to the number of individuals who are members of the population involved" (42 U.S.C. 295). Adoption of this definition would acknowledge the substantial demographic changes that have occurred and the lack of significant progress in the integration of these groups in medical education. If approved, the AAMC could then establish targeted enrichment programs and promote affirmative action admissions programs designed to fully integrate these groups in the medical profession.

Persistent Socioeconomic and Educational Inequities

Although the Civil Rights movement of the 1960s and 1970s outlawed overt barriers to admission, it did not rectify the legacy of discrimination that persists. Major obstacles remain for students living in homes and communities with high rates of poverty. These students lack access not only to quality educational programs but also to advanced placement programs, college-level courses, quality advising, role models, and mentors. Students whose parents have lower levels of educational achievement, who live in low-income households, or who are exposed to violence and racism in the community face increased challenges in reaching their full potential. Exclusion from educational and professional opportunities experienced over several generations persists because there are fewer well-trained teachers in rural and inner city public schools than in middle- and upper class communities. The stereotype of lower expectations for minority students by teachers and other adults also has negative self-fulfilling effects for those who do not believe in their own potential. This widespread lack of support for disadvantaged students who wish to excel makes peer pressure to join gangs, use drugs, and drop out of school a frequent choice for many students living in America's inner cities and poorest communities.

Inadequate Advising

While inequities in educational opportunities for many URM students contribute to the small size of the health professions applicant pool, inadequate advising creates other less obvious dilemmas even for those students who go on to college with an interest in the health sciences. Students who experience academic difficulty in science and nonscience courses during their first year of college often seek help from premedical advisors at a critical stage in their education. While some receive the advice they need to pursue their goals, others are discouraged from a career in medicine or science on the basis of grades received in one or two courses. Turnover among health sciences advisors creates further challenges in ensuring that all students have access to reliable information about admissions and the full range of resources that are available to help them (UCOP, 2000).

Data provided by the AAMC to the University of California's Medical Student Diversity Task Force in 2000, for example, suggest that California undergraduate health sciences majors enter college in a ratio of three non-URM students to one URM student. The UC task force examined these data and found that the differences and changes in the sizes of these groups during the college years were substantial. The final report of the task force stated that if "attention is focused on those freshmen health science majors who score well on the Scholastic Aptitude Test (SAT), the picture becomes more encouraging. Among this group, the 'attrition rate' of URM health sciences majors is about the same as for non-URM students. And, if acceptance to medical school is taken as the end point, these URM students do slightly better. It is therefore particularly noteworthy that among the pool of URM students that enter college with an interest in a health career, the majority who change career goals do so during (or shortly after) their freshman year" (UCOP, 2000, p. 27).

Because URM students are less likely than their majority peers to have role models in the health professions and a support system that encourages their educational interests, access to quality advising services is essential. Improved quality and consistency of premedical advising is thus a viable mechanism for encouraging those students with interest to continue and for providing students with access to resources that will enhance their preparation.

THE ADMISSIONS PROCESS

The goal of the admissions process is to identify candidates who will be successful in their individual careers and collective contributions as future clinicians, teachers, researchers, and leaders. For committees making these choices, the challenge is to select an entering class that reflects the mission of the school and is capable of outstanding performance and future success. The process typically involves the review of applications from thousands of students who are competing for admission to an average entering class of 90 to 140 students. For any given school, a look at its mission and mission statement and in-depth review of the actual process and factors that are valued for admission will provide a strong indication of its commitment to diversity. The composition of admissions committees and the orientation provided to members about the value of diversity will influence the choices made about whom to admit. Then, in turn, tangible evidence of diversity on campus—or the lack thereof—will influence the choices made by students about where to enroll.

Medical School Missions and Mission Statements

The mission of a medical school is a statement of purpose. Because each school has its own history and set of institutional values, the missions of U.S. schools vary considerably. At any given school, however, its mission shapes the role of that institution in the educational community. It often drives the admissions process to identify and accept applicants who reflect its values and will embrace its educational goals and contribute to the desired learning environment. The mission will impact curricular design to enhance the likelihood that a student will learn concepts and participate in professional activities, such as research, public service, teaching, and advocacy, that reflect the school's core values. The net effect tends to be the graduation of students whose careers are influenced by the faculty from whom they learn and whose choices of professional activities are transformed through their educational experiences.

Choosing Students

Although the predominant major of medical school applicants is still in the biologic sciences, this is not required nor is it necessarily ideal. Data from the AAMC show, for example, that English majors achieve the highest scores on the biological science section of the MCAT. The AAMC's Medical School Admissions Requirement indicates that schools are responding to these and other findings by focusing on the personal attributes of students in their admissions decisions. Most committees use some mechanism to assess the qualifications of each applicant's academic preparation, aptitude for science, enthusiasm for learning, evidence of outstanding interpersonal and communication skills, and motivation for a career in medicine. The details of the selection process, however, and the weight and value assigned to particular academic and nonacademic factors vary widely across schools; these, in turn, affect the diversity of students admitted.

Role and Relevance of Grades and MCAT Scores

There is ample evidence that undergraduate science GPA and MCAT scores are predictors of grades and performance on standardized tests during medical school. The individual MCAT scores and the undergraduate GPA in science and nonscience courses contribute something unique to the prediction of medical school grades, and the combination is more powerful than either alone. Results of the MCAT are also good predictors of test scores on the United States Medical Licensing Exam (USMLE); by contrast, the GPA adds little additional predictive value (Julian, 2000). Despite this evidence, a base multiple regression model considering gender, URM status, science GPA, and MCAT scores in physical sciences and biological sciences explained only 29.1 percent of the variation in USMLE Step 1 test scores (Basco et al., 2002). Most variation in standardized test scores is not predicted by either demographic information or traditional measures of academic performance; grades in the clinical years are least well predicted by either MCATs or GPAs.

Medical schools also consider potential variables that suggest that a student may encounter academic difficulty—traditionally defined as withdrawal from school, a nonmedical leave of absence, dismissal, or delay of graduation date. Most studies have found that an increased risk of encountering academic difficulty is associated with low MCAT scores (particularly biological sciences scores), low science GPAs, low selectivity of the undergraduate institution, female gender, being an URM member, or older age. The majority of students who experience academic difficulty, however, eventually graduate from medical school, and the risk and timing of these episodes has been found to vary among the different groups of students studied (Huff and Fang, 1999).

Standardized test results and grades are thus useful but not exceptional or unique predictors of medical school performance. They are designed and validated by their ability to predict future test scores. GPAs and MCAT scores are not useful in predicting clinical performance, even when adjusting for the students' undergraduate institution (Silver and Hodgson, 1997). Standardized tests measure already developed skills but not the mastery of a particular curriculum or a student's innate ability. Experiences that are closely tied to an individual's racial and ethnic identity can lower the results of standardized tests independent of socioeconomic status. This outcome is more likely to occur for a minority or other student whose abilities are negatively stereotyped by society; this is particularly true for the student who is deeply invested in achieving good results on a test. This "stereotype threat" may interfere with test performance for any student (or group of students) for whom abilities are negatively stereotyped in the larger society (Steele and Aronson, 1995). Admissions committees that place the greatest weight on standardized test scores limit the opportunities of minority students to participate in the medical profession.

Personal Characteristics

Academic success during the first 2 years of medical school is not, in and of itself, predictive of success in meeting the clinical training and patient care requirements of the third and fourth years of medical school and future practice. To be successful in clinical settings, students must demonstrate an ability to apply what they have learned and communicate and interact effectively with patients, faculty and staff, peers, and others. Good judgment, common sense, maturity, compassion, and professionalism are among the qualities that are expected, valued, and routinely evaluated as part of student performance during the clinical years of medical school and residency training.

Defining the desirable traits of physicians is best accomplished by relying on the measures of professionalism being developed by medical associations and translating them into attributes that can be measured at the time of application to medical school. Such definitions should factor in the health needs of society and the means to create a workforce that will meet those needs. By considering patient care a first priority, physicians are expected to be ethical, honest, and dedicated. In making decisions for their patients, they should be knowledgeable, willing to learn, and able to use newly acquired knowledge to modify their practice to ensure optimal patient care. Not surprisingly, "good doctors" are considered those who relate well to their patients, possess good communication skills, and understand the cultural context in which they deliver medical care (Leahy et al., 2003).

Motivation for the medical profession is assessed through a track record that reflects the desire to positively affect the health care of individuals and communities through public service, cultural activities, educational endeavors, and scholarly activities. Many schools seek evidence of leadership, with awareness and participation in activities that are intended to have a positive influence on others. Competitive applicants will have a record of activities and leadership roles in which they are perceived as innovators in their chosen field, advocates for the communities they serve, and contributors toward a legacy that reflects their creativity and drive.

Attention to Details

Recruitment of a diverse class requires that admissions committees take into account the "distance traveled" by each applicant. Certain characteristics are important to consider, particularly for those students who have not had optimal access to educational opportunities. The following characteristics are among those that merit careful attention.

Parental income, education, and occupation. The lack of role models in the applicant's home and family, or the possibility that they may be the first in their family to achieve a college or professional degree may limit their contact with people who can help them navigate the challenges of higher education.

Precollege education. The quality of teachers, curriculum, and available resources varies tremendously across high school districts and is closely tied to educational outcomes.

Hours worked while attending college. Applicants who made a significant commitment to a part-time job during their undergraduate years to support themselves or their families cannot be expected to have participated in extracurricular activities to the same degree as those applicants without similar obligations.

Cultural barriers. Expected educational outcomes vary among racial and ethnic groups. The applicant may have been subject to an environment in which high levels of educational achievement were neither expected nor valued.

Geographic location or neighborhood where applicant was raised. The location in which a student was raised and attended schools directly affects the number and quality of his or her educational opportunities.

Prior experience with prejudice. Underperformance on standardized tests based on stereotype threat is a frequent outcome for students whose abilities have been persistently questioned or challenged by the society at large.

Special family obligations and other circumstances. Minority students from poor families are frequently asked to contribute to the finances of their household or obliged to provide supervision and assistance to siblings or disabled relatives.

Appointment and Training of Committee Members

Admissions committees consist of individuals, appointed by their schools, to review applications and make determinations about which students they will admit. An admissions dean, and his or her staff, assist committees with this work. In the not-too-distant past, committees were often composed of basic sciences faculty who were (primarily) academically distinguished white men. Over time, the composition of many medical school admissions committees has changed to reflect changes in the curriculum as well as changing expectations of accreditation bodies, graduate medical education programs, and the public. Although most committees now include basic sciences and clinical faculty, alumni, medical students, and residents, the lack of diversity of most medical school faculties is also a characteristic of their admissions committees.

The education and training of admissions committees regarding the value of diversity and the relevance of a diverse health workforce for improving access to health services and reducing health disparities are suspected to vary widely across institutions. Increased awareness by committees of research findings and relevant literature would be appropriate for this purpose. Examples include findings showing that physicians are more likely to treat higher proportions of patients from their own racial and ethnic groups (Keith et al., 1985; Komaromy et al., 1996); minority physicians have higher percentages of patients covered by Medicaid in their practices (Davidson and Montoya, 1987); minority patients who have a regular physician are four times as likely to report care from a minority physician than white patients (Moy et al., 1995); and increased diversity more effectively engages health professionals in a biomedical and public health research agenda that addresses health disparities and other public health needs (Cohen, 2003).

Recruitment Efforts

While the admissions process determines who is admitted to medical school, the small size of the national URM applicant pool creates the situation that many top minority students will receive more than one offer about where to enroll. In making their choices, students will consider a number of factors. The number of minority students and faculty on campus, for example, is an obvious sign of the extent to which an institution supports a culture of diversity. The presence of targeted enrichment and support programs for minority faculty and students also gives a view of the institutional climate and support for diversity. Correspondingly, the absence of a critical mass of minority students and faculty, and the absence of dedicated enrichment and academic support programs, may be deterrents for minority students who have more than one choice about where to enroll. Active recruitment efforts dedicated to welcoming and encouraging admitted students to enroll are a factor in making a final choice for some students.

CLINICAL PSYCHOLOGY, DENTISTRY, AND NURSING

Clinical Psychology

The number of ethnic minority students enrolled in graduate programs in psychology has been increasing steadily over the past two decades. In 2002–2003, 14.3 percent of 39,672 full-time students enrolled in doctoral-level departments of psychology described themselves as black, Hispanic, Native American, or multiethnic; of 6,411 students enrolled in master departments of psychology, the equivalent statistic is 11.3 percent (APA, 2003a). The number of Ph.D. degrees awarded to all ethnic minorities (including Asian students) rose from 6.3 percent in 1978 to 8.1 percent in 1988 to 15.5 percent in 1998 (APA, 2003b). Because psychology is a field in which ethnic minority psychologists make up only 7.5 percent of full-time faculty in graduate departments of psychology and 6 percent of the total, the profile of the profession is that of relatively more ethnic minority psychologists in training than in the profession or academia, a situation parallel to that in medicine.

This growth in minority enrollment has resulted from institutional commitments and recruitment programs started by the professional graduate schools and strong support from professional associations. The American Psychological Association (APA) has had a significant track record of attention to multicultural awareness and competence, recruiting of ethnic minority students, and career guidance, even before the establishment of the APA Office of Ethnic Minority Affairs in 1979. In February 1994, the APA Council of Representatives passed a resolution placing a "high priority on issues related to the education of ethnic minorities. These issues include planning appropriately diverse curricula, promoting psychology as a course of study and career option, as well as recruitment, retention, advising and mentoring students at all levels of education" (Holliday et al., 1997, p. 3). Also in 1994, a Commission on Ethnic Minority Recruitment, Retention and Training in Psychology (CEMRRAT) was established with the aim, among others, to promote an educational pipeline for ethnic minority students. CEMRRAT's Work Group on Student Recruitment and Retention has prepared two booklets to assist ethnic minority students and admissions officers in the application process: *How to Apply to Graduate and Professional Programs in Psychology* and *Minority Student Recruitment Resources Booklet*. A subsequent CEMRRAT task force (CEMRRAT2 TF) has continued this process for the APA.

The ambivalence or resistance of psychology faculty to the need and value of diversity in the student body, faculty, and curriculum is considered a major barrier to effective minority student recruitment and training. In response, the APA has promoted initiatives that provide incentives to psychology programs for ethnic minority recruitment, retention, and graduation activities. These activities include, among others, securing grants to support students in historically black colleges and universities and to establish regional centers of excellence in the recruitment, retention, and training of ethnic minority students. Other activities involve developing publications that address best practices in recruitment and retention of ethnic minority students and recognizing graduate programs in psychology with demonstrated excellence in the recruitment and retention of ethnic minority students through their annual APA Suinn Minority Achievement Awards.

Efforts by individual schools are outlined in *Model Strategies for Ethnic Minority Recruitment, Retention and Training in Higher Education*, which was published in May 2000 by the APA Office of Ethnic Minority Affairs (APA, 2000). This document details 13 model strategies to enhance recruitment and retention of ethnic minority students and faculty. The strategies, based on the assumption that students of color bring an added value to the educational program and institution, range from course development to enrichment programs for undergraduates and mentoring and social or community services for enrolled students. Strategies for admissions officers emphasize the use of a holistic or comprehensive review of applications rather than the setting of thresholds for academic and test performance. Although this report does not highlight programs at all graduate schools, it summarizes well the types of initiatives that are in place.

Finally, the APA has encouraged and supported stronger linkages among institutions with varying missions at different points in the educational pipeline (high schools, community colleges, and 4-year colleges). Characteristic of this support is its provision of funding and technical assistance necessary for encouraging psychology programs to develop multicultural curricula and academic and social climates that are supportive of diversity. These efforts include the dissemination of information related to diversity and multicultural education strategies; outcomes in postsecondary education; and evaluative processes that document the impact of the new initiatives on both the institutional climate and the numbers of ethnic minorities that have participated in the process.

Dentistry

The first report on oral health ever issued by a U.S. Surgeon General reported dramatic improvements in the overall oral health status of Americans and recognized the contributions of the dental profession in making this progress (DHHS, 2000). The report, however, identified major disparities in the oral health status of some populations and disproportionate disease of individuals living in poor and underserved communities. In 2002, the American Dental Education Association (ADEA) appointed a group of national experts to examine the roles and responsibilities of academic dental institutions in improving the oral health of all Americans. The report of the ADEA president's commission, *Improving the Oral Health Status of All Americans: Roles and Responsibilities* (Haden et al., 2003), summarized these disparities and cited data concerning Dental Health Professions Shortage Areas issued by the Health Resources and Services Administration's Bureau of Health Professions. These data show that during the years 1993–2002, the number of designated shortage areas grew from 792 to 1,892 nationally, and more than 40 million Americans reside in these areas (HRSA, 2002b).

The ADEA report concluded with a series of recommendations for improving the oral health of the public, with a focus on meeting the needs of underserved communities. In addition to urging dental schools to monitor workforce needs and increase the cultural competency of all students, the report recognized the importance of increasing the diversity of the workforce as a strategy for meeting the needs of the increasingly diverse public. Expanding outreach programs, identifying best practices for recruiting and retaining URM students and faculty, and reviewing and amending admissions criteria were among the recommendations cited.

Accredited dental education programs in the United States are offered by 56 dental schools. Although the closure of five dental schools between 1986 and 1993 contributed to the 37 percent decline in first-year enrollments that occurred in the 1980s, the opening of three new schools since 1997 enabled the total number of first-year positions to increase from a low of 3,573 in 1989 to an average of 4,100–4,300 during the 1990s (Valachovic et al., 2001; Weaver et al., 2000). During the same period, the total number of applicants to U.S. schools increased nearly 100 percent to a peak of approximately 9,800 in 1997. For the next several years, and despite relatively stable enrollments, the total number of applicants declined.

Although these overall trends apply to total applications and enrollments for all students, it is important to emphasize that trends for URM applicants, defined as black/African American, Hispanic/Latino, and Native American, differ in critical ways. Data reported by the ADEA show that between 1980 and 1999, URM applicants increased slightly from 8 percent to 10.5 percent of total applicants and 10.2 percent of first-year enrollees. A careful look at data for the past decade, however, shows that the number of first-time, first-year URM enrollees in U.S. dental schools declined by 23 percent between 1990 and 1998 (Weaver, 2003). Although the ADEA is pursuing a number of initiatives to increase diversity in U.S. dental schools, it is nevertheless astonishing to note that its December 2000 report stated that among the nation's (then) 55 dental schools, half of all schools had one or no black/African American first-year students, and nearly half had one or no Hispanic/Latino enrollees. Although gains have been made since then, the 2001 nationwide enrollment of 499 URM dental students is a reminder that despite ongoing efforts, total URM enrollments have not increased appreciably in more than a decade.

In 2002, with a goal of improving these numbers, the Robert Wood Johnson Foundation (RWJ) implemented a new grant program entitled "Pipeline, Profession, and Practice: Community Based Dental Education." Through a competitive process, a total of 11 U.S. dental schools were granted approximately $1.5 million per dental school over a 5-year period. In their grant applications, each school identified goals for increasing its URM enrollments. If each school reaches its goals, total URM enrollment would increase by 90 new first-year students—representing a 20 percent increase over the total number of first-year URM students in all U.S. dental schools. The California Endowment is funding California dental schools to conduct the same type of programs; if these schools increase their enrollments to the same extent as those funded by RWJ, the ADEA estimates that total URM dental student enrollment could increase by 25 percent nation-wide.

Through the leadership of the ADEA, foundation partners, and various associations and health professions coalitions, U.S. schools have the opportunity to be active partners in increasing the diversity of their future dental student classes. Like medicine, the track records of individual dental schools vary; schools with poor prior records will require new efforts and institutional commitment if they wish to make change. New York University's College of Dentistry provides a recent example. In fall 1997, the school's entering class of 230 students included only one African American student. Determined to promote change, the recently appointed dean, Dr. Michael Alfano, appointed a committee that made recommendations addressing the need for leadership, increased outreach to students and patients, creation of multiyear partnerships with undergraduate schools, development of recruitment and retention efforts for faculty, and outreach to community leaders requesting their support in encouraging qualified URM students to apply. The majority of the committee's recommendations were implemented, along with others identified by the faculty, dean, and staff. The results of these efforts are reflected in the entering class of 2003, where nine African American students are currently enrolled as first-year students (Personal communication, M. Alfano, New York University, September 2003).

Nursing

The enumeration and examination of the deepening nursing shortage nationwide highlight the need in nursing, as in the other health professions, to increase the diversity of its workforce as it ensures adequate supply. In 2002, the *National Sample of Registered Nurses* revealed that of the estimated 2,694,540 registered nurses (RNs) in the United States in 2000, only 331,428 (12.3 percent) represented racial or ethnic minority groups: 133,041 were African American/black (non-Hispanic); 93,415 were Asian; 54,861 were Hispanic/Latino; and 13,040 were American Indians/Alaskan Natives (HRSA, 2002a). Although the 12.3 percent figure represents an increase from 7 percent in 1980, it is still well below the 30 percent of the general population identified as being from a racial or ethnic minority group.

One solution to correcting this disparity is to prepare a more diverse group of men and women to meet the health-care needs of an increasingly diverse population. The importance of achieving this goal was highlighted in a report prepared by the National Advisory Council on Nurse Education and Practice, which showed that minority nurses, despite their low numbers, are integral to developing and implementing models of care that address the unique needs of minority populations. To do so, however, requires continued efforts in nursing schools and training programs to correct their own lack of diversity. While the minority student population in U.S. nursing schools approaches 26 percent, as compared with 10.5 percent in medical schools and 11 percent in dental schools, 73.5 percent of nursing students in baccalaureate programs are from nonminority backgrounds.

In their efforts to attract and retain minority students, nursing schools face profession-specific challenges in addition to those common to many of the health science professions. Commonly cited reasons why members of minority groups do not pursue nursing range from the public perception of the field (lack of mentors, gender biases, confusion and misunderstanding about nursing practice, and role stereotypes) to economics (costs of training programs, future earnings compared with other health disciplines). The lack of ethnic and gender diversity in nursing faculty further compounds real and perceived difficulties in recruiting qualified minority students.

The variability of the nursing educational programs leading to a degree and licensure poses a particular challenge to consistent and effective minority student recruitment and retention that is unique to nursing. Training to become a practicing RN is accomplished by completing a 3-year diploma program typically administered in hospitals; a 2- to 3-year associate degree usually offered at community colleges; or a 4-year baccalaureate degree offered at senior colleges and universities. Unlike other health professions, which draw generally from a pool of baccalaureate-trained, academically advanced students, many nursing schools draw from a pool of applicants with a wider range of skill and experience to bring to an increasingly demanding regimen of courses and requirements. Even when nursing programs successfully draw a diverse group of applicants through outreach efforts in their local communities, academic disadvantage and inability to master the coursework often lead to failure rates as high as 50 percent.

A national effort to address these challenges is ongoing. In December 2001, the American Association of Colleges of Nursing published *Effective Strategies for Increasing Diversity in Nursing Programs* (AACN, 2001). This report includes a summary of the successful efforts by more than 10 nursing programs in the United States that, through innovative and effective recruitment strategies, measurably improved their student ratios. Examples of strategies in practice include:

• Investment of nursing students in community care programs in the region surrounding the school. Nursing students of diverse backgrounds who train and work in community clinics, local high schools, and health service programs function as both mentors and recruiters to the field of nursing. Such exposure also contributes to students' preparation for practice in a variety of settings.

• Outreach and recruitment in diverse communities. Students inter-

ested in nursing training through diploma and associate degree programs typically enroll in local programs offered in the community college system. Drawing from within the community, those schools in racially diverse regions recruit student populations that reflect regional demographics.
 • Supporting students from within the student population. Peer support of minority students encourages academic success and increases the likelihood of retaining the student within the training program.

In several areas of the country, state legislatures have mandated that health professions schools increase the diversity of their student populations, prompting analysis and change at all points of the educational pipeline. In June 2003, DHHS awarded $3.5 million in grants to support nursing education opportunities for disadvantaged students. Finally, leaders in the nursing education community state a collective awareness of the "need to do better" and continue to share resources and strategies (Personal communication, C. Waltz, University of Maryland, August 28, 2003). Accelerated programs to prepare nurses for practice and further study are increasing in number and scope and student support and mentoring efforts are increasingly the likelihood of success for students enrolling in nursing degree and training programs.

STRATEGIES AND BEST PRACTICES

Attorney Maureen Mahoney of the University of Michigan Law School stated clearly the reason for affirmative action and integration of the school by saying that the state has "a compelling interest in having an institution that is both academically excellent and racially diverse" (University of Michigan, 2003).

Health professions programs committed to increasing the diversity of their future classes must be committed to the principal of diversity and its value; to be successful, schools require strong, active leadership and development of comprehensive strategies addressing both current and future applicants. For individual schools, articulation of a mission statement and cultivation of an institutional culture that supports diversity are essential to creating a foundation on which to base campus policies, practices, and programs to enhance diversity. Carefully tailored admissions strategies, including affirmative action programs where lawful, will increase the likelihood that a school is successful. Attention to the selection and education of admissions committee members, together with careful consideration during the admissions process of factors predictive of academic success *and* supportive of diversity, will contribute to improving admissions outcomes. Recruitment efforts for students already admitted, but not yet enrolled, will also make a difference. Finally, and although not part of the actual admissions process, improved outreach to students, communities, and health professions advisors are among the activities that should be supported by and linked to admissions offices.

This section identifies recommended strategies and best practices for health professions schools seeking to increase and maintain diversity in their classes. While these recommendations are based largely on medicine, similarities exist for many health professions programs, particularly those with substantial basic science prerequisites and standardized tests requirements such as the MCAT. The following suggestions and commentary thus apply broadly across the health professions and may be adapted and tailored to meet various profession-specific needs. Where applicable, distinctions are noted for public institutions subject to legal prohibitions banning the consideration of race or ethnicity as part of the admissions process.

Recommendation: Demonstrate institutional commitment to diversity through strong and active leadership.

University leaders committed to diversity should select deans of their health professions programs with a record of active support in this area. Health professions programs, through their leaders, must support diversity initiatives by making personal statements of support, by cultivating and funding programs that support a culture of diversity on campus, and by recruiting faculty and staff who share this goal.

Stanford University President John Hennessey voiced his support for affirmative action and the need for admissions processes tailored to achieve this goal in these remarks:

> The consideration of race and ethnicity as one factor among many in the admissions process is consistent with our history as an institution and our belief that the next generation of leaders must reflect the strengths and talents of all our nation's citizens. . . . We remain committed to affirmative action, to the importance of diversity broadly defined, and to the principles set forth in the Supreme Court's 1978 decision in the *Bakke* case as practical and appropriate means to achieve such diversity (Hennessey, 2003).

Public health professions schools in states where race-conscious admissions policies have been forbidden are unable to use race-conscious affirmative action programs to achieve a diverse student body. For these schools, strong and active leadership is even more critical. In his farewell remarks to the University of California's board of regents on September 18, 2003, President Richard C. Atkinson discussed his commitment to diversity and concern for the future: "I came into office just after The Regents approved Resolution SP-1 and as voters were preparing to approve Proposition 209, forbidding the consideration of race and ethnicity in university admissions, among other things. I continue to believe those were the wrong decisions. As I wrote in *The Washington Post* not long ago, 'We have pursued both excellence and diversity because we believe they are inextricably linked, and because we know that an institution that ignores either of them runs the risk of becoming irrelevant in a state with the knowledge-based economy and tremendously varied population of California.'"

Recommendation: Develop mission statements that reflect institutional commitment to diversity.

Health professions programs committed to increasing the diversity of their faculty and students must adopt mission statements that explicitly support the goal of campus diversity. From such statements of purpose, admissions policies, educational programs, and practices of individual schools should be developed and aligned to support this goal.

Recommendation: Select "well-rounded" students by evaluating both academic factors and personal attributes within the context of the "distance traveled" by the applicant.

Admissions committees should evaluate academic and nonacademic factors with a goal of selecting bright and multidimensional individuals. This effort should include a definition of "ideal candidates" for admission, the factors to be assessed, and the delineation of an admissions process that is consistent with institutional goals and desired outcomes. The process should be developed with outcomes in mind and should be consistent and reproducible. At each step of the admissions process, careful consideration and attention should be given to "the distance traveled by the applicant."

Ideal candidates will have completed a broad undergraduate education, satisfied medical school science requirements, and excelled in the other coursework. They also, through their experiences, will have demonstrated leadership, teamwork, compassion, altruism, friendliness, and interest in their neighbors and communities.

Recommendation: Ensure that admissions committees understand the role and relevance of grades and test scores in predicting future success in clinical settings.

The admissions process is inherently prone to bias that may disfavor disadvantaged and minority students by the "ease" of measuring variables related to knowledge (grades and MCAT scores) and the "difficulty" inherent in assessing the personal attributes that make an applicant particularly well suited for admission.

It is important to note that aptitude tests such as the SAT or the MCAT were not designed as tools to evaluate a specific curriculum nor do they measure students' aptitude in subjects they intend to study. Rather, they are predictors of performance in subsequent standardized tests. There have been attempts to create an admissions process that does not consider the MCAT scores, which present a large hurdle for many otherwise qualified applicants. As an example, the Texas A&M College of Medicine program called Partnerships for Primary Care encourages applicants to medical school who are likely to practice primary care medicine in underserved areas of Texas. Eligible applicants must earn the equivalent of a GPA of 3.50 on a 4.00 scale; be predicted to graduate in the top 10 percent of their class; achieve a minimum of 1200 on the SAT or 26 on the ACT; have a legal residence in a rural or underserved area, or health profession shortage area as defined by the Health Professions Resource Center, Texas Department of Health; be a U.S. citizen or permanent resident; be a resident of the state of Texas; and commit to attend one of the seven partner universities in the Texas A&M University system. College students need to maintain a 3.50 GPA on a 4.00 scale annually and complete the required medical school prerequisite courses with no grade below a "C." They must also remain in good standing at all times, participate in community service and medically related activities, demonstrate leadership, and complete a baccalaureate degree within a standard acceptable time frame (usually four years).

Based on these performance criteria, the student is guaranteed a position at Texas A&M College of Medicine. There is no requirement for the MCAT in this program. Its purpose is to eliminate the MCAT as a hurdle for medical school candidates who live in underserved areas. These applicants are more likely to be a member of a minority group and more likely to return to underserved areas to practice, both important educational goals for the school and the state. Since the program's inception, this and other race-neutral measures have increased the number of minority students in their entering classes in the post-*Hopwood* era to levels that exceed those prior to 1996. Further details are available at the Texas A&M College of Medicine website, http://medicine.tamu.edu/studentaffairs/pcc01.htm.

Although there have been other proposals to ignore the results of standardized tests in the medical school admissions process, the frequent use of tests for institutional accreditation and professional licensure makes such changes unlikely unless national credentialing systems change drastically.

For schools prohibited from the use of affirmative action, a series of race-neutral alternatives for admissions and the granting of financial aid have been proposed to enhance diversity. Virtually all of these use another variable or set(s) of variables to define a group that will yield a diverse group of students but that is not determined by race. One such approach is to use class-conscious, rather than race-conscious, affirmative action. Many schools already give consideration to economic hardship and poverty as well as race. These models provide short-term solutions to enhancing diversity by race-neutral means, yet they provide only a partial solution with several adverse effects. Although minority families are more likely to be among the poorest Americans than the richest, socioeconomic hardship is an inefficient route to integration if racial and ethnic diversity is the ultimate goal. Middle-class and upper class minorities who have not had significant economic disadvantages would not be considered under this approach, yet they may be among the strongest candidates for success in medical school. Ultimately, these models are flawed in that they depend on the effects of disparities in educational opportunities, the core objective of which is ostensibly to end such disparity.

A preferred admissions approach is to use standardized test results as a dichotomous variable and to decide on a threshold value below which a student is not believed to be competitive for admission to medical school and above which factors other than the test scores will determine eligibility for school. With such an approach, the initial screen will be strongly weighted by standardized test scores, but the ultimate decision will rest on other measures of knowledge, skills, and personal qualities. Students who have performed well in college and have acquired the skills and attitudes that will serve them well in medicine will have a strong chance of acceptance to medical school, even in the presence of less than stellar MCAT scores.

Schools that have adopted this approach find and accept candidates whose performance in college is exceptional and have a track record of activities that reflect the expectations derived from the mission of the school, even though the MCAT scores of those students are not in the highest percentile. Because many URM students may find themselves in this group, an environment that recognizes their strengths and supports them through the future testing requirements by teaching test-taking and other skills is most likely to help students succeed.

Recommendation: Ensure that careful assessment of personal qualities is a priority consideration for each candidate.

Evaluating students on their personal qualities and their acquisition of skills useful in the medical profession necessitates a method to categorize these variables and determine their relative value. This method should be consistent with the mission of the school and the expectations derived from that mission. Research-intensive medical schools should look for a track record of and a desire to continue productive and creative scholarly activities. Public-service-oriented schools will look for evidence of participation in activities intended to improve the health of needy communities and an indication of leadership and innovative approaches to service. Schools with missions to serve specific communities—described in religious, geographic, or racial/ethnic terms—will look for evidence of prior and future service to these communities. The decision by the University of California-Irvine College of Medicine to develop a program dedicated to improving the health of the Latino community in California is a good example. This newly proposed program seeks to identify and recruit talented students with Spanish-language ability and a prior record of service to the Latino community—both race-neutral variables that are likely to enrich the applicant pool and ultimately their entering classes.

Many schools will find that their missions encompass research, teaching, public service, or other particular goal. Development of an evaluation process that will assess each goal will increase the likelihood that the admissions process will achieve its intended result for each campus. Creating evaluation forms for each major goal helps to categorize these elements in the admissions process. In one model currently used by a California medical school, the knowledge assessment form evaluates the results of the MCATs and the GPA as well as the actual transcript to assess academic trends. Another form allows the educational context or "distance traveled" to be studied and actual performance to be adjusted. In some schools, each file reviewer and interviewer is asked to evaluate the elements of the distance traveled so that each evaluator may place the applicant's accomplishments in context. The skill assessment form evaluates the "tools set" that the student has acquired in his or her extracurricular activities and how these skills will help the student's career.

Value is given to depth of study and achievement rather than superficial sampling, accomplishments rather than future plans, and demonstrated ability rather than aptitude. The attitude assessment form depends on the description in the letters of recommendation about each candidate's determination, dedication, and desire to learn and serve. Sample forms that rate these elements are enclosed in this paper and are currently used by one school.

Using summary forms that are devoid of grades and test scores is labor intensive and requires a large cadre of well-motivated and trained volunteer faculty and students. However, analyzing and ranking the personal attributes of the candidates and how the candidate's knowledge, character, and accomplishments fit the mission of the school are vital for selecting a diverse class. The executive admissions committee at one school ultimately will make a decision based on two simple questions:

1. How will this candidate contribute to and benefit from your medical school?
2. Will accepting this candidate be in keeping with the mission of your medical school?

Other schools use similar questions, including an assessment of the extent to which an applicant is predicted to be a leader and to contribute substantially to his or her community. The institution that embraces the diversity of the student body as a significant educational goal and the diversity and cultural competence of the medical workforce as an important societal goal will value a process that yields a class that embraces these values. The process will define excellent academic preparation as necessary but not sufficient for a successful career and will value those qualities that give the future physician the right "toolbox" for future success.

> **Recommendation: Appoint admissions committee members who reflect the diversity that is sought in the student body.**

Medical schools have different systems for appointing faculty to serve on their admissions committees. Some schools recruit faculty volunteers, others rely on candidates appointed by their department chairs; many use a blend of these approaches. Committee members should include a diverse group of individuals who share a clear understanding of the mission of the school, its societal commitment, and how these missions are reflected in the admissions process. They should be willing to embrace the core values of the institution, evaluate candidates for admission with those values in mind, and appreciate how their own biases may affect their admissions recommendations.

> **Recommendation: Educate committee members about societal health needs and the role of a diverse health workforce in meeting those needs**

Ongoing support and education of committee members should be provided in a variety of areas. This should include provision of an orientation manual that explains the admissions process and desired outcomes in detail with illustrations, case studies, and simulated admissions exercises. Awareness of public health needs and familiarity with predictors of good performance, the educational context, stereotype threat, and other challenges of minority and disadvantaged applicants are necessary for faculty to understand fully the nature of their task. The expanded minority admissions exercise developed by the AAMC includes case studies that allow faculty to practice and score their performance. An updated version is currently under development.

> **Recommendation: Actively recruit disadvantaged and minority students who have been accepted but have yet to enroll.**

For many medical students, the final step in the admissions process is based on personal choice. For students receiving offers of admission from more than one medical school, a number of factors are considered before making a final choice. Data provided by the AAMC indicate that among first-year URM students admitted to at least one California medical school in the fall of 1998, more than 95 percent received more than one offer.

Although the factor(s) considered most important by an individual student may differ, most students consistently identify the following as among the most important: academic reputation of the school, anticipated costs of attendance, financial aid offered, location of the school (e.g., urban versus suburban or rural settings), and diversity of the student body, faculty, and surrounding community.

Recruitment efforts for students already admitted involve simultaneously putting the school's "best face" forward and providing an honest assessment of the learning climate and institutional culture on campus. At some schools, this is likely to occur during the interview process itself, with seasoned interviewers recognizing the opportunity to begin recruiting their applicants as soon as they have identified them as highly desirable. Often, this project involves the faculty, students, and staff of the school, all of whom are stakeholders in creating an ideal learning climate that is both excellent and diverse. Different approaches are used, but typical strategies include pairing current students with an accepted applicant to maintain communications and answer questions and inviting accepted applicants to a preview weekend when the school can optimally display its learning climate and diverse community. It is important to note, however, that most applicants will assess the school's commitment to diversity by looking at the numbers of minority students and faculty and the quality of enrichment and support programs in place and by considering the mission and goals of the institution.

Recommendation: Develop educational programs that allow disadvantaged and minority students to succeed.

Successful in this regard are early matriculation programs that allow students who have had little exposure to research to establish a relationship with a research mentor, develop skills for research endeavors, and learn leadership skills. One of these programs (the Stanford Early Matriculation Program) has been shown to enhance the likelihood that a minority medical student will have a competitive research grant funded (from 42 percent to 65 percent), that a minority student will publish a manuscript in a peer-reviewed journal (from 16 percent to 22 percent), and that a minority student will graduate from medical school (from 90 percent to 98 percent).

Students who enter medical schools with limited prior educational opportunities may have had limited didactic preparation in upper level science courses. These students benefit greatly from schools that provide an environment in which learning skills are assessed and taught, the option to take required courses ahead of schedule is available, and the flexibility to decelerate their coursework is permissible to allow mastery of the curriculum at their own pace. It is important for all medical schools to allow all students to succeed, and this requires the need to accommodate varying levels of achievement and different learning styles.

Medical schools should enhance the ability of their students to choose from all careers in medicine to determine those that best fit their skills and interests. Research-intensive medical schools should create an educational environment that encourages participation in scholarly activities, ensures mentorship by faculty, stimulates interest in academic medicine, and enables the student to develop the skills necessary for a career as an educator and researcher. Public-service-oriented schools should teach students how to translate new medical knowledge into effective medical care to all citizens in the community. Faculty should be encouraged to lead by example in teaching students to deliver culturally respectful and competent care to all patients and to work toward reducing the disparities in health status that exist.

Recommendation: Establish and maintain outreach programs to increase student interest in the health professions and their eligibility for admission.

Many schools have programs that span the educational pipeline, beginning in elementary school and continuing through high school, into college, and beyond. Successful programs should include efforts to provide information to prospective applicants and be tailored appropriately to various educational levels. Medical, dental, and other health professions schools should send representatives to other campuses and undergraduate institutions as well as to community forums and fairs that hold informational sessions for prospective applicants, making special efforts to reach disadvantaged and underrepresented students. These efforts will help to ensure that students identify a health professions career as an option and that they have access to reliable information when preparing for and applying to medical school.

For students who apply, but are not initially accepted, many medical schools and some dental schools offer postbaccalaureate programs to help students prepare and reapply. These programs are available to students who seek to improve their application; some are available to those making a career change. These programs typically offer programs that can be adjusted to meet the needs of individual students; most, however, offer MCAT (or other standardized test) preparation, additional science coursework, and support with the application process for disadvantaged students who are reapplying. Many postbaccalaureate programs have had highly successful records in helping promising young students gain admission. Health professions schools that do not offer a postbaccalaureate program should consider creating a program or partnering with a school that has an existing program with a record of success.

Recommendation: Improve and maintain active partnerships with undergraduate health sciences advisors.

The academic and personal advising that many students receive in high school and college plays an influential role in building confidence and in determining whether many students will go on to apply to medical or health professions programs. For those experiencing academic difficulties at an early stage, tutoring and advising by knowledgeable teachers or advisors often make the critical difference in developing the skills and confidence needed for success. Many students believe that science grades are the exclusive or primary factor considered in the admissions process. As a result, poor grades or difficulty with an introductory undergraduate course such as inorganic chemistry or physics may deter an otherwise promising undergraduate from giving further consideration to the health sciences as an educational option. For students with relatively poor high school preparation, such as those entering college with few opportunities to have taken advanced placement courses, these perceptions can play a powerful role at an early stage in their decision making relative to a future career in medicine.

REFERENCES

AACN (American Association of Colleges of Nursing). 2001. *Effective Strategies for Increasing Diversity in Nursing Programs*. [Online]. Available: http://www.aacn.nche.edu/Publications/issues/dec01.htm [accessed August 26, 2003].

AACOM (American Association of Colleges of Osteopathic Medicine). 2003. *AACOMAS Update*. [Online]. Available: http://www.aacom.org/data/advisorupdate/ [accessed August 21, 2003].

AAMC (Association of American Medical Colleges). 1970. *Report of the Association of American Medical Colleges Task Force to the Inter-Association Committee on Expanding Educational Opportunities in Medicine for Blacks and Other Minority Students*, April 22, 1970. Washington, DC: AAMC.

AAMC. 1998. *Report I. Learning Objectives for Medical Education: Guidelines for Medical Schools*. Washington, DC: Medical School Objectives Project.

AAMC. 2000. *Minority Graduates of U.S. Medical Schools: Trends, 1950–1998*. Washington, DC: Association of American Medical Colleges.

AAMC. 2003. *Medical School Profile System*. [Online]. Available: http://services.aamc.org/msps/report.cfm [accessed August 21, 2003].

APA (American Psychological Association). 2000. *Model Strategies for Ethnic Minority Recruitment, Retention and Training in Higher Education*. Washington, DC: APA Office of Ethnic Minority Affairs.

APA. 2003a. 2004 Graduate Study in Psychology, Research Office, APA. Washington, DC: American Psychological Association.

APA. 2003b. *Summary Report: Doctorate Recipients from United States Universities* (selected years). Washington, DC: APA Research Office.

Basco WT Jr., Way DP, Gilbert GE, Hudson A. 2002. Undergraduate institutional MCAT scores as predictors of USMLE Step 1 performance. *Academic Medicine* 77:S13–S16.

BHPR (Bureau of Health Professions). 2003. *Health Professional Shortage Areas: Shortage Designation.* Health Resources and Services Administration. [Online]. Available: http://bhpr.hrsa.gov/shortage/index.htm [accessed August 21, 2003].

Callahan D. 1996. The goals of medicine: Setting new priorities. *The Hastings Center Report* 26:S1-S27.

CMS (Centers for Medicare & Medicaid Services). 2003. *Highlights—National Health Expenditures, 2001.* [Online]. Available: http://cms.hhs.gov/statistics/nhe/ [accessed August 20, 2003].

Cohen JJ. 2003. The consequences of premature abandonment of affirmative action in medical school admissions. *Journal of the American Medical Association* 289:1143–1149.

Davidson RC, Montoya R. 1987. The distribution of medical services to the underserved: A comparison of majority and minority medical graduates in California. *Western Journal of Medicine* 146:114–117.

DHHS (Department of Health and Human Services). 1985. *Health, United States, 1983 and Prevention Profile.* Publication number (PHS) 84-1232. Pp. 1–256. [Online]. Available: http://www.cdc.gov/nchs/data/hus/hus83acc.pdf [accessed July 13, 2003].

DHHS (Department of Health and Human Services). 2000. *Oral Health in America: A Report of the Surgeon General.* Rockville, MD: U.S. Department of Health and Human Services, National Institute of Dental and Craniofacial Research, National Institutes of Health. Pp. 1–332.

Grumbach K, Coffman J, Liu R, Mertz E. 1999. *Strategies for Increasing Physician Supply in Medically Underserved Communities in California.* San Francisco: University of California, California Policy Research Center.

Haden NK, Catalanotto FA, Alexander CJ et al. 2003. *Improving the Oral Health Status of All Americans: Roles and Responsibilities of Academic Dental Institutions. The Report of the ADEA President's Commission.* Washington, DC: American Dental Education Association. Pp. 1–22.

Hennessey J. 2003. Statement on Affirmative Action. Meeting of the Stanford University Faculty Senate, Stanford, CA, January 23, 2003.

Holliday BG et al. 1997. *Visions and Transformations: The Final Report.* American Psychological Association, Washington, DC, January 1997. [Online]. Available: http://www.apa.org/pi/oema/visions/resolution.html [accessed December 16, 2003].

HRSA (Health Resources and Services Administration). 2002a. *The Registered Nurse Population: March 2000. Findings from the National Sample Survey of Registered Nurses.* Washington, DC: Bureau of Health Professions, Division of Nursing. Pp. 1–125.

HRSA (Health Resources and Services Administration). 2002b. *Shortage Designation Branch, Bureau of Health Professions.* [Online]. Available: http://bphc.hrsa.gov/databases/newhpsa/newhpsa.cfm [accessed November 26, 2002].

Huff KL, Fang D. 1999. When are students most at risk of encountering academic difficulty? A study of 1992 matriculants to U.S. medical schools. *Academic Medicine* 74:454–460.

IPEDS. 1999. *1997 Fall Enrollment.* Barron's Profiles of American Colleges.

Julian E. 2000. The predictive ability of the Medical College Admissions Test. *Contemporary Issues in Medical Education* 3(2):1–2.

Keith SN, Bell RN, Swanson AG, Williams AP. 1985. Effects of affirmative action in medical schools: A study of the class of 1975. *New England Journal of Medicine* 313:1519–1525.

KFF (Kaiser Family Foundation). 2002. *Underinsured in America: Is Health Coverage Adequate?* Menlo Park, CA: Kaiser Commission on Medicaid and the Uninsured.

Komaromy M, Grumbach K, Drake M, Vranizan K, Lurie N, Keane D, Bindman AB. 1996. The role of black and Hispanic physicians in providing health care for underserved populations. *New England Journal of Medicine* 334:1305–1310.

Leahy M, Cullen W, Bury G. 2003. "What makes a good doctor?" A cross sectional survey of public opinion. *Irish Medical Journal* 96(2):38–41.

MedPAC (Medicare Payment Advisory Commission). 1998. *Rethinking Medicare's Payment Policies for Graduate Medical Education and Teaching Hospitals.* Report to the Congress. Washington, DC: Medicare Payment Advisory Commission. Pp. 1–19.

Mills R. 2002, September 30. Health insurance coverage: 2001. *Current Population Reports.* Washington, DC: U.S. Census Bureau, U.S. Department of Commerce, Economics and Statistic Administration. Pp. 1–24.

Moy E, Bartman BA, Weir MR. 1995. Access to hypertensive care. *Archives of Internal Medicine* 155:1497–1502.

Powell L. 1978. *Bakke,* 438 U.S. at 312–13 n.48.

Shea S, Fullilove M. 1985. Entry of blacks and other medical students into U.S. medical schools: Historical perspective and recent trends. *New England Journal of Medicine* 313:933–940.

Silver B, Hodgson CS. 1997. Evaluating GPAs and MCAT scores as predictors of NBME I and clerkship performances based on students' data from one undergraduate institution. *Academic Medicine* 72:394–396.

Steele CM, Aronson J. 1995. Stereotype threat and the intellectual test performance of African Americans. *Journal of Personality and Social Psychology* 69:797–811.

UCOP (University of California Office of the President). 2000. *Special Report on Medical Student Diversity.* Medical Student Diversity Task Force, Office of Health Affairs, University of California. Oakland, CA: UCOP. Pp. 1–75.

University of Michigan. 2003. University Record. [Online]. Available: http:/www.umich.edu/ ~urecord/0203/June16_03/19_mahoney.shtml [accessed June 23, 2003].

U.S. Census Bureau. 1999. *U.S. Population by Race: 1980, 2000, and 2020.* U.S. Population Trends. [Online]. Available: http://www.census.gov/mso/www/pres_lib/poptrnd/ sld023.htm [accessed August 21, 2003].

U.S. Census Bureau. 2003. *Population Briefing: National Population Estimates for July 21, 2002.* [Online]. Available: http://eire.census.gov/popest/data/national/popbriefing.php [accessed August 21, 2003].

U.S. Department of Education. 2000. National Center for Education Statistics. [Online]. Available: http://nces.ed.gov/ [accessed August 21, 2003].

Valachovic RW, Weaver RG, Sinkford JC, Haden NK. 2001. Trends in dentistry and dental education. *Journal of Dental Education* 65(6):539–563.

Weaver RG. 2003. *Priming the Pipeline II: Recruiting Dental Professionals for the Future.* Presentation to the National Dental Association's 2003 Minority Faculty and Administrators' Forum. New Orleans, August 1, 2003.

Weaver RG, Haden NK, Valachovic RW. 2000. U.S. dental school applicants and enrollees: A ten-year perspective. *Journal of Dental Education* 64:867–868.

APPENDIX TO COMMISSIONED PAPER A

DISADVANTAGED STATUS EVALUATION FORM

This form is included in the folders of applicants who consider themselves disadvantaged according to the following American Medical College Application Service (AMCAS) question: "Do you wish to be considered a disadvantaged applicant by any of your designated medical schools which may consider such factors (social, economic, or educational)?"

APPLICANT'S NAME: _____

Average parental education *(See AMCAS "Parent Information" Section— Pg. 2):*
  1 Elementary school or less
  2 High school
  3 Some college, no degree (Q: fix vertical alignment)
  4 College, advance degree (Q: advanced?)

Parental occupation (Please fill in):

Geographic location where applicant was raised *(See AMCAS "Bio. Info." Section—Pg. 2):*
Inner City   Rural   Suburban or City

Hours per week applicant worked for self-support during school year *(See AMCAS "Experience" Section—Various Hrs.):*
20 or more   15–20   <15

English is applicant's second language *(See AMCAS "Bio. Info." Section— Pg. 2):*
     Yes   No

Additional factors indicated (e.g., physical handicap, immigrant, experience with prejudice, special family situation/responsibilities, cultural differences)?
(*See AMCAS "Bio." Section for Hardships & Family Income*)

Please list:_____

Please circle which best describes your assessment of this applicant as *Disadvantaged*:

1	2	3	4
Very	Somewhat	Little Evidence of	No Evidence of
Disadvantaged	Disadvantaged	Disadvantaged	Disadvantaged
		Status	Status

2002–2003 ADMISSIONS SEASON – MD FILE REVIEW FORM

Please circle your scores for each category.   **HIGH**   **LOW**

**RESEARCH OR OTHER
SCHOLARLY PROJECTS**   1   2   3   4

(1) In-depth experience with significant productivity (e.g., publication). Evidence of critical independence and outstanding scholarship.

(2) In-depth (>1 year) experience in a single area. Letters suggest above average scholarship and potential as an independent investigator.

(3) Some experience (<1 year), usually in nonindependent or technical capacity. Or, may have short experiences (e.g., in summers) in different fields. May be seen as "industrious, learns techniques quickly," etc., but no suggestion of scholarly independence.

(4) Little (3 months or less) or no experience.

LEADERSHIP   1   2   3   4

(1) Outstanding in all areas. Demonstrated clear evidence of innovative thinking, left a <u>legacy</u> of her/his work.

(2) Held a leadership position <u>of consequence</u>, elected or appointed. <u>Sustained</u> commitment to activities.

(3) Felt to be a strong team player and/or congenial and mature.

(4) Showed up for activities as a member but added little value to them beyond his/her participation (or less).

ORIGINALITY, CREATIVITY   1   2   3   4

(1) Everyone comments on it—unusual accomplishment in science, fine arts, etc.

(2) Comments by more than one person—may have substantial musical, artistic, literary, organizational, etc., talents.

(3) One person comments (usually a research advisor)—no, or little, other evidence for it.

(4) No mention in letters; no evidence in research or otherwise (music, art, organizational talents, etc).

270IN THE NATION'S COMPELLING INTEREST

NONACADEMIC ACCOMPLISHMENTS   1   2   3   4
(includes working)

(1) Outstanding accomplishments (national recognition in sports, artistic endeavors, established business or program, etc.).
(2) Above-average skill/achievement in an extracurricular area (e.g., varsity sports, arts, editor of yearbook, etc.) plus participation in other areas. Heavy work load (>15 hrs/wk) during academic year required for self-support.
(3) Participation in routine extracurricular activities (intramurals, premed club, etc.), routine jobs.
(4) Few, if any, extracurricular activities—routine jobs, few hours.

We interview to confirm that an applicant is outstanding, not just to gain more info. not evident in the Supplemental Application.

1	2	3	4
INTERVIEW	PROBABLY	PROBABLY	DO NOT
(Most impressive	INTERVIEW	DO NOT	INTERVIEW
type of candidate)	*(Interview if*	INTERVIEW	*(Fine person*
	there are not	*(Very good*	*but not*
	500 candid.	*but not*	*competitive*
	in Group 1)	*outstand.)*	*with others)*

Please circle one. Why <u>YOU DO</u> or <u>DO NOT</u> favor an interview? Please explain below.

Indicate specific aspects of the application that an interviewer should clarify during the interview.

INTERVIEW FORM

Name of Candidate:_____ Date of Interview: _____
Undergraduate University:_____Time of Interview: _____
Interviewer:_____Place of Interview: _____

Note: The interview report should provide the Admissions Committee with more information about the candidate's apparent strengths and weaknesses and should supply information that is not evident from the file. It is most important that you give evidence (i.e., SPECIFIC DETAILS OF YOUR

CONVERSATION) *rather than mere impressions. We request that you address at least the following issues in your interview:*

1) Does your interaction with the candidate conform to expectations derived from reading the application? If not, what are the discrepancies, re: major commitments, scholarly interests, and long-range goals?

2) In the candidate's research, are you able to determine the motivation, persistence, level of independence—i.e., range from talented technician, to independent execution of a research protocol established by others, or to responsibility for developing an original research proposal and execution thereof? What role did the candidate play in interpretation and reporting of results? Does the candidate have an appreciation of how the results of the research project(s) fit into a larger field of knowledge? What are the candidate's plans for research in the future?

3) Do you think the letters of support fairly represent the candidate?

4) Does the candidate have a lively interest in the world outside of academics and an interest in the welfare of others?

5) Does the candidate have any significant knowledge of our school and how it would benefit him/her in pursuit of stated goals?

6) Has the candidate volunteered any consideration for exploring a career in academic medicine? Do you consider that a career in academic medicine will be likely for this candidate?

7) Do you think the candidate has a reasonable understanding of the positive and the negative aspects of a career in medicine?

8) Please evaluate the educational context of this applicant with respect to high school education; parental income, education, and occupation; hours per week of work during college; geographic location where applicant grew up; prior experiences with prejudice; cultural and language barriers or other special family circumstances.

9) Have you explored answers to questions raised by file reviewers?

10) Do you detect any characteristics that cause you to question the candidate's suitability for a career in medicine or the ability to think logically and critically?

11) Are there specific concerns the candidate may have about our school?

12) Is follow-up necessary by the Admissions Office or Committee? Yes___ No___ (If yes, please specify: e.g., "Solicit further information from Dr. X on candidate's research role," etc.)

13) <u>Summary Statement</u>:
We will only interview the most compelling 8–10 percent of our applicant pool. We will only make an initial offer of acceptance to one-third (1/3) of applicants interviewed. Please rank this applicant with an "X" anywhere along this scale based on your review of the file and your interview. If you interview a random pool of applicants, you should only score 1/3 of your interviewees in the top group.

1   **2**   **3**

1   A must-have candidate, with evidence of independent thinking and creativity, potential for an academic medicine career or leadership role, outstanding depth of education and community service activities, and a contribution to the learning environment and diversity of the school.

2   An excellent candidate who may have an outstanding track record in one or more areas of interest to us but lacks the special qualities of our top applicants.

3   Capable of the intellectual demands of medical school but whose accomplishments and potential for success in scholarly, educational, or service activities are not exceptional.

14) Briefly state the most significant item in this application that resulted in this ranking.

Paper Contribution B
The Role of Public Financing in Improving Diversity in the Health Professions

Karen Matherlee

Public financing of the health professions in the United States is a labyrinth of federal and state initiatives, a maze of both "discretionary" and "mandatory" pathways. This paper follows that labyrinth to examine federal and state health professions programs that affect or encourage the participation of underrepresented minorities (URMs)[1] in certain professions in the health workforce. Responding to the mandate of the Institute of Medicine's (IOM's) "Strategies for Increasing the Racial and Ethnic Diversity of the U.S. Health Care Workforce" project, the paper focuses on four health professions: medicine (allopathic and osteopathic), dentistry (general and pediatric), nursing, and professional psychology (clinical and counseling). In tracing public funding sources, the paper identifies barriers to and opportunities for changing financial incentives in order to expand URM participation in the four health professions.

---

[1]URM, a term established in 1970 by the Association of American Medical Colleges, refers to "the disparity between the proportion of health care providers from certain racial and ethnic groups and their total proportion in the U.S. population" (COGME, 1998). The term, as currently used by the U.S. Department of Health and Human Services, includes "Blacks or African Americans, Hispanics or Latinos, American Indians or Alaska Natives, Native Hawaiians or other Pacific Islanders, and Asian subpopulations (any Asians other than Chinese, Filipino, Japanese, Korean, Asian Indian, or Thai)" (U.S. DHHS, 2003b). Although the AAMC originally used the term to recognize the underrepresentation of certain ethnic groups, it recently revised its definition to refer to underrepresented in medicine: "those racial and ethnic populations that are underrepresented in the medical profession relative to their numbers in the general population" (AAMC Executive Council, June 26, 2003).

"Following the dollars" is a straightforward way of checking out government's commitment to encouraging diversity in the health workforce. For the most part, that means following the dollars that flow to health professions training, with its links to delivery of health services and conduct of biomedical research. However, because of the nature of the payment flows and unevenness of the available data, the dollars are not easy to follow.

On the federal side, funding for health professions programs comes from congressionally authorized and appropriated legislation—labeled "discretionary"—as well as from the "mandatory" Medicare entitlement program. The Department of Health and Human Services (DHHS) and Departments of Defense (DoD) and Veterans Affairs (VA) administer discretionary health professions programs, while DHHS is also responsible for the Medicare graduate medical education (GME) program. Various states spend grant and Medicaid funds on the health professions, while localities provide some support as well. (See Table PCB-1 for an overview of federal and state health professions funding.)

Although precise figures are difficult to obtain, there is a clear consensus in the health care field that minorities are underrepresented in the health professions. For example, according to the 2000 Census, African Americans made up 12.8 percent of the total U.S. population (U.S. Census Bureau, 2001) but, by the end of 2001, accounted for 2.5 percent of physicians in this country (AMA, 2001). Similarly, persons of Hispanic origin made up 11.8 percent of the population, but only 3.4 percent of physicians, and Native Americans were 0.9 percent of the population, but only 0.06 percent of physicians (U.S. Census Bureau, 2001; AMA, 2001). (The American Medical Association indicates, however, that race and ethnicity are unknown for a large number of physicians, so the percentages of URMs are probably higher.) Of dentists, according to data from the end of the 1990s, only 6.8 percent of U.S. dentists were African American, Hispanic, or Native American (Mertz and O'Neil, 2002).

In ferreting out URM participation in the field of nursing, the data also present a challenge. The summary, *The Registered Nurse Population: Findings from the National Sample Survey of Registered Nurses,* issued in March 2000, indicates that approximately 12 percent of the total number of registered nurses (RNs) "came from racial and ethnic minority backgrounds": African American/black (non-Hispanic), Asian, Hispanic/Latino, American Indian/Alaska Native, Native Hawaiian/Other Pacific Islander, and non-Hispanic of two or more races (Spratley et al., 2000).

The document also states that approximately 7.3 percent of the 2,694,540 RNs in the survey could be classified as advanced practitioners: clinical nurse specialists, nurse anesthetists, nurse midwives, and nurse practitioners (Spratley et al., 2000). Although these data do not indicate the percentage of advanced practice nurses from racial and ethnic minority backgrounds (or, more pertinently, those characterized as URMs), they do point to underrepresentation. At the same time, the document notes that "Native Hawaiian and Other Pacific Islander, African American/Black, and white nurses were the racial/ethnic groups with the highest percentages of master's or doctoral degrees" (Spratley et al., 2000).

For professional psychology, the American Psychological Association (APA) has data indicating that "racial and ethnic minority students represented approximately 18 percent of first-year enrollments" in graduate programs in psychology in 1999–2000 (Pate, 2001). Another study reported by the APA—on persons receiving doctorates in psychology and entering the workforce—found that the number of respondents self-reporting as minority rose from 7 percent in 1985 to nearly 15 percent in 1996. Hispanics and Asians made up about 4 percent each, African Americans fewer than 4 percent, and American Indians "or other" 1 percent, with about 1 percent "multiple race or ethnicity" (Kohout et al., 1999).

Although reams have been written on why underrepresentation is a problem, Jordan Cohen, M.D., president of the Association of American Medical Colleges (AAMC), and two AAMC colleagues recently summed up the "practical reasons" for greater health workforce diversity in a few lines: "(1) advancing cultural competency, (2) increasing access to high-quality health services, (3) strengthening the medical research agenda, and (4) ensuring optimal management of the health care system" (Cohen et al., 2002).

FEDERAL HEALTH PROFESSIONS FUNDING SOURCES

Discretionary Funds

Department of Health and Human Services

The Health Resources and Services Administration (HRSA) is the most prominent public funder of health professions programs in which URM participation is a direct goal or a grant factor. When the goal is direct, it is included in the legislation that authorized HRSA to implement the program. When the goal is a factor—whether a preference, a priority, or a special consideration (sometimes incorporated into grant review criteria)—it is one of several review criteria in HRSA's grant process (Advisory Committee on Training in Primary Care Medicine and Dentistry, 2001).

HRSA administers Titles VII and VIII of the Public Health Service (PHS) Act. The titles authorize discretionary funds for a variety of programs affecting URM participation in medicine and dentistry (Title VII) and nursing (Title VIII). However, HRSA is dependent on Congress (with the approval of the President) for appropriations, so that specific programs

TABLE PCB-1 An Overview of Federal and State Health Professions Funding That Directly or Indirectly Affects Diversity in the Health Professions

Originating Source	Forms of Payment	Recipients
Department of Health and Human Services' (DHHS') Health Resources and Services Administration		
Health Careers Opportunities Program	Grants	Medical, dental schools; programs in clinical psychology; other (but not nursing)
Centers of Excellence	Grants	Schools with URM enrollments above national average—medical, dental schools; clinical and counseling psychology; other (but not nursing)
Scholarships for Disadvantaged Students	Scholarships	Medical, dental, nursing, behavioral health (including clinical psychology), and various other schools
Faculty Loan Repayment Program	Loan repayments	Degree-trained health professionals
Nursing Workforce Diversity Program	Grants	Health professions schools
Nursing Education Loan Repayment Program	Loan repayments	Registered nurses
Area Health Education Center	Grants	Schools of medicine and (sometimes) nursing, consortia, parent institutions
Health Education Training Center	Grants	Schools of medicine and (sometimes) nursing

Intended Beneficiaries	Payback (if any)	Total Dollars*
Persons from disadvantaged backgrounds		FY 2002: $34.6 million
Minority individuals (students and faculty)		FY 2002: $32.7 million
Persons from disadvantaged backgrounds		FY 2002: $46.2 million
Persons from disadvantaged backgrounds	Service commitment of up to 2 years	FY 2002: $1.3 million (up to $20,000 a year paid on loans)
Persons from disadvantaged Backgrounds		FY 2002: $6.2 million
Areas of nursing shortage	Service commitment of up to 3 years	FY 2002: $10.2 million (60 percent of loan for 2 years; 25 percent more for third year)
Delivery of care in underserved areas through improvement of health workforce		FY 2002: $33.3 million
Improvement of health care of low-income racial and ethnic minorities in severely underserved areas		FY 2002: $4.4 million

Continued

IN THE NATION'S COMPELLING INTEREST

TABLE PCB-1 Continued

Originating Source	Forms of Payment	Recipients
National Health Service Corps	Scholarships and loan repayments	Scholarships: persons pursuing medicine, dentistry, nurse practitioner, nurse midwife, physician assistant, psychology careers; loan repayment: same as above plus additional health professions
Children's Hospitals Graduate Medical Education Program	Grants	Children's hospitals
DHHS' National Institutes of Health		
Minority Access to Research Careers	Grants and fellowships	Research institutions with substantial minority enrollments
Minority Biomedical Research Support	Grants	Higher education institutions with 50 percent or more minority enrollment underrepresented in biomedical or behavioral research
Loan Repayment Program for Health Disparities Research	Loan repayments	Lenders (half of loan repayments earmarked for URMs)
Research Supplements for URMs	Grants	Research institutions
Extramural Loan Repayment for Individuals from Disadvantaged Backgrounds Conducting Clinical Research	Loan repayments	Persons with advanced health professions degrees who come from disadvantaged backgrounds
Undergraduate Scholarship Program	Scholarships	Persons from disadvantaged backgrounds

Intended Beneficiaries	Payback (if any)	Total Dollars*
Expansion of health care to persons in need (rural and inner city)	Scholarships: year of service for each year of support, with minimum of 2 years and maximum of 4 years; loan repayment: 2-year service requirement, with possibility of additional service	FY 2002: $46.2 million (field operations)
Training of pediatric and other residents in GME programs		FY 2002: $284.9 million
Increase in number and capabilities of URMs in biomedical research		FY 2002: About $3 million
Strengthen URM faculty, research environment, URM student capabilities		FY 2002: About $92 million
Conduct of research related to minority health disparities	2 years of research related to disparities, with possibility of extension	FY 2002: About $2 million (up to $35,000 a year, depending on loan debt)
Recruitment, and retention, of minority individuals to research		Unavailable
Recruitment and retention of health professionals from disadvantaged backgrounds to conduct clinical research	2 years of clinical research, with possibility of extension	FY 2002: Slightly more than $1.9 million
Pursuit of careers in research at NIH	1 year of employment at NIH for each scholarship year	FY 2002: $620,000 (up to $20,000 per year for up to 4 years)

Continued

TABLE PCB-1 Continued

Originating Source	Forms of Payment	Recipients
Department of Defense		
Health Professions Scholarship Program	Scholarships	Persons joining Army, Navy, Air Force
Graduate Medical Education	Graduate training costs (in addition to salary)	Interns, residents, and fellows in Army, Navy, Air Force
Health Professions Loan Repayment Program	Loan repayments	Health professionals in Army
Department of Veterans Affairs		
Clinical Training	Direct grants to students and indirect support to VA medical centers	Students and trainees in 4,000 education programs at 1,200 colleges and universities affiliated with VA
Mentored Minority Research Enhancement Coordinating Center	Grants	Minority-serving institutions
Mentored Minority Supplemental Award	Grants	VA-funded research projects
Mentored Minority Career Enhancement Award	Salaries	Mentored researchers in VA
National Science Foundation		
Louis Stokes Alliances for Minority Participation	Grants	Research institutions
Alliances for Graduate Education and the Professoriate	Grants	Research institutions

Intended Beneficiaries	Payback (if any)	Total Dollars*
Ensurance of adequate number of active-duty health professionals	Up to 4 years and longer for graduates of Uniformed Services University of the Health Sciences	Not available (each service has its own budget)
Ensurance of adequate number of active-duty health professionals	Service commitment	FY 2002: Estimated $86 million in training costs ($222.4 million for salaries)
Ensurance of adequate number of active-duty health professionals	Service commitment (1 year for each annual loan repayment)	Not available
Ensurance of adequate number of health professionals to treat patients in VA facilities		FY 2002: $786 million ($438 million in direct costs and $348 million in indirect costs)
Mentoring		New program
Applied research training to students, high school through postdoctoral		New program
Nurturing of researchers		New program
Strengthen preparation of minority students in science, math, engineering, and technology		FY 2003: Approximately $6 million
Increase in number of URMs receiving doctorates in science, math, engineering, and technology		FY 2002: Approximately $1 million to $2 million

Continued

TABLE PCB-1 Continued

Originating Source	Forms of Payment	Recipients
Centers of Research Excellence in Science and Technology	Grants	Research institutions (minority serving)
Medicare Graduate Medical Education	Direct and indirect payments	Approximately 1,200 teaching hospitals (and limited other facilities)
States		
Grants	Various grant initiatives for family physicians, rural underserved programs	Considerable variation from state to state
Medicaid Graduate Medical Education	Various forms of payment (e.g., direct and indirect, per case or per diem)	Teaching hospitals, medical schools; in some cases, managed care organizations

*FY 2002 figures are used when available for purposes of comparability.
SOURCE: Drawn from various online federal program descriptions and budget documents, including some of the references listed at the end of this paper.

in its budget (a Bush administration request of $6.4 billion for all HRSA operations in fiscal year 2004) (U.S. DHHS, 2003b) are often at risk.

According to HRSA Administrator Elizabeth M. Duke, Ph.D., "HRSA-supported training programs in the health care professions graduate two to five times more minority and disadvantaged students than training programs that receive no HRSA funds. And we know that these minority health care providers are more likely to practice in underserved areas" (Duke, 2002). HRSA's Office of Minority Health is involved in the four White House initiatives on Historically Black Colleges and Universities, Educational Excellence for Hispanic Americans, Tribal Colleges and Universities, and Asian Americans and Pacific Islanders, as well as the White House's Hispanic Agenda for Action Initiative, Association of Hispanic-Serving Health Professions Schools, Minority Health Knowledge Management Initiative, Minority Management Development Program, Minority Training Programs Tracking System, and Cultural Competence Initiative (HRSA, 2003i).

Intended Beneficiaries	Payback (if any)	Total Dollars*
Development of outstanding research centers		FY 2003: Approximately $5 million
Recognition of costs of training physicians and limited other practitioners primarily in inpatient setting		FY 2002: Estimated $9 billion
Mainly expansion and distribution of practitioners to underserved areas		Not available
Primary care training, preparation of practitioners for underserved areas; New York: increase in number of URMs		Last estimate (1998) as result of survey: $2.3 to $2.4 billion

The most recent study of HRSA diversity programs, *Strategies for Improving the Diversity of the Health Professions,* was conducted by Kevin Grumbach, Janet Coffman, Claudia Muñoz, and Emily Rosenoff of the Center for California Health Workforce Studies, University of California at San Francisco (UCSF), and Patricia Gándara and Enrique Sepulveda of the Education Policy Center, University of California, Davis, and published by The California Endowment (Grumbach et al., 2003). Because most of the programs focus on "disadvantaged" students, the research team addressed whether or not there is a correlation between "disadvantaged" and "URM." The researchers concluded that lack of basic educational opportunities for many minority groups leads fundamentally to the underrepresentation of these groups in the health professions. They also indicated that "URM students are more likely than non-URM students to come from low-income families, and are therefore disproportionately affected by the rising costs of higher education and adverse trends in the availability of financial aid" (Grumbach et al., 2003).

Following are HRSA programs in which URM participation is either a direct goal or an influence on funding, such as a "disadvantaged/minority funding factor," preference, or priority:

• The Health Careers Opportunity Program (HCOP) is aimed at drawing a more diverse applicant pool to the health professions by providing students from disadvantaged backgrounds with opportunities to receive degrees from health professions programs. HCOP accounted for $36 million in FY 2003, with the funds awarded to allopathic and osteopathic schools of medicine, dental schools, and graduate programs in clinical psychology, as well as to other health institutions (HRSA, 2003b).

• The Centers of Excellence (COE) program awards grants to health professions schools (allopathic and osteopathic medicine, dentistry, and graduate programs in clinical and counseling psychology, as well as clinical social work, marriage and family therapy, and pharmacy) with enrollments of URMs that are significantly above the national average. The COE program enables the schools to address their applicant pools, engage in faculty development, focus on minority issues in clinical education, promote faculty and student research in minority health, provide community-based clinical training involving significant numbers of racial and ethnic minorities, and offer stipends to URMs. The program also requires the grantee institutions to improve their recruitment and retention of URM faculty and to open up research opportunities for faculty as well as students (HRSA, 2003a). The COE program in FY 2003 accounted for approximately $34 million.

• The Scholarships for Disadvantaged Students (SDS) program makes grants to health professions schools (allopathic and osteopathic medicine, dentistry, nursing, and behavioral health, including clinical psychology, as well as various other disciplines) to provide assistance to disadvantaged students (HRSA, 2003e). The SDS program was funded at nearly $48 million in FY 2003.

• The Faculty Loan Repayment Program (FLRP) provides funds directly to degree-trained health professionals to pursue careers in academia. Directed at disadvantaged individuals (with "minority status in and of itself not a factor in determining disadvantaged background"), the program requires a service commitment of up to 2 years; HRSA pays up to $20,000 a year on the person's educational loans in return (HRSA, 2003c). FLRP accounted for slightly over $1 million of HRSA's budget in FY 2003.

A 2001 evaluation by the DHHS Office of Inspector General (OIG) revealed that FLRP routinely waives the institutional matching requirement, which has "the potential impact of reducing the effectiveness of federal funds." Participating institutions are supposed to match the federal loan repayment amount, unless they can demonstrate financial hardship.

"OIG found that waivers are routinely granted without an in-depth review of the institutions' financial condition" (HRSA, 2003c).

• The Nursing Workforce Diversity Program is HRSA's principal program for "improving the racial and ethnic diversity of the basic nursing workforce." The program is aimed primarily at expanding nursing education opportunities at the baccalaureate level for persons who come from disadvantaged backgrounds ("including racial and ethnic minorities underrepresented among registered nurses") (HRSA, 2003h). In some respects, it parallels the HCOP, which is not open to nursing. Schools of nursing, nursing centers, academic health centers, state and local governments, and others receive funds to support academic preparation activities, retention efforts, and student stipends. The program received nearly $10 million in FY 2003.

• The Nursing Education Loan Repayment Program (NELRP) offers registered nurses opportunities to pay back educational loans in exchange for service in health facilities in areas with nursing shortages. In return for a 2-year commitment, HRSA will pay 60 percent of a nurse's loan. If the nurse serves a third year, HRSA pays an additional 25 percent. Among the approved health facilities are Indian Health Service and Native Hawaiian health centers, community health centers, migrant health centers, rural health clinics, and public health clinics (HRSA, 2003g). HRSA's budget for NELRP was nearly $20 million in FY 2003.

• The Area Health Education Center (AHEC) and Health Education and Training Center (HETC) programs are closely aligned. While the major mission of the AHEC program is "to improve the supply, distribution, quality, utilization, and efficiency of the health workforce to ultimately improve delivery of quality health care in underserved areas," it has the related objective of improving health workforce diversity (Grumbach et al., 2003). The HETC program, which has the same mission as the AHEC program, focuses on Florida and states along the border between the United States and Mexico (Grumbach et al., 2003). HRSA uses minority and disadvantaged student funding factors in its grant processes for both. AHECs received approximately $33 million and HETCs obtained more than $4 million in FY 2003.

• The National Health Service Corps (NHSC) has a scholarship program for individuals entering medical, dental, family nurse practice, and certified nurse-midwifery programs (among others) and a loan repayment program for "a long list of medical professionals, among them physicians, nurses, and dentists" (Thompson, 2002). Reauthorization of the NHSC program in 2002 resulted in psychologists being listed as "primary care providers" in the scholarship program, along with physicians, dentists, and nurses (APA, 2002). (Practicing psychologists remained eligible for the loan repayment program.)

NHSC accounted for a total of $171 million of HRSA's FY 2003 budget. Field operations amounted to nearly $46 million and NHSC recruitment to slightly more than $125 million.

While NHSC's main purpose is to expand access to health services to persons most in need (especially in rural and inner city settings), the organization offers service opportunities to providers. HRSA reserves some of its funding to target recruitment of "URMs and other students and professionals from disadvantaged backgrounds into the program" (Duke, 2003). In its 2001 annual report, HRSA indicated that 25 percent of NHSC scholarship and loan repayment awards had gone to URMs (HRSA, 2001a).

An evaluation of the NHSC program in 2000 by researchers at the Cecil G. Sheps Center for Health Services Research at the University of North Carolina at Chapel Hill and at Mathematica Policy Research, Inc., did not address the topic of URM inclusion and retention in NHSC. However, it did look at affirmation of cultural competence and cultural concordance in NHSC practice:

> Over the years, NHSC clinicians have come to accept the affirmation of cultural competence as an important element in health care practice. On the other hand, they have been less receptive to the notion of cultural concordance through the matching of clinicians to communities. Nonetheless, cultural concordance finds greater support among members of racial and ethnic minority groups that have been historically underrepresented in the health professions. Moreover, women (compared with men) are also more likely to affirm the importance of cultural concordance and cultural competence (Konrad et al., 2000).

• Some other HRSA programs affecting the four professions also take into account disadvantaged/minority funding factors in their grant processes. For example, the Geriatric Education Centers program grants 10 points if an applicant's project has the potential to recruit and retain minority faculty members and trainees and improve access to a diverse and culturally competent workforce, according to HRSA's FY 2003 application kit for the program. The Primary Care Medicine and Dentistry Grant Program grants 20 points for diversity, in terms of an applicant's racial and socioeconomic makeup of trainees and faculty and its goal of increasing the proportions of both in the health professions workforce, according to that program's application kit.

The Children's Hospitals Graduate Medical Education (CHGME) program is a recently enacted initiative given to HRSA to administer. Congress authorized the program in 1999 in response to complaints that children's hospitals received "$374 per resident in Medicare funds versus an average of $87,034 per resident for a non-children's hospital" because of their low proportion of Medicare patients. CHGME provides funds to children's hospitals "to support the training of pediatric and other residents in GME programs" (Advisory Committee on Training in Primary Care Medicine and Dentistry, 2001). Rather than making CHGME permanent or mandatory (like Medicare GME), Congress established it as an interim discretionary program while it "examines the medical education funding system." CHGME received $40 million in 2000, $235 million in 2001, $285 million in 2002, and $292 million in 2003. The President is requesting $199 million in 2004 (U.S. DHHS, 2003b).

The National Institutes of Health, through its National Institute of General Medical Sciences (NIGMS), has administered two programs for more than 20 years to increase the number of minority biomedical scientists. The programs support graduate and postdoctoral (as well as undergraduate) students, faculty members, and education and research infrastructure improvements in institutions in the United States. They are directed toward, but not limited to, "African Americans, Hispanic Americans, Native Americans (including Alaska Natives), and natives of the U.S. Pacific Islands" (NIGMS, 2002). Following are descriptions of the two programs:

• Minority Access to Research Careers (MARC), one of the NIGMS programs, includes postbaccalaureate research education program awards, predoctoral fellowships, faculty predoctoral fellowships, and faculty senior fellowships, as well as an undergraduate student training award. The MARC program budget has been running at nearly $31 million a year. In 2001 (in addition to 647 students at undergraduate institutions), the program supported 45 students with MARC predoctoral fellowships and 75 NIH predoctoral fellows and 2 faculty members (NIGMS, 2002).
• Minority Biomedical Research Support (MBRS), the other NIGMS program, makes awards to "two- or four-year colleges, universities, and health professional schools with 50 percent or more enrollments of minorities that have been determined by the grantee institution to be underrepresented in biomedical or behavioral research." It may also provide awards to institutions that have enrollments of less than 50 percent if they "have a demonstrated commitment to the special encouragement and assistance of minority students" (NIGMS, 2002). The MBRS program, which operates with an approximate annual budget of $92 million, has three components: Support of Continuous Research Excellence (SCORE), which is faculty oriented; Research Initiative for Scientific Enhancement (RISE), which is environment centered; and Initiative for Minority Student Development, which is focused on undergraduate, graduate, and postdoctoral students (NIGMS, 2003).

In addition to being reviewed by Grumbach and his colleagues, the

MARC and MBRS programs are cited in the Council on Graduate Medical Education's (COGME's) *Twelfth Report: Minorities in Medicine,* issued in 1998. In addition, the MARC program was the subject of a lengthy evaluation covering cohorts for 1981–1985, 1986–1990, and 1991–1993 (NIGMS, 2000). The NIH also has the following programs:

• The Loan Repayment Program for Health Disparities Research, a program administered by the NIH National Center on Minority Health and Health Disparities, provides educational loan repayment to qualified individuals to engage in basic, clinical, or behavioral research that is related to minority health disparities. Half of the program's awards are earmarked for persons from populations with health disparities. Participants may receive up to $35,000 per year, with the awards going directly to lenders.

• This program emphasizes the recruitment of racial and ethnic minorities and other underrepresented individuals to conduct research because such emphasis "promotes a diverse and strong 21st century workforce" that is able to address society's diverse needs. The program enables the NIH to support and facilitate the development of research programs that reflect an understanding of the variety of issues and problems associated with disparities in health status (National Center on Minority Health and Health Disparities, 2003). The Extramural Loan Repayment for Individuals from Disadvantaged Backgrounds Conducting Clinical Research program encourages qualified health professionals from minority backgrounds to enter and remain in clinical research careers. Participants commit to at least 2 years of conducting clinical research in return for having payments made to pay off their educational debts (Catalog of Federal Domestic Assistance, 2003).

• The Extramural Associates Research Development Award program provides grants to minority and women's educational institutions that are seeking to increase their participation in biomedical and behavioral research and training. Since 1994, the NIH has made grants to 44 institutions in this country. An evaluation of the program—due September 30, 2004—is under way (U.S. DHHS, 2003a).

• Research Supplements for Underrepresented Minorities, a program initiated by the NIH in 1989, is designed to increase the number of URM scientists in biomedical research and the health-related sciences. The NIH established the program to encourage principal investigators with NIGMS grants to request supplemental funds to attract and retain minority individuals in biomedical research careers. Then, in 2001, the NIH, acknowledging that the need to expand research opportunities for URMs was as great as ever, renewed its call. The agency provided contacts for interested investigators in 18 of its institutes and the National Library of Medicine,

National Center for Research Resources, Fogarty International Center, National Center for Complementary and Alternative Medicine, and Office of Behavioral and Social Sciences Research (NIH, 2001).

• The Undergraduate Scholarship Program is aimed at students who want to pursue "careers in biomedical, behavioral, and social science research at the NIH." The program pays up to $20,000 per year (for a maximum of 4 years, with annual renewal required) (NIH, 2003). The program has a service commitment of a year's employment at the NIH for each scholarship year. The program is for persons from disadvantaged backgrounds. "Disadvantaged" is defined as coming from a low-income family. The program is neutral as to race and ethnicity.

Department of Defense[2]

DoD provides support for health professions education through the Armed Forces Health Professions Scholarship Program (HPSP), authorized by the Uniformed Services Health Professions Revitalization Act of 1972. The purpose of the program is to obtain adequate numbers of qualified active-duty health professionals (U.S. Navy Medical Education and Training Command, 2003). Up to 5,000 HPSP scholarships are authorized across the Army, Navy, and Air Force, with each of the services having its own budget allocation, operating its own HPSP, and determining the disciplines to be eligible and the number of scholarships to be made available. These parameters may vary over time.

HPSP scholarships provide full tuition, laboratory fees, books, insurance, and a living stipend for education in medicine, dentistry, nursing, and other health professions such as veterinary medicine, optometry, psychology, pharmacy, and clinical psychology (U.S. Navy Medical Department, 2003). For example, the Army currently sponsors 1,511 HPSP scholarships in five disciplines, of which 1,065 (about one-third) are in medical training (personal communication, K. Raines, Director, Medical Education, Medical Corps, Department of the Army, August 28, 2003). Scholarships are granted to participants in return for their performing subsequent service as active-duty health professionals on a year-for-year basis, with up to 4 years of commitment beyond training and a longer period for graduates of the Uniformed Services University of the Health Sciences.

DoD also carries out a significant program in GME. It is responsible for

---

[2]The author gratefully acknowledges the contributions (research and writing) of F. Lawrence Clare, M.D., a private consultant, to the Department of Defense section of this paper.

about 3 percent of all U.S. medical residents. The department currently supports 2,965 interns, residents, and fellows in military GME programs, at an annual level of $104,000 each. While that support amounts to $308.4 million per year, $70,000 to $80,000 per individual is for salary, which DoD does not consider to be part of graduate training costs. When $222.4 million (based on $75,000 each) is subtracted, DoD estimates its annual training cost at $86 million (personal communication, J. Powers, Director, Clinical and Medical Education, Assistant Secretary of Defense for Health Affairs, June 3, 2003).

A considerable portion of the new entrants in military GME programs are there because they have HPSP scholarship obligations. In the Navy's 58 in-service GME programs, for example, graduating HPSP scholarship recipients fill about 200 of the service's 258 first-year GME positions. The Navy has more than 900 total in-service positions and another 120 in civilian GME programs (U.S. Navy Medical Department, 2003).

The Army also uses a Health Professions Loan Repayment Program to enhance recruitment of needed health professionals. The program provides annual grants to qualified practitioners in many health professions to help them repay their educational loans, in exchange for a year of service commitment for each grant (U.S. Army, 2003b).

At the college or undergraduate level, each service has a Reserve Officer Training Corps (ROTC) program, which can help facilitate entry into health professions education through ROTC scholarships. The Army, for example, provides ROTC scholarships at more than 600 schools. The scholarships provide payments for tuition and fees, monthly stipends, and book allowances, in return for a service commitment after completion of education (U.S. Army, 2003c). Graduating ROTC cadets may apply for HPSP scholarships, and HPSP recipients receive delays in entering required service. Air Force ROTC "pre-health" scholarship recipients are specifically guaranteed HPSP scholarship awards after acceptance to medical school. In addition, it is not necessary for a graduating ROTC cadet to have an HPSP scholarship to receive a delay in the service obligation if he or she enters health professions training. Specific nurse ROTC programs are available from both the Army and the Navy (U.S. Army, 2003c).

Because DoD's health professions programs are insular—conducted for the purpose of having sufficient numbers of health professionals for the various services—and because they are compartmentalized by service, it is difficult to get a profile of the numbers of URMs participating in the programs. However, minorities are overrepresented in the military relative to their share of the overall population: They account for 40.8 percent of Army, 35.6 percent of Navy, 32.4 percent of Marine Corps, and 29.4 percent of Air Force personnel, according to 2000 data. African Americans, for example, make up 26.4 percent of Army personnel, compared to 12.8

percent of the general population. However, African Americans constitute only 11.3 percent of Army officers (physicians, dentists, nurses, and other health professionals tend to be in the officer ranks). Overall, omitting warrant officers, 20.6 percent of Army, 16.9 percent of Navy, 14.8 percent of Marine Corps, and 14.1 percent of Air Force officers are minority (Minorities in Uniform, 2000).

Department of Veterans Affairs (VA)

The VA, which serves a veteran population of more than 25 million men and women, has been training health care professionals for more than 50 years, in part to recruit personnel to and retain them in the VA health care system. The VA is the largest single provider of clinical health services in the United States and is second only to DHHS' Centers for Medicare and Medicaid Services (CMS), which administers Medicare GME, as a federal funder of health professions education. The VA supports 8,800 physician resident positions and accounts for approximately 9 percent of GME in this country (U.S. VA, 2003a).

"Each year, over 76,000 students and trainees receive some or all of their clinical training in VA through affiliations with over 4,000 education programs at 1,200 colleges and universities"(personal communication, G. J. Holland, Special Assistant to the Chief Academic Affiliations Officer, VA, April 4, 2003). Those in training include medical, dental, nursing, and clinical psychology interns, as well as other health professionals. Rather than providing awards to the institutions themselves, the VA provides direct support for students receiving training in the VA. Direct support includes the salary and fringe benefits paid directly to medical residents and associated health trainees. The VA also provides indirect support in its medical centers through VA staff who serve as instructors and through various administrative costs that are associated with its health professions programs. In 2002, the VA's education and training budget was $786 million: $438 million in direct costs and $348 million in indirect costs (personal communication, Holland, 2003).

The VA generally does not have breakdowns by race and ethnicity for participants in its clinical training programs. However, the VA does have statistics for participants (all of whom, of course, are not URMs) from the historically black colleges, historically Hispanic-serving institutions, and tribal colleges and universities with which it has affiliation agreements. Thirty-two historically black colleges have affiliations with the VA, resulting in 1,102 of their students having received clinical training in VA facilities in 2002. These included 166 medical residents, 5 specialized fellows, and 78 medical students. They also included 22 dental residents, 457 professional nurses, and 1 in mental health (not otherwise specified). Thirty-four historically Hispanic institutions have affiliations with the VA, with 3,395 of their students having gotten part of their clinical training in VA facilities in 2002. These included 1,283 medical residents, 1 specialized fellow, and 471 medical students; 32 dental residents; 694 professional nurses; and 53 in mental health. Two tribal colleges and universities have VA affiliations, resulting in 10 of their students having received clinical training in 2002. Of these, 9 were professional nurses (personal communication, Holland, 2003).

The VA is unveiling three new research training programs in 2003. The programs expand the collaboration between VA health facilities and historically black colleges and universities, Hispanic-serving institutions, and tribal colleges and universities to include several minority-oriented national organizations and "institutions of higher education with sizeable concentrations of Asian Americans, Pacific Islanders, Native Hawaiians, Native Americans, Alaskan Natives, or persons with disabilities" (U.S. VA, 2002).

The three new programs (U.S. VA, 2002) include the following:

• Mentored Minority Research Enhancement Coordinating Center, to support collaboration between the VA and minority-serving institutions, with students and faculty from the institutions partnering with mentors from the VA.
• Mentored Minority Supplemental Award, to provide applied research training with investigators on VA-funded research projects, with high school, undergraduate, graduate, and predoctoral students eligible.
• Mentored Minority Career Enhancement Award, to provide full salary for 3 years to mentored researchers in the VA.

National Science Foundation

The National Science Foundation (NSF), a freestanding entity in the federal budget, funds basic research as an underpinning of other science and engineering government functions. "Although the NSF represents less than 4 percent of the total federal budget for research and development, it accounts for approximately 13 percent of all federal support for basic research and 40 percent of non-life-science basic research at U.S. academic institutions." About 95 percent of the NSF's budget goes directly to educational and research institutions and contractors (OMB, 2003).

The NSF's efforts "include the recruitment and retention of minority students into doctoral science, mathematics, engineering, and technology programs, recruitment of minority faculty, and the strengthening of research capabilities of historically African American colleges and universities." Its programs include the Louis Stokes Alliances for Minority Participation, Alliances for Graduate Education and the Professoriate, and Centers of Research Excellence in Science and Technology, plus an undergraduate-level program at historically black colleges and universities (Grumbach et al., 2003).

Mandatory Funds: DHHS' Medicare GME Program

The premier health professions program in terms of dollars spent is Medicare GME, administered by CMS.[3] Because Medicare is a service delivery program for eligible persons 65 and older and for younger people with disability determinations, its GME program is viewed within the rubric of patient care. Outlays for the GME program are estimated at $9 billion for FY 2002 (CMS, 2002). Medicare GME funding, paid to teaching hospitals under Part A of the Medicare program, has two components: direct and indirect. Direct GME funds cover allopathic, osteopathic, podiatric, and dental residents' salaries and fringe benefits; allocated hospital overhead connected with training programs; and other costs (such as teaching physicians' supervisory costs). Although podiatrists and dentists (for example, those doing inpatient surgery) who choose hospital residencies and those that may be part of certain ambulatory arrangements are included in Medicare GME, the program centers predominately on physicians.

Indirect GME funds recognize the added costs teaching hospitals incur as a result of their teaching programs. Indirect medical education payments began in FY 1984, as part of the new inpatient prospective payment system (PPS). Add-ons to the diagnosis-related-group rates upon which the inpatient PPS operates, indirect payments are currently paid at the rate of 5.5 percent per 0.1 intern/resident per bed (IRB).

Medicare GME funds, which go to approximately 1,200 teaching hospitals across the country, are concentrated in about 120 major teaching hospitals that have high IRB ratios. These hospitals have about half of all residents and receive approximately two-thirds of all indirect payments. There are some nursing and allied health expenditures in the Medicare GME program, but they are modest amounts (approximately $300 million), given the billions in outlays for the program. As hospitals close diploma schools of nursing and related educational programs, the amounts are dwindling rather than growing.

---

[3]For a description of Medicare GME within the context of the Medicare program, see Matherlee K. 2003. *The U.S. Health Workforce: Definitions, Dollars, and Dilemmas.* Washington, DC: National Health Policy Forum, George Washington University. Pp. 6-11. Much of the Medicare GME description is drawn from that document.

The Medicare GME program has not been involved in efforts to increase the participation of URM physicians, podiatrists, or dentists—or any other URM health professionals—in the health workforce. From a policy standpoint, however, Congress has linked the program to attempts to control physician supply by capping the number of physician residents per teaching hospital effective the start of each hospital's 1996 fiscal year (with podiatric and dental residents excluded from the cap). Congress has also linked the program to efforts to shift training from inpatient hospital to outpatient settings by authorizing direct (but not indirect) payments to organizations such as community health centers, rural health clinics, and certain managed care organizations if they incur the costs of operating approved residency programs. Moreover, Congress has linked the program to primary care training incentives.

STATE HEALTH PROFESSIONS FUNDING SOURCES

Various states have health professions initiatives, both in grant form and as part of Medicaid, the federal-state program that provides health services to certain persons and families with low incomes and assets. Although the challenge of keeping up with health professions programs that vary state by state is daunting, Tim Henderson, director of the Institute for Primary Care and Workforce Analysis, National Conference of State Legislatures, has tracked them for more than a decade. He was joined several years ago by HRSA's National Center for Health Workforce Analysis, which has Regional Centers for Health Workforce Studies at UCSF, State University of New York at Albany (SUNY at Albany), University of Illinois at Chicago (UIC), University of Washington (UW), and University of Texas (UT) to collect data on state practices and policies. The National Center for Health Workforce Analysis is tracking activities in 10 states: California, Connecticut, Florida, Illinois, Iowa, Texas, Utah, Washington, West Virginia, and Wisconsin.

Grant Funds

Data from the Institute for Primary Care and Workforce Analysis

The Institute for Primary Care and Workforce Analysis distinguishes three states that are using innovative financing approaches in addressing state health workforce needs. They are Arkansas, Colorado, and Texas. The states use appropriated funds for family practice residencies aimed at increasing the number of physicians who provide primary health care in underserved areas. Although the programs do not have explicit goals regarding URM physicians, they do exemplify the use of funds to address specific workforce goals.

Arkansas has had a program of community family physician residency programs for more than 25 years. The goal of the program is to distribute physicians to underserved populations throughout the state. Developed in collaboration with the state's AHEC, the program has six community-based family medicine residency practices outside Little Rock, the state's largest city. Credited with providing most of the state's rural physicians, it provides opportunities for 45 percent of graduating medical residents to practice in communities with populations of less than 20,000.

The Arkansas state legislature recently agreed to appropriate $4 million of the state's tobacco settlement to support the community residency programs. According to Henderson, the legislature is interested in tying the program to the state's Medicaid GME program in order to receive additional federal Medicaid matching funds for the teaching hospitals that are affiliated with the community residencies.

Colorado, which has had a program for 25 years, directs its efforts to the needs of rural and urban underserved communities for family physicians. Run by a committee of academic, provider, and consumer representatives, the program includes 10 family practice residencies that currently train approximately 200 residents. While 80 percent of the residents in the program are from medical schools outside Colorado, two-thirds of the graduates remain in the state to practice, with about 25 to 30 percent opting for a rural or urban underserved area practice. The Colorado legislature makes an annual appropriation of about $2.4 million to the program.

Texas has a program, also 25 years old, to fund postgraduate training in family medicine. By the late 1990s, the state provided approximately $11 million to 26 programs for more than 700 positions, sponsored by medical schools in the state. It requires the schools to have substantial support from other sources, such as patient revenues and local funds.

Statistics from the National Center for Health Workforce Analysis

The National Center for Health Workforce Analysis offers the following statistics for 1994–1998 on allopathic medical school graduates characterized as URMs, with 10.5 being the U.S. average and Texas providing the only overlap with Henderson's analysis (National Center for Health Workforce Analysis, 2001):

- California—16.7
- Connecticut—13.1
- Florida—7.6
- Iowa—8.0
- Illinois—8.8
- Texas—12.7
- Utah—2.5
- Washington—7.4
- West Virginia—1.0
- Wisconsin—8.3

Medicaid GME

Even before the Medicaid program was enacted in the mid-1960s, most states had some expenditures for medical education, mainly for under-graduate training. After Medicaid's inception, states became contributors of the second largest amount of explicit GME funding. According to a study that Henderson conducted for the AAMC in 1998 and 1999:

- A total of 45 states and the District of Columbia paid for GME at some level.
- Of the 45 states and the District of Columbia, 43 paid for GME in their fee-for-service (FFS) programs. Of these, 24 made both direct and indirect payments and 11 did not distinguish between the two. Thirty-five of the states that paid for GME under FFS did so through hospital per-case or per-diem rates.
- Of the 42 states and the District of Columbia that reported capitated Medicaid arrangements, 16 states and the District of Columbia made ex-plicit Medicaid GME payments to teaching hospitals or teaching programs. Seventeen other states included the payments in managed care organiza-tions' capitated rates. Teaching hospitals were the recipients of most states' GME payments, although, in Oklahoma and Tennessee, medical schools were the only training programs to receive them directly under managed care.
- While medical residents were predominantly eligible for Medicaid GME payments, nurses and other health professions students were eligible under managed care (or there was no distinction among the health profes-sions) in eight states and the District of Columbia.
- Of the five states—Alaska, Idaho, Illinois, Montana, and South Da-kota—that either did not report or indicated they did not provide Medicaid GME support, only Illinois had significant residency programs. (In the case of Illinois, how the state labels "Medicaid GME support" may mask funds that go to support GME.) South Dakota did not report any GME payments

to its teaching hospital or medical school. Puerto Rico also indicated no Medicaid GME support (Henderson, 2000).

Henderson estimated total state Medicaid expenditures on GME in 1998 at $2.3 to $2.4 billion.

In a summary prepared earlier this year, Henderson singled out four states—Georgia, Michigan, Tennessee, and Utah—as particularly noteworthy relative to their linking Medicaid payments to state workforce goals, and two states—Minnesota and New York—for being especially creative in pooling Medicaid and other payment sources:

• Georgia's Medicaid program began paying a lump sum to the Medical College of Georgia in 2000 to support core clinical training activities in the state's five AHECs. Through an intergovernmental transfer (IGT), the sum—part of an appropriated budget for the AHEC program—was used to draw down additional federal Medicaid matching funds for clinical training of physician residents needed by the state's medically underserved regions. Currently the total value of this "new money" is $1.45 million.

• Michigan established three Medicaid GME pools in 1997 in order "to bring physician education more in line with its specific public policy goals to train appropriate numbers of primary care providers, enhance training in rural areas, and support education in ways of particular importance in the treatment of the Medicaid-eligible population." For the first 3 years, there were a historic cost pool to reimburse each hospital based on what it had received in 1995; a primary care pool to encourage the training of young physicians in primary care fields (general practice, family practice, preventive medicine, obstetrics, and geriatrics) based on a hospital's residents in primary care and its share of Medicaid patients; and an Innovations in Health Professions Education Grant Fund.

The innovations fund, financed with GME dollars that formerly were included in capitation payments to managed care organizations, was designed to foster innovations in health professions education. Funds are available only to consortia consisting of at least a hospital, a university, and a managed care plan. Examples of initiatives funded include curriculum changes to add exposure to managed care, development of evidence-based-medicine teaching experiences, and interdisciplinary efforts among different health professions.

The state started using a new Medicaid GME formula that considered characteristics of the state's Medicaid population. It also began to require hospital participation in a managed care plan in order to receive GME funds. In addition, it opened the program to third- and fourth-year dental students to increase the participation of dentists in Medicaid and agreed to use the IGT mechanism to develop physician residency programs in psychiatry to provide training in community mental health settings.

• When Tennessee replaced its Medicaid program with TennCare in 1996, it became the only state to require that Medicaid GME funds go directly to medical schools. Under this stipulation, GME funds follow residents to training sites and are distributed by the state's medical schools to pay residents' basic stipends and supplements for primary care training in community sites (as well as underserved areas). By July 1, 2000, half of the aggregate residency positions under the sponsorship of the state's four medical schools were to be in one of the primary care specialties.

Although the program has experienced problems in recruitment and retention, TennCare has extended the program through 2007. It has set aside $2 million to support new efforts by the state's medical schools to recruit and retain residents interested in rural practice. Other uses that have been suggested include support for training other health professionals that are in short supply, such as dentists, advanced practice nurses, and psychologists.

• Utah has a federal waiver from CMS to conduct a Medicare GME demonstration. Originally, the state proposed that it include Medicaid and other state funds as well, but CMS limited the demonstration to Medicare. Effective January 2003, all Medicare funds for direct and indirect Medicare GME are paid to a statewide council. The council is responsible for creating a new formula for distributing indirect GME payments based on actual documented costs and development of a statewide physician resident rotation information system to assist with payment verification.

On the Medicaid side, the state is using the IGT mechanism—with state medical school funds as the state share—to draw down federal matching funds to increase Medicaid support for GME at its three teaching hospitals. The total amount in the Medicaid GME pool is estimated at close to $20 million. Funds in the pool are used not only for medical but also for dental and podiatry residents at the hospitals. They are also weighted toward physician specialties that are in short supply.

• Minnesota established a Medical Education and Research Cost (MERC) trust fund in 1996 to capture new and existing state sources of medical education funds. The state legislature appropriated $5 million in new funding from the state's general fund and took $3.5 million from an existing state health-care provider tax pool for the fund (there was some IGT federal matching for one year only). Institutions that receive financing from the trust fund distribute the money to the more than 300 training sites, including nonhospital settings, that train physicians, dentists, advanced practice nurses, and some other health professionals. GME funds have also been carved out from Medicaid managed care rates. The trust fund has experienced increased funding, with its current sources including tobacco settlement dollars, Medicaid matching funds, state general fund payments, and Medicaid managed care carve-out amounts.

MERC funds support 2,000 full-time-equivalent trainees at 400 training sites. To date, the distribution of payments is not linked to state workforce goals because state officials do not believe they have enough good data to determine objectives and incentives.

• New York is the only state that explicitly ties its GME payments to increasing the number of URMs. The state's GME Reform Incentive Pool also seeks to reduce the number of physician trainees, increase the number of primary care physicians, and promote residency training in ambulatory sites. Distribution of the funds, which may be to individual hospitals or a consortium of hospitals, is based on performance in meeting the goals. Increasing the proportion of URMs has a weight of 0.15, while expanding the proportions of minority faculty and linkages with pipeline programs have weights of 0.75 each (personal communication, J. Betancourt, Senior Scientist, Institute for Health Policy, and Director, Multicultural Education, Massachusetts General Hospital, May 23, 2003).

PUBLIC FINANCING BARRIERS TO URM HEALTH PROFESSIONS DEMAND INITIATIVES

Scarcity of Evaluations on Effectiveness of Initiatives to Increase URMs in the Health Professions

Evaluative studies of programs to increase the numbers of URM health professionals do not seem to be a public priority. At DHHS, for example, the Office of the Assistant Secretary for Planning and Evaluation (ASPE) has responsibility for "policy coordination, legislation development, strategic planning, policy research and evaluation, and economic analysis." A review of the ASPE Policy Information Center website (http://aspe.hhs.gov/pic/), which indexes studies, turns up a handful of evaluations in the past 5 years, four of which are cited in this paper:

• "Historically Black Medical Colleges' Participation in HRSA-Supported Health Professions Training Programs," September 30, 2000;
• "Evaluation of the Health Resources and Services Administration's National Health Service Corps Program," September 30, 2000;
• "Faculty Loan Repayment Program—Making More Effective Use of Program Funds," January 29, 2001; and
• "Evaluation of the Extramural Associates Research Development Award Program" (in progress).

The other key evaluations include the following:

- "Strategies for the Recruitment, Retention, and Graduation of Hispanics into the Baccalaureate Level of Nursing," September 30, 1998 (U.S. DHHS, 1998);
- "Midcourse Assessment of the Research Infrastructure in Minority Institution Programs," January 30, 2000 (NIH, 2000b);
- "Evaluation of the Research Centers in Minority Institutions Program: Final Report," April 30, 2000 (NIH, 2000a); and
- "Professional Nurse Traineeship Grants: Who Gets Them and Where Do They Work After Graduation?" July 31, 2001 (HRSA, 2001b).

Public sources such as the Bureau of the Census, General Accounting Office (GAO), Office of Management and Budget, and individual agencies (through, for example, annual reports and internal evaluations, such as the 2001 review of Title VII by the HRSA Advisory Committee on Training in Primary Care Medicine and Dentistry) provide valuable information on the operations of federal programs. However, evaluations of specific URM programs, the roles of specific agencies in administering programs targeted at URMs, and especially cross-cutting or comprehensive federal efforts to address URMs in the health professions are rare.

Unpredictability of Health Professions Discretionary Funding

The distinction between discretionary and mandatory funding is extremely important, especially because success in achieving a policy goal tends to take a considerable period of time. Most of the federal government's programs to increase the participation of URMs in the health professions are in HRSA, which must seek periodic reauthorization of its programs and undergo annual appropriations struggles for its funding. This tends to be an annual budget game in which the President—Republican or Democrat—zeroes out or reduces certain HRSA programs in the administration budget proposal and defers to interest groups to lobby Congress for their reinstatement. When Congress responds, it takes responsibility for the additional dollars.

A review of HRSA's FY 2003 grants website (last updated November 4, 2002, more than a month after the beginning of federal FY 2003) was particularly telling. While some programs had application due dates, others, such as HCOP, COE, and Basic/Core and Model AHECs, had the following message: "This program is not included in the President's budget for FY 2003 and is provisional until final Congressional action on appropriations is taken" (HRSA, 2002). This injects uncertainty into HRSA's commitment to URM progress in the health professions, despite the intent and rhetoric of the programs.

"Siloing" of Small Discretionary URM Programs

Former Senator Everett Dirksen (R–IL) is well known for having said something like "a billion here, a billion there, and pretty soon you're talking about real money." Unlike the Medicare GME program, where billions of dollars are concentrated in a mandatory program, efforts to increase URMs in the health professions are "siloed" in HRSA, the National Institutes of Health, the National Science Foundation, and other agencies of the federal government and represent relatively small efforts from state to state.

Given the existence of various pots of money—many of them modest—and the lack of incentives for coordination, it is difficult to see the impact of the federal commitment to increasing URM participation. This is apparent in the Grumbach et al. evaluation that is cited numerous times in this paper and in some of the less comprehensive examinations that are available.

For example, a 1998 evaluation of historically black medical schools' participation in HRSA-supported health professions training programs says that "both within HRSA and the black medical schools, there is a lack of communication, coordination, and resources to encourage and maintain teamwork." The evaluation compares the various components of the agency to a medical school, where "faculty in one department may not know what is occurring in another department" (Distributed Communications Corporation, 1998).

Lack of Recognition of the Importance of DoD and VA Health Professions Programs

Although DoD and the VA have significant health professions programs of potential benefit to URMs, the programs' purposes are to recruit and retain health professionals to care for military and veteran populations, respectively, not to address URM workforce goals. However, the three new initiatives that the VA announced this year (Mentored Minority Research Enhancement Coordinating Center, Mentored Minority Supplemental Award, and Mentored Minority Career Enhancement Award) reflect the department's growing awareness of the importance of URMs in its workforce.

The federal dollars expended on the DoD and VA health professions education and training programs are considerable and should be recognized for the influence they have in shaping the health workforce. For example, as noted earlier, DoD trains 3 percent of U.S. medical residents and the VA trains 9 percent. As the proportions of URMs serving in the military and subsequently becoming veterans swell, the policy issue of having health professionals who reflect the minority populations needing health services becomes ever more important.

Compartmentalization, whether by agency or congressional staff or by health researchers, often leads to tunnel vision, with those involved with HRSA's discretionary health professions programs or Medicare's GME program generally focusing only on their own areas, with little recognition of other federal contributions (such as those of DoD and the VA) to health professions training. This precludes any sort of coordination or collaboration, which suits agencies' and congressional committees' tendencies to protect their jurisdictions but places a heavy burden on URMs and others interested in finding out the options open to them.

Absence of Health Workforce Goals in the Medicare GME Program

Because the Medicare GME program has such a large pot of money, it tends to be targeted by various advocates of reform. Thus far, the teaching hospitals that receive Medicare GME funds and their proponents in Congress and the White House have resisted most attempts at reform. While the number of medical residents has been capped and there have been some inroads toward ambulatory training and managed and primary care, the program has, for the most part, remained as it was established by the Social Security Amendments of 1983.

Medicare is payment oriented, administered by CMS and Medicare fiscal intermediaries and carriers as a public insurance program. Although the program, because of its size, helps to define the health workforce by its coverage and benefit policies, it has not made overt attempts, through GME or other mechanisms, to influence workforce policy. Medicare GME is hospital based, physician focused, and service oriented, with patient care and medical training dollars commingled.

One area of controversy is the amount of money that Medicare GME devotes to training of international medical graduates (IMGs), who tend to boost the IRBs of teaching hospitals, particularly in states such as New York and Massachusetts. According to COGME, 2001 National Resident Matching Program data show that IMGs filled approximately 36 percent of family medicine positions and 36 percent of general internal medicine positions. COGME points out that "IMGs, compared with U.S. medical graduates, consistently fill gaps in the physician workforce in counties having poor scores on a number of health status and economic indicators" (COGME, 2002). While some argue that IMGs increase the diversity of the health professions (although few fit the definition of URM), others say that they take places that might otherwise go to the native born, including URMs.

*Uneven Efforts from State to State in Using Grant and Medicaid Funds
to Achieve URM Policy Goals*

Just as states vary in their grant programs and in the levels of poverty
and optional benefits in their Medicaid programs, they differ significantly
in their support of the health professions and in their efforts to increase
health workforce diversity. While some states' grant and Medicaid initiatives may indirectly affect the participation of URMs in the four professions, only New York explicitly weights its GME pool dollars to URM
residents and faculty.

In view of changing demographics, it remains to be seen whether New
York will serve as a model for other states, or whether states that have clear
policy aims in increasing certain types of practitioners (for example, primary care physicians and advanced practice nurses) will adopt URM initiatives.

High Debt Loads of Newly Trained Physicians and Dentists

The costs of higher education pose an obvious barrier to URM health
professions participation; provision of financial aid is a strategy to leap the
barrier. As pointed out by Grumbach et al., most of the studies that have
focused on the cost barrier have looked at college entry and retention rather
than health professions training for physicians, nurses, and others in this
IOM study on diversity. It is important to note, as Grumbach and colleagues do, that "low income" is not synonymous with "minority" or
"URM," so that "financial aid based on economic need is not a strategy
that selectively targets URMs. . . . Need-based financial aid will benefit
many students who are not URMs, and will not reach those URMs who are
not from lower income families" (Grumbach et al., 2003).

Medical school graduates have debts of between $70,000 and
$100,000, and one in four has debt that exceeds $100,000, according to an
IOM report (IOM, 2001a). URM graduates tend to have higher debt levels.
COGME pointed out that "the average debt for both URMs and white
indebted students was nearly $20,000 in 1981." It increased by approxi-
mately 250 percent by 1995, "reaching an average $71,364 debt for URMs
and $68,910 for nonminorities." COGME indicated that URM students'
"greater length of time between matriculation and graduation is one of the
factors contributing to the differential in debt level for URM students."
COGME also indicated that, while 35 percent of all students rely on high-
cost unsubsidized loans, 40 percent of URMs do.

In addition, COGME reported that "more than 83 percent of graduating URMs, compared with 51 percent of non-URMs" said they had received scholarships or grants during medical school. Whereas URMs were

more likely than non-URMs to receive assistance from "School-Based Scholarships for the Disadvantaged, Financial Aid for Disadvantaged Health Professions Students, National Medical Fellowships, the Exceptional Financial Need program, and the NHSC," non-URM students tended to draw upon "need-based school scholarships, school merit scholarships, and Armed Forces scholarships" (COGME, 1998).

HRSA's Advisory Committee on Training in Primary Care Medicine and Dentistry reports that dental tuition and fees "have risen annually by an average of 5 percent per year for residents and nearly 6 percent for nonresidents." They were 55 percent higher in 1997–1998 than in 1989–1990. "The average dental graduate with debt in 2000 had a debt load of $106,000" (Advisory Committee on Training in Primary Care Medicine and Dentistry, 2001). In large part because of the debt load, only a third of dental graduates go on to postgraduate training.

Reluctance to Fund New URM Initiatives Due to the Rising Federal Budget Deficit and State Budget Crises

As this country has moved from a balanced budget to deficit financing and to priority status for Department of Homeland Security and DoD spending, funds for various initiatives, particularly for social spending, have become increasingly competitive at the federal level. The same is true at the state level, where rising deficits are resulting in budget downsizing and, at times, tax increases. Existing programs designed to increase the participation of URMs in the health professions seem either stagnant or at risk in terms of their funding levels, and the possibility of public financing for new initiatives appears to be low.

OPPORTUNITIES FOR CHANGING FINANCIAL INCENTIVES TO INCREASE URM HEALTH PROFESSIONS PARTICIPATION

Conduct of Studies to Evaluate Federal URM Workforce Initiatives

The paucity of studies on federal strategies to increase URM participation in the health professions hinders policy makers. Whether due to lack of funding, absence of political will, opposition to affirmative action, or other reasons, lack of evidence on the efficacy of public incentive programs and the transfer of private incentive models, such as the AAMC's "Project 3000 by 2000 Health Professions Partnership Initiative" (AAMC, 2003), to the public sector takes the winds out of the sails of the proponents of such activities. However, the mechanisms exist for a research agenda to be undertaken and funded.

For example, at DHHS, evaluation may be done either directly through program funds or through a legislatively mandated set-aside. The most significant set-aside

> is one established for evaluations conducted by several agencies of the . . . PHS (Agency for Healthcare Research and Quality, Centers for Disease Control [and Prevention], HRSA, NIH, and Substance Abuse and Mental Health Services Administration), ASPE, and the Office of Public Health and Science in the Office of the Secretary. The mechanism is called the PHS evaluation set-aside legislative authority, which is provided for in Section 241 of the PHS Act. This authority was established in 1970, when the Congress amended the Act to permit the HHS Secretary to use up to 1 percent of appropriated funds to evaluate authorized programs. Section 206 of the FY 2002 Labor, HHS, and Education Appropriations Act increases the amount the Secretary may use for evaluation to 1.25 percent. Section 241 limits the base from which 1.25 percent of appropriated funds can be reserved for evaluations of programs authorized by the PHS Act (Policy Information Center, 2002).

For another DHHS example, at CMS, evaluation of the role of URM health providers in serving an increasingly diverse Medicare population could be conducted by the Office of Research, Development, and Information, which carries out various studies and demonstrations on the agency's programs. Bureau of the Census predictions on diversity show that, by 2025, "racial and ethnic minority Americans will more than double as a share of the elderly, rising from 14 percent to 35 percent and representing one in three seniors." Latinos are expected to account for 18 percent, African Americans for 10 percent, and other races for 7 percent of the minority elderly population (Henry J. Kaiser Family Foundation, 1999).

For a final example, evaluation at the VA is the responsibility of the Office of Policy, Planning, and Preparedness. None of the recent evaluations completed by the office dealt with URMs in the health professions, although one ("An Evaluation of Leadership VA") touched on changing veteran demographics and leadership responses (U.S. VA, 2003b).

Private as well as public funders should recognize the importance of conducting high-quality studies and evaluations that rigorously examine federal URM health professions programs. Studies are needed to document the programs' effectiveness or lack of effectiveness over time and their outcomes relative to program participants' lives and contributions to the health professions.

Greater Support for the National Center for Health Workforce Analysis and Its Regional Centers in URM Data Collection and Analysis

Obtaining data to provide supporting documentation for initiatives to increase URM participation in the health professions has been a major barrier. Establishment of the National Center for Health Workforce Analysis and its regional centers at UCSF, SUNY at Albany, UIC, UW, and UT is a significant step forward in collecting and analyzing data on national and state practices and policies. The center's mission is to collect and analyze health professions data, assist in state and local workforce planning efforts, conduct workforce issues analyses, evaluate health professions training programs, and develop tools for and conduct research on the health workforce. It is the only federal effort that focuses on health workforce supply, demand, and related issues.

The National Center for Health Workforce Analysis has ambitious goals, given its modest budget ($819,000 for FY 2003, down from $824,000 in FY 2002). These goals are the following (HRSA, 2003f):

• Assess the nation's supply of and requirements for health professionals and paraprofessionals and analyze how they are affected by internal and external changes in the health care system.
• Carry out technical and analytic activities regarding the adequacy of the health professions workforce in meeting the nation's need for an appropriately sized and trained health workforce that is suitably diversified by specialty, race, and gender, and is geographically balanced.
• Conduct research studies, data collection, and technical modeling.
• Assist regional workforce planning efforts.
• Evaluate the success of HRSA Bureau of Health Professions training programs.
• Include physicians, registered nurses, licensed practical nurses, certified nursing assistants, pharmacists, optometrists, chiropractors, allied health personnel, and public health personnel.
• Compile limited data on national health expenditures.

Obviously, if the center is to fulfill its promise, its budget, which competes with various other activities in HRSA, agencies in DHHS, and departments in the federal government for funds, has to be sufficient for its staff and subcontractors to gather the needed data and analyze them. Instead, the budget seems to be on a downward, rather than upward, trajectory, at a time when having and assessing workforce data have never been more important.

Improved Response to Demographic Changes by Federal and State Health Agencies

Just as various agencies at DHHS and the VA are aware of the growing burden on their health and social insurance resources caused by aging of the baby boomers (people born between 1946 and 1964), their administrators are becoming increasingly sensitive to the racial and ethnic demographic changes occurring in this country. Given the prediction that, by 2050, "one of every two U.S. workers [of all types] will be African American, Hispanic, Asian American, Pacific Islander, or Native American" (IOM, 2001b), officials in both the federal and state governments face a number of challenges. One challenge is the significance of cultural competence—and perhaps cultural concordance—in the delivery of quality care. Another is the disproportionate impact of certain illnesses—hypertension, diabetes, heart disease, and asthma, for example—in certain minority groups. Still another is preparation of a health workforce to care for an increasingly diverse population.

Various efforts are underway to respond to the challenges—providing patients who have limited English skills with access to interpreters or native-speaking providers; tying health status goals and indicators to ethnicity (as in *Healthy People 2000* and *2010*); assessing cultural competency of providers in government-funded health settings; conducting clinical and quality studies of services provided to individuals in various racial and ethnic groups; making sure that Medicaid managed care contractors meet culturally appropriate standards; and tracking Medicaid patients relative to demographic data on ethnicity and cultural characteristics. Crucial as well are broad-based efforts to project the needs of increasingly diverse Medicare and Medicaid beneficiaries and discretionary program clients; to provide incentives to attract URMs to health professions careers; to strengthen scholarship, loan, mentoring, and other aspects that relate to health professions education and training; and to put greater emphasis on nurturing URM health professions faculty, administrators, researchers, and other health leaders.

Strategies such as multiyear authorizations and appropriations to give greater certainty to program funding, interagency coordinating councils to share information and seek common threads among compartmentalized programs, and joint efforts (such as the clinical partnership that DoD and the VA have in sites such as Albuquerque) would enhance federal responses to the demographic evolution that the United States is undergoing.

Initiation of Research and Demonstrations by CMS on URM Relationships to the Medicare and Medicaid Programs

Although DHHS' Health Care Financing Administration (now CMS) waxed and waned over time regarding Medicare and Medicaid waiver authority, there seems to be greater receptivity at this time to demonstrations in both programs. CMS can grant waivers applicable to both Medicare and Medicaid regarding provider reimbursement, prospective payment, and social health maintenance organization projects. Under Medicaid alone, CMS can give states program flexibility: "freedom of choice" waivers for development of case management and managed care arrangements and home- and community-based waivers for provision of services outside hospital and nursing-home settings. Under Medicaid, CMS can also encourage states to experiment and conduct research through Section 1115 waivers that allow them to depart from federal Medicaid requirements; states have been pushing the envelope in using the waivers to address innovative policy goals.

It is unclear how far CMS might go in the testing of new policy approaches in the Medicare program, such as in targeting some Medicare GME funds to increasing URM participation in medical residencies, perhaps by developing additional incentives for teaching hospitals that have been successful in mentoring URM residents. Nevertheless, CMS has the tools for experimentation, although it may take congressional bill or report language to give priority to it.

Action on Medicare GME Proposals by the Council on Graduate Medical Education and the Medicare Payment Advisory Commission

Both COGME and the Medicare Payment Advisory Commission (MedPAC) have proposals on the table to address discretionary and Medicare GME financial incentives. COGME, authorized in 1986 to advise both Congress and the Secretary of Health and Human Services and housed in HRSA's Bureau of Health Professions, has made various recommendations over the years in a series of reports. COGME dealt specifically with minority representation in the physician workforce in 1990 and 1998. Its recommendations on minority representation are summarized in COGME's *2002 Summary Report*. In addition to suggesting supply approaches, COGME "urged that federal funding priority be given to medical schools and teaching hospitals that have demonstrated success in recruiting and retaining underrepresented minority students." It also urged expansion of public- and private-sector scholarship and loan programs and of the NHSC "to allow targeted opportunities for minority students."

Noting that "Native Americans, Blacks, Hispanics, or Latinos comprise only 6.2 percent of faculty in U.S. medical schools," COGME also recommended that the federal government "support programs that encourage minorities to pursue careers in academic medicine and provide incentives to medical schools that are successful in recruiting and retaining minority faculty" (COGME, 2002).

MedPAC, an amalgam of the Prospective Payment Assessment Commission and Physician Payment Review Commission that was created in 1997, is responsible for reporting to Congress and the Secretary of Health and Human Services on Medicare payment policies. It recommended a couple of years ago that Medicare GME policy be reformed, especially in terms of combining direct and indirect Medicare GME payments to hospitals to encompass patient care and teaching physician expenses. At the same time, it has shied away from targeting specific health professions workforce goals, such as physician supply or specialty mix, through the Medicare program. Nonetheless, opening the door to changes in how Medicare direct and indirect dollars are dispersed would mean opportunities to tie the payment of funds to specific workforce goals, including those involving URMs.

Development of Clearinghouse on Federal Program Options for URMs in the Health Professions

The lack of centralization, coordination, and collaboration among public funding entities involved in initiatives that directly or indirectly affect URMs in the health professions has a chilling effect on opportunities for individuals interested in, training for, or entering medical, dental, nursing, psychology, and other health careers. Having a clearinghouse of information on federal program criteria, key contact persons, evaluative studies, workforce data, and other topics would be one means of addressing the problem.

A model for such a clearinghouse might be the IOM's Clinical Research Roundtable, which has as one of its aims developing the clinical research workforce (IOM, 2001a). Spurred by the AAMC and leaders in the medical community and housed at the IOM, the roundtable's mission is to explore challenges facing clinical research, including workforce issues.

Leadership of Key Organizations

Several organizations have worked to spearhead public-private partnerships committed to increasing URM participation in the health professions. Both the W.K. Kellogg Foundation and the Robert Wood Johnson Foundation, at times working with the AAMC, Association of Academic Health Centers, American Association of Colleges of Nursing, the IOM, and other organizations, have funded initiatives on the supply and demand sides to increase minority representation in medicine, nursing, dentistry, and other health professions. Other national foundations, such as the Henry J. Kaiser Family Foundation and Pew Charitable Trusts, have also provided leadership. In addition, state-focused foundations, such as the California HealthCare Foundation and The California Endowment, have been involved, especially in states in which minorities have become or are about to become majorities.

Given key foundations' interest in URM health workforce issues, public-private partnerships should be encouraged. Such partnerships might include hosting conferences to bring private initiatives to the attention of federal and state officials, researching and demonstrating model incentive programs, disseminating information on federal health professions options of all types for URMs, or other initiatives.

Responses to GAO Recommendations to Increase Diversity of the Senior Executive Service

In increasing URM participation in the health professions, leadership is clearly important to the formulation of goals, development of programs, and directing of dollars. The GAO reported on diversity—defined by race, ethnicity, and gender—in the federal "senior corps," the Senior Executive Service (SES), in a January 2003 report (GAO, 2003), concluding that efforts need to be made to make it more diverse. GAO indicated that "more than half of the 6,100 career SES members employed on October 1, 2000, will have left service by October 1, 2007."

Of the 6,100, minority women and men made up about 14 percent, "white women about 19 percent, and white men about 67 percent." Based on current SES employment trends, GAO projected what the employment profile would be if appointment trends do not change. It found that "the only significant changes in diversity will be an increase in the number of white women and an essentially equal decrease in white men. The proportions of minority women and men will remain virtually unchanged in the SES corps." The increase in racial and ethnic minorities is only 0.7 percent, with that of white women at 4 percent; the decrease in white men is projected at 5 percent.

While commitment to goals of diversity in the health professions goes beyond race and ethnicity, there is reason to question federal dedication to the goals if its own leadership is so skewed. The GAO study implies that it is skewed and is likely to remain so. Although GAO likely will monitor development of the workforce over time, the topic of URM participation in SES needs to be addressed as quickly as possible, with a focus on recruitment, leadership training, mentoring, and retention issues. Although the project might fall within the rubric of a public–private partnership or a foundation program, it has ramifications not only for 2007 but also for the years that follow.

CONCLUSION

This paper provides an overview of various programs in the federal government and in the states that address the health professions, particularly medicine, nursing, dentistry, and professional psychology. It seeks to follow the financial trails of these federal and state programs: to indicate direct URM goals, when they exist, and indirect URM goals, when they are apparent. It also seeks to identify health professions programs that might serve as models and policies that might be pursued to increase the participation of URMs in the health professions.

The paper relies on various evaluations of federal health professions programs, some of which are URM centered and some of which are not. It also draws from numerous other sources, including program descriptions and overviews from both public and private sources, many drawn from the World Wide Web. An analysis of the evaluations and sources reveals various barriers to increasing URM participation in the health professions. The opportunities section provides pathways that might be taken to expand such participation:

- By using existing authorities and pursuing new funding sources to conduct studies at the federal level on increasing URM participation in the health professions, particularly medicine, dentistry, nursing, and professional psychology.
- By providing greater support to the National Center for Health Workforce Analysis and its regional centers to address URM health professions issues at both the national and state levels.
- By strengthening existing and developing new public programs—federal and state—dedicated to educating, training, and nurturing URMs in medicine, dentistry, nursing, professional psychology, and other health professions.
- By encouraging and perhaps mandating CMS to do research and demonstrations on the relationship between URM health professionals and its programs.
- By adopting COGME's recommendations for improving the participation of URMs in medicine and responding to MedPAC's criticisms of current Medicare GME policy.
- By creating a clearinghouse to collect and disseminate information on various aspects of URM preparation for and participation in the health professions.
- By seeking public-private partnerships and foundation initiatives that relate to URM participation in the health workforce.
- By undertaking an initiative that focuses on increasing URM entry into and retention in SES in order to strengthen the leadership that is essential to making federal government officials more representative of the population they serve.

GLOSSARY

AAMC = Association of American Medical Colleges
AHEC = Area Health Education Center
APA = American Psychological Association
ASPE = Assistant Secretary for Planning and Evaluation
CHGME = Children's Hospitals Graduate Medical Education
CMS = Centers for Medicare and Medicaid Services
COE = Centers of Excellence
COGME = Council on Graduate Medical Education
DHHS = Department of Health and Human Services
DoD = Department of Defense
FFS = fee for service
FLRP = Faculty Loan Repayment Program
GAO = General Accounting Office
GME = Graduate Medical Education
HCOP = Health Careers Opportunity Program
HETC = Health Education and Training Center
HPSP = Health Professions Scholarship Program
HRSA = Health Resources and Services Administration
IGT = intergovernmental transfer
IMG = international medical graduate
IOM = Institute of Medicine
IRB = intern/resident per bed
MARC = Minority Access to Research Careers
MBRS = Minority Biomedical Research Support
MedPAC = Medicare Payment Advisory Commission
MERC = Medical Education and Research Cost
NELRP = Nursing Education Loan Repayment Program
NHSC = National Health Service Corps
NIGMS = National Institute of General Medical Sciences
NIH = National Institutes of Health
NSF = National Science Foundation
OIG = Office of Inspector General
PHS = Public Health Service
PPS = prospective payment system
RISE = Research Initiative for Scientific Enhancement
RN = registered nurse
ROTC = Reserve Officer Training Corps
SCORE = Support of Continuous Research Excellence
SDS = Scholarships for Disadvantaged Students
SES = Senior Executive Service
SUNY = State University of New York

UCSF = University of California, San Francisco
UIC = University of Illinois at Chicago
URM = underrepresented minority
UT = Utah or University of Texas (depending on context)
UW = University of Washington
VA = Department of Veterans Affairs or Virginia (depending on context)

REFERENCES

Advisory Committee on Training in Primary Care Medicine and Dentistry. 2001. *Comprehensive Review and Recommendations, Title VII, Section 747 of the Public Health Service Act*. Report to Secretary of the U.S. Department of Health and Human Services, and Congress. [Online]. Available: http://www.bhpr.hrsa.gov/medicine-dentistry/ actpcmd/report2001.htm [accessed March 29, 2003]. Pp. 19 67, 69.

AAMC (Association of American Medical Colleges). 2003. *AAMC's Project 3000 by 2000 Announces New Grants to Prepare Minorities for Health Professions Careers*. [Online]. Available: http://www.aamc.org/newsroom/pressrel/1999/990209.htm [accessed August 28, 2003].

AMA (American Medical Association). 2001. *Total Physicians by Race/Ethnicity—2001*. [Online]. Available: http://www.ama-assn.org/ama/pub/article/168-187.html [accessed May 18, 2003].

APA (American Psychological Association). 2002. *National Health Service Corps Reauthorization*. [Online]. Available: http://www.apa.org/ppo/issues/enhscupd.html [accessed May 19, 2003]. P. 1.

Catalog of Federal Domestic Assistance. 2003. *Extramural Loan Repayment for Individuals from Disadvantaged Backgrounds Conducting Clinical Research*. [Online]. Available: http://www.cfda.gov/static/93308.htm [accessed August 29, 2003].

CMS (Centers for Medicare and Medicaid Services), U.S. Department of Health and Human Services. 2002. November 12. *Health Care Industry Market Update. Acute Care Hospitals, Vol. 2. Appendix: Medicare Payment Systems*. [Online]. Available: http://www.cms .hhs.gov/reports/hcimu/hcimu_04292002_append.pdf [accessed August 28, 2003]. P. 6.

COGME (Council on Graduate Medical Education). 1998. *Twelfth Report*. Rockville, MD: Health Resources and Services Administration, U.S. Department of Health and Human Services. P. 19.

_____. 2002. *2002 Summary Report*. Rockville, MD: Health Resources and Services Administration, U.S. Department of Health and Human Services. Pp. 6-7, 8–9.

Cohen JJ, Gabriel BA, Terrell C. 2002. The case for diversity in the health care workforce. *Health Affairs* 21(5):91.

Distributed Communications Corporation. 1998. *Health Resources and Services Administration: Assessment of Historically Black Medical Schools; Participation in HRSA-Supported Health Professions Training Programs*. [Online]. Available: http://www.hrsa.gov/ OMH/HBMS/cover-contents-execsummary.doc [accessed May 23, 2003]. P. xv.

Duke EM. 2002. *Remarks to a Meeting of Health Careers Opportunity Program Directors*. [Online]. Available: http://newsroom.hrsa.gov/speeches/2002speeches/hcop.htm [accessed May 19, 2003]. P. 4.

_____. 2003. *Statement on Fiscal Year 2004 President's Budget Request for the Health Resources and Services Administration*. [Online]. Available: http://www.hhs.gov/budget/ testify/b20030326c.html [accessed May 21, 2003]. P. 3.

GAO (General Accounting Office). 2003, January 17. *Senior Executive Service: Enhanced Agency Efforts Needed to Improve Diversity as the Senior Corps Turns Over.* GAO-03-34. [Online]. Available: http://www.gao.gov/ [accessed May 21, 2003].

Grumbach K, Coffman J, Muñoz C, Rosenoff E, Gándara P, Sepulveda E. 2003, August. *Strategies for Improving the Diversity of the Health Professions.* The California Endowment. [Online]. Available: http://www.calendow.org/pub/publications/Strategiesfor Improving11-03.pdf [accessed December 20, 2003].

Henderson T. 2000. Medicaid's role in financing graduate medical education. *Health Affairs* 19(1):223–225. In: Matherlee K. 2001. *Federal and State Perspectives on GME Reform.* Washington, DC: National Health Policy Forum, George Washington University. P. 7.

Henry J. Kaiser Family Foundation. 1999, July 1. *The Faces of Medicine: Medicare and Minority Americans.* [Online]. Available: http://www.kff.org/content/1999/1481/minorities.pdf [accessed January 29, 2003].

HRSA (Health Resources and Services Administration), U.S. Department of Health and Human Services. 2001a. *Annual Report 2001.* [Online]. Available: http://www.hrsa.gov/annualreport2001/part6.html [accessed May 21, 2003]. P. 6.

_____. 2001b. *Professional Nurse Traineeship Grants: Who Gets Them and Where Do They Work After Graduation?* [Online]. Available: http://bhpr.hrsa.gov/nursing/pntreport.htm [accessed August 26, 2003].

_____. 2002, November 4. *FY 2003 Applications.* [Online]. Available: http://www.bhpr.hrsa.gov/grants/ [accessed March 20, 2003].

_____. 2003a. *Bureau of Health Professions Programs: Diversity—Centers of Excellence.* [Online]. Available: http://bhpr.hrsa.gov/diversity/coe/default.htm [accessed August 26, 2003].

_____. 2003b. *Bureau of Health Professions Programs: Diversity—Health Careers Opportunity Program.* [Online]. Available: http://bhpr.hrsa.gov/diversity/hcop/default.htm [accessed August 26, 2003].

_____. 2003c. *Faculty Loan Repayment Program.* [Online]. Available: http://bhpr.hrsa.gov/DSA/flrp/ [accessed August 26, 2003].

_____. 2003d. *FY 2003 Application Kit: Training in Primary Care Medicine and Dentistry Grant Program.* [Online]. Available: http://www.bhpr.hrsa.gov/grants/applications/03dentpc.htm [accessed March 29, 2003].

_____. 2003e. *Health Professions: Scholarships for Disadvantaged Students.* [Online]. Available: http://bhpr.hrsa.gov/dsa/sfag/health_professions/bk1prt6.htm [accessed August 26, 2003].

_____. 2003f. *National Center for Health Workforce Analysis Areas of Focus.* [Online]. Available: http://bhpr.hrsa.gov/healthworkforce/about/default.htm [accessed August 16, 2003].

_____. 2003g. *Nursing Education Loan Repayment Program.* [Online]. Available: http://bhpr.hrsa.gov/nursing/loanreehf.htm [accessed August 26, 2003].

_____. 2003h. *Nursing Workforce Diversity Program.* [Online]. Available: http://bhpr.hrsa.gov/kidscareers/nursing_workforce.htm [accessed August 26, 2003].

_____. 2003i. *Office of Minority Health Projects and Initiatives.* [Online]. Available: http://www.hrsa.gov/OMH/OMH/main2_projects.htm [accessed March 20, 2003]. P. 1–7.

IOM (Institute of Medicine). 2001a. *Developing the Clinical Investigator Workforce: Clinical Research Roundtable Symposium I.* [Online]. Available: http://www.iom.edu/includes/dbfile.asp?id=4127 [accessed August 28, 2003]. P. 2.

_____. 2001b. In: Smedley BD, Stith AY, Colburn L, Evans CH, eds.. *The Right Thing to Do, The Smart Thing to Do: Enhancing Diversity in Health Professions—Summary of the Symposium on Diversity in Health Professions in Honor of Herbert W. Nickens, M.D.* Washington, DC: National Academy Press. P. 1.

Kohout J, Wicherski M, Woerheide K. 1999. *1996 Doctorate Employment Survey.* [Online]. Available: http://research.apa.org/des96contents.html#demographic [accessed May 18, 2003]. P. 3.

Konrad T, Leysieffer K, Stevens C, Irvin C, Martinez RM, Nguyen TTH. 2000. *Evaluation of the Effectiveness of the National Health Service Corps: Executive Summary of the Final Report.* [Online]. Available: http://216.239.33.100/search?q=cache:-VkoIcF7BAgJ:www.shepscenter.unc.edu/research_programs/primary_care/nhscsum.pdf+Evaluation+of+the+Effectiveness+of+the+National+Health+Service+Corps&hl=en&ie=UTF-8 [accessed May 21, 2003]. P. xxi

Mertz E, O'Neil E. 2002. The growing challenge of providing oral health care services to all Americans. *Health Affairs* 21(5):68.

Minorities in Uniform as of September 5, 2000. 2000, September 5. [Online]. Available: http://www.defenselink.mil/pubs/almanac/almanac/people/minorities.html [accessed August 29, 2003].

National Center for Health Workforce Analysis, Health Resources and Services Administration. 2001. *The Health Care Workforce in Ten States: Education, Practice, and Policy.* Rockville, MD: Bureau of Health Professions. P. 20.

National Center on Minority Health and Health Disparities. 2003. *Loan Repayment Program for Health Disparities Research.* [Online]. Available: http://ncmhd.nih.gov/our_programs/loan/index.asp [accessed August 29, 2003].

NIGMS (National Institute of General Medical Science), National Institutes of Health. 2000, May. *News and Events: The Careers and Professional Activities of Former NIGMS Minority Access to Research Careers Predoctoral Fellows.* [Online]. Available: http://www.nigms.nih.gov/news/reports/marcstudy.html [accessed May 21, 2003]. P. 1.

_____. 2002. *MARC and MBRS Programs. Update.* [Online]. Available: http://www.nigms.nih.gov/news/mpusummer02.pdf [accessed May 21, 2003]. P. 1, 5.

_____. 2003. *Research Funding: Research Grant Mechanisms.* [Online]. Available: http://www.nigms.nih.gov/funding/grntmech.html [accessed May 21, 2003]. P. 1–2.

NIH (National Institutes of Health). 2000a. *Evaluation of the Research Centers in Minority Institutions Program. Final Report 2000.* [Online]. Available: www.ncrr.nih.gov/newspub/apr00rpt/News.asp [accessed August 29, 2003].

_____. 2000b. *Midcourse Assessment of the Research Infrastructure in Minority Institutions Program.* [Online]. Available: http://www.ncrr.nih.gov/newspub/apr00rpt/News.asp [accessed August 29, 2003].

_____. 2001, April 9. *Program Announcement: Research Supplements for Underrepresented Minorities.* [Online]. Available: http://grants1.nih.gov/grants/guide/pa-files/PA-01-079.html [accessed May 21, 2003].

_____. 2003. Undergraduate Scholarship Program. [Online]. Available: http://ugsp.info.nih.gov/exesumfaq.htm#exesum_awards [accessed August 29, 2003].

OMB (Office of Management and Budget). 2003. National Science Foundation. *Budget of the United States Government.* [Online]. Available: http://www.whitehouse.gov/omb/budget/fy2004/pdf/budget/nsf.pdf [accessed May 21, 2003]. P. 279.

Pate WE II. 2001. *Analyses of Data from Graduate Study in Psychology: 1999–2000.* [Online]. Available: http://research.apa.org/grad00contents.html [accessed May 18, 2003].

Policy Information Center, Office of the Assistant Secretary for Planning and Evaluation, U.S. Department of Health and Human Services. 2002. *Performance Improvement 2002. Appendix A: Evaluation in the Department of Health and Human Services.* [Online]. Available: http://aspe.hhs.gov/pic/perfimp/2002/appendixa.htm#eval [accessed August 29, 2003].

Spratley E, Johnson A, Sochalski J, Fritz M, Spencer W. 2000. *The Registered Nurse Population: Findings from the National Sample Survey of Registered Nurses.* [Online]. Available: http://bhpr.hrsa.gov/healthworkforce/rnsurvey/ [accessed May 18, 2003]. Pp. 17, 20.

Thompson TG. 2002, February 28. NHSC press release [untitled]. [Online]. Available: http://bhpr.hrsa.gov/dsa/pages/hot.htm [accessed March 20, 2003]. P. 1.

U.S. Army. 1982, June 1. *Army Regulation 601-141, U.S. Army Health Professions Scholarship Program.* [Online]. Available: http://www.usapa.army.mil/pdffiles/r601_141.pdf [accessed August 21, 2003]. P. 1.

_____. 2003a. *Army ROTC Nurse Officer Program.* [Online]. Available: http://www.armyrotc.com/scholar_pgs/scholar_nurse.html [accessed August 18, 2003].

_____. 2003b. *Health Professions Loan Repayment Program.* [Online]. Available: http://meded.amedd.army.mil/pages/health.htm [accessed August 18, 2003].

_____. 2003c. *ROTC Officership: To Help You Finance Your College Years.* [Online]. Available: http://www.armyrotc.com/scholar.html [accessed August 18, 2003].

U.S. Census Bureau. 2001. *Statistical Abstract of the United States, 2001.* Section 1: Population, Table 10. [Online]. Available: http://www.census.gov/prod/2002pubs/01statab/pop.pdf [accessed March 10, 2003]. P. 13.

U.S. DHHS (U.S. Department of Health and Human Services). 1998. *Strategies for the Recruitment, Retention, and Graduation of Hispanics into Baccalaureate Levels of Nursing.* [Online]. Available: http://www.aspe.hhs.gov/pic/perfimp/1998/appendixb.htm [accessed August 29, 2003].

_____. 2002, January. *Faculty Loan Repayment Program—Making More Effective Use of Program Funds, January 29, 2001.* [Online]. Available: http://aspe.hhs.gov/pic/display.cfm?varID=7778 [accessed August 29, 2003].

_____. 2003a. *Evaluation of the Extramural Associates Research Development Award Program.* [Online]. Available: http://aspe.hhs.gov/pic/display.cfm?varID=7627 [accessed January 29, 2003].

_____. 2003b. *FY 2004 Budget in Brief.* HRSA section. [Online]. Available: http://www.hhs.gov/budget/04budget/fy2004bib.pdf [accessed May 20, 2003]. P. 14.

U.S. Navy Education and Training Command. 2003. *Naval Reserve Officers Training Corps. Nursing Option.* [Online]. Available: https://www.nrotc.navy.mil/nursingoption.cfm [accessed August 18, 2003].

U.S. Navy Medical Department. 2003. *Navy Medical Department GME Overview 2003.* [Online]. Available: http://nshs.med.navy.mil/gme/NAVMEDGME.htm [accessed August 18, 2003].

U.S. Navy Medical Education and Training Command. 2003. *Armed Forces Health Professions Scholarship Program.* [Online]. Available: http://nshs.med.navy.mil/hpsp/Pages/HPSPHome.htm [accessed August 18, 2003].

U.S. VA (U.S. Department of Veterans Affairs). 2002. *For Researchers: Minority Research Training Programs.* [Online]. Available: http://www.va.gov/resdev/fr/minority_training.cfm [accessed August 28, 2003].

_____. Office of Academic Affiliations. 2003a. *Graduate Medical Education.* [Online]. Available: http://www.va.gov/oaa/gme_default.asp [accessed September 3, 2002].

_____. 2003b. *Office of Policy, Planning, and Preparedness Program Evaluation Service.* [Online]. Available: http://www.va.gov/OPP/organizations/progeval.htm [accessed August 28, 2003].

Paper Contribution C
The Role of Accreditation in Increasing Racial and Ethnic Diversity in the Health Professions

Norma E. Wagoner, Ph.D., Leon Johnson, D.Ed., M.B.A., and Harry S. Jonas, M.D.

The authors will review accreditation from a historical and process-oriented vantage point and examine various health professions standards relating to diversity. Because our expertise lies in the field of medical student education, we will closely analyze those standards promulgated by the Liaison Committee on Medical Education (LCME), including a discernment of the impact the LCME standards have had on U.S. medical school programs. As background for the role of accreditation, the authors review the social contract that the health professions have with the public. Background information also includes looking at ways in which accrediting bodies can assist through standards to achieve diversity in student bodies and faculties. Within this context, we examine the recent Supreme Court decision to determine the latitude now allowed to develop new standards for admissions. Throughout this commissioned paper the authors will make recommendations as to the development of new accreditation standards, strengthening of existing ones, and ways in which accreditation, with effort and collaboration among health care leaders, will ultimately result in a diverse U.S. health-care workforce commensurate with a diverse population.

THE ROLES AND REPSONSIBILITIES OF ACCREDITING BODIES

The Goal of Accreditation

The U.S. Department of Education (ED) defines accreditation as "a status granted to an institution that indicates it is meeting its mission and the standards of the [accreditation] organization and seems likely to continue to meet that mission for the foreseeable future" (U.S. Department of State, 2003, p. 2). Accreditation is the primary means by which the federal government ensures that U.S. institutions and programs of higher education maintain and improve their quality standards of education. It has been in place for nearly a century. Those institutions/programs that meet and maintain specified educational standards are deemed "accredited," or as holding "accreditation."

Although accrediting bodies have their own specific standards, they may require that institutions and programs that seek accreditation have an overall stated purpose (or mission) that defines the students it serves and delineates the objectives of the institution's or program's activities. In addition, accrediting organizations direct each educational institution/program to show evidence that it accomplishes the following:

• Provides adequate resources necessary to achieve its purposes; that is, financial resources, sufficiently prepared faculty and instructional staff, clearly defined admissions policies, and a coordinated and coherent curriculum;
• Defines educational objectives; and
• Demonstrates evidence that those objectives are being achieved.

A private form of self-regulation, accreditation offers a strong incentive to institutions/programs to improve academic quality as they go through the required periodic reviews. Accreditation's most critical responsibility is to sustain and enhance the quality of higher education. In so doing, it protects the public by identifying institutions/programs that have yet to establish "sound academic and fiscal practices leading to quality operations" (Eaton, 2003, p. 1). In addition to serving the public's interest and needs, accreditation acts as a protective barrier against the undue pressures of politics. Accrediting organizations have adopted this role in part because of the willingness of the federal government to rely on accreditation to guarantee academic quality rather than directly assuming responsibility. Each of the 50 states has a system of licensing institutions of higher education that allows them to conduct business and issue degrees legally in that state. The determination of how institutions/programs meet minimum education standards primarily falls on the accreditation body.

Through their domains and standards, accrediting bodies encourage institutional freedom in developing programs that secure sound educational experimentation and constructive innovation (APA, 2002).

Inherent in their overall goal, accrediting organizations assume the responsibility of making certain that institutions/programs pursue and achieve diversity both in accordance with their individual mission statements and educational objectives, as well as with the standards of the accrediting body (CCNE, 1998). Their purpose further includes the improvement of institutions or programs relevant to resources invested, processes followed, and results achieved. The monitoring of certificate, diploma, and degree offerings ties closely to state and national examinations, licensing rules, and the oversight of preparation for work in the profession (NLNAC, 1999).

What Constitutes an Accrediting Body

In accordance with their mission, accrediting organizations determine and oversee compliance of standards. Furthermore, they provide mechanisms to perform an evaluation of an institution's/program's mission, educational philosophy, and goals/objectives, as well as to assess the performance of the program in achieving these goals. Currently 19 nongovernmental organizations accredit approximately 6,300 institutions, and an additional 60 (e.g., law, medicine, business) accredit approximately 17,500 programs (Eaton, 2003). Institutional accreditation deals with the quality and integrity of the total institution, while program accreditation evaluates programs in the various specialized professional or occupational fields.

Who Governs Accrediting Bodies

The ED oversees all accrediting bodies, including specifying and approving the role and scope of their activities (Commissioned Paper C). ED performs a periodic review of each organization to determine the merit of its continuation as the accreditation body. ED activities in this regard are determined by federal legislation known as the Higher Education Act. The reauthorization of that legislation, currently under consideration, should focus on the importance of increasing racial and ethnic diversity in the health professions. Although not directly involved in the process of accreditation, ED does publish a list of accrediting organizations that it recognizes as reliable authorities on the quality of education or training provided by institutions of higher education and their educational programs. Should an accrediting association fail to achieve ED recognition, students under the jurisdiction of that association no longer would be eligible for certain federal loan programs.

Accrediting bodies oversee (1) general, liberal education; (2) technical and vocational education and training; and (3) education and training for the professions. Accrediting bodies generally belong to one of two organizations:

- The Council for Higher Education Accreditation (CHEA), which ensures the quality and integrity of the total institution in its efforts to meet stated mission, goals, and objectives; or
- The Association of Specialized and Professional Accreditors (ASPA), which oversees programs of study in professional or occupational fields (e.g., law, medicine, dentistry).

Nongovernmental organizations such as CHEA and ASPA align closely with public interest. While maintaining a "suitable distance from the political realm" (Eaton, 2003, p. 6), they serve in a critical capacity in their commitment to regulating academic values.

How the Accreditation Process Works

The accreditation process consists of a review and assessment of an institution or program relevant both to the accrediting body's standards as well as to the institution's/program's mission, educational philosophy, and goals/objectives. Accrediting organizations also evaluate evidence regarding the application of available resources, programs, and administration in assisting the students in attaining their educational goals. Medical institutions usually acknowledge that, without being proscriptive, the accreditation process has served as a powerful influence in shaping the medical education experience. Accrediting organizations initiate the accreditation process every 5 to 10 years or sooner, depending on the success of the institution/program in demonstrating continuing compliance and improvements in the quality of its educational program.

THE HISTORICAL AND CURRENT ROLE OF THE LIAISON COMMITTEE ON MEDICAL EDUCATION

Historical Perspective

Assessment of the quality of medical education programs began in the United States more than 150 years ago, when a group of physicians who were frustrated and discouraged about the lack of educational excellence of these programs decided to address the issue. Prior to this time, the quality of medical education in the United States was so poor that those U.S. residents who desired a first rate medical education attended European institutions. The hundreds of so-called medical schools in this country, mostly proprietary, provided little in the way of a formal education and for the most part consisted of storefront operations that awarded the degree of doctor of medicine primarily to those willing to pay for it.

With the improvement of American medical education as their focus, this group of early-day physicians founded the American Medical Association (AMA) in 1847. This effort prompted the Carnegie Foundation to fund a study of U.S. medical education, conducted by Abraham Flexner. Flexner's landmark report, published in 1910 (Flexner, 1910), resulted in the closure of the vast majority of the poor-quality medical schools. Among those closed were five of the seven medical schools that admitted black applicants. The report also led to the development of a process to set standards to guarantee higher quality education, including periodic review of medical schools to ensure compliance with established standards. The process of accreditation now extends to all levels and types of educational programs.

In the early part of the twentieth century, two organizations, the AMA and the Association of American Medical Colleges (AAMC), conducted the accreditation of U.S. medical schools. In 1942, because of both wartime constrictions in resources and the objections of medical school deans to the efforts required to undergo two accreditation reviews, the AMA and the AAMC formed an accreditation partnership. This became known as the Liaison Committee on Medical Education, or LCME, with the AMA representing rank-and-file practicing physicians and the AAMC representing academic physicians.

The LCME assumed full responsibility for accreditation of medical education programs leading to the M.D. degree in the United States. Subsequently the organization, in cooperation with the Committee on Accreditation of Canadian Medical Schools (CACMS), expanded its scope to include accreditation of Canadian programs leading to the M.D. degree. CACMS is structured similarly to the LCME, with equal representation from the Association of Canadian Medical Colleges and the Council on Medical Education of the Canadian Medical Association, making it a joint venture between the organization representing academic medicine and the organization representing organized medicine. Although the committees function independently and meet separately, cross-representation occurs at both the membership and the secretariat levels. The LCME consists of 17 members: 6 appointed by the AMA, 6 appointed by the AAMC, 2 students selected from the student organizations of the two sponsors, 2 public representatives, and 1 CACMS representative.

In the introduction to the LCME standards document, *Functions and Structure of a Medical School,* updated in June 2002, the organization defines accreditation as a "voluntary, peer-review process designed to attest to the educational quality of new and established educational programs" (LCME, 2002, p. ii). The introduction continues (*and this is key to the subject being addressed in this paper*): "By judging the compliance of medical education programs with nationally accepted standards of educational quality, these accrediting agencies serve the interest of the general public and of the students enrolled in those programs" (LCME, 2000, p. ii).

Development of Accreditation Standards

The four sponsoring organizations that constitute North American accreditation for the M.D. degree develop the actual accreditation standards by consensus. Standards typically are broadly drawn up and not overly proscriptive to allow more innovative approaches throughout 152 very different U.S. and Canadian medical schools. Accreditation standards are written in narrative fashion and divided into two categories, "musts" and "shoulds." The "musts" standards require compliance regardless of circumstances. Although accrediting bodies expect institutions/programs to comply with "should" standards, they allow them to be modified by extenuating circumstances. The sponsoring organizations do not incorporate numerical standards and, in fact, only one number appears in the entire LCME standards document, and that is the minimal number of time in weeks required to obtain the M.D. degree.

Changing accreditation standards involves a rather complicated, lengthy process that requires a public hearing and approval by the accrediting organizations, CACMS and the LCME, and their sponsors. Once the accreditation standard has been changed, ED reviews it and may make recommendations regarding the wording or the use of such standards.

The Present Role of the LCME

Today LCME's accreditation of educational programs leading to the M.D. degree involves visits to the 126 U.S. medical schools on an 8-year cycle. Approximately 18 months prior to the visits, the LCME asks the institution/program to select an internal task force, various committees that broadly represent faculty, students, administration, teaching hospital representatives, and support staff to conduct an Institutional Self-Study. The purpose of the self-study is "to promote institutional self-evaluation and improvement" (LCME, *Guide to Institutional Self-Study*, 2002, p. 1). In addition, this experience affords medical schools/programs the opportunity to establish objectives, as well as the proposed means of achieving those objectives relative to its mission.

The LCME chooses a team of medical educators consisting of administrators, faculty members of U.S. medical schools, and/or practicing physicians, usually five in number, to visit the school. On occasion, the team might also include one of the two LCME public members or one of the two student members. The team meets with administrators, faculty, and students to examine all aspects of the educational program, including governance and administration, the academic environment, medical student issues, faculty issues, and educational resources, including finances, general facilities, clinical teaching facilities, information resources, and library services. The LCME requires each school, prior to the team visit, to prepare a comprehensive database that includes detailed information about each of the above listed areas. The school is required to mail this to the LCME team members well in advance of the site visit.

At the end of the two-and-one-half-day site visit, the team chairperson presents an oral report at an exit interview with the dean of the medical school and the university president or chancellor. This report covers three areas: Areas of Strength, Areas of Partial Compliance or Non-Compliance With LCME Standards, and Areas in Transition. Following this oral exit interview, the team departs and each member prepares a segment of the report that the team's secretary later compiles into a full-text written document submitted to the dean for editing of any factual errors. This is then sent to the full membership of the LCME. At the next regular meeting of the LCME, the report is presented, discussion ensues, and after discussion, members decide what action to take regarding accreditation of the educational program. Such action may consist of extending full accreditation for an 8-year term, extending full accreditation pending a return limited visit to determine whether the program has come into compliance with specified standards, or placing the program on probation. If the LCME grants accreditation for an 8-year term, it usually asks the school to submit periodic written reports indicating its progress in addressing any issues identified in the report.

HEALTH PROFESSIONS'/MEDICAL EDUCATION'S RESPONSIBILITY WITHIN THE SOCIAL CONTRACT

The concept of the social contract dates back to the seventeenth-century writing of Hobbes and Locke and the later works of Rousseau. In more recent times, various authors writing about medicine's contract with society have advanced two general themes: First, the responsibility of medical schools to society arises from the nature of the profession itself. That is, by virtue of being a helping profession, all those involved in medicine have an obligation to produce maximum benefit not only to individual patients, but also to society as a whole. Second, because medical schools receive public funds and benefit from public exemptions, they are morally obligated to act in the public interest, which entails taking societal needs into account.

John Colloton, in his 1988 chairman's address to the AAMC, reiterated the first of these contentions: "The traditional covenant between academic medicine and society had its origin in trust. It was based on the premise that academic medicine's unique programs and commitments constituted substantial societal contributions, and thus justified generous support and the *privilege* of self regulation" (Colloton, 1989, p. 55). In a 2003 article from the Association of Canadian Medical Colleges' Working Group on Social Accountability. Parboosing (2003, p. 852) contends:

> Society provides medical schools and the medical profession with certain privileges and resources; these are justified only insofar as they are placed unambiguously in the service of those in need and their community. The public and patients expect that governments and the health care professions will work collaboratively to ensure that the Canadian health care system continues to provide the necessary access and quality to meet the needs of the population. . . . Canadian medical schools along with their partners, such as academic health centers, governments, communities and other relevant professional organizations, have a major role to play in influencing the changes in the health care system that are necessary to ensure an effective, efficient, accessible, equitable and sustainable system.

The World Health Organization has defined the social accountability of medical schools as "the obligation to direct their education, research and service activities towards addressing the priority health concerns of the community, region, and/or nation that they have a mandate to serve" (Borsellino, 2003, p. 1). In a speech in 1989, the then-president of the Robert Wood Johnson Foundation, Dr. Steven Schroeder, reinforced the second premise of accountability: "Because academic medical centers are supported primarily by public funds, and their educational, patient care, and research missions are delegated by society, the health needs of the general population must be considered in decisions about program development" (Schroeder et al., 1989, p. 803).

Although few would argue with the concept of medicine's responsibility to society, various opinions have been voiced as to how institutions/programs should meet this responsibility. Thus no conclusive standard of action has been created that the health professions can adopt. The AAMC and its President, Dr. Jordan Cohen, have clearly articulated the importance of medical schools' responsibility to society and their requirement to fulfill a social contract, particularly in regard to meeting society's need for a diverse health care workforce (Cohen et al., 2002). Indeed, serving public interest and need have been "fundamental to establishing and maintaining a system of higher education that proves responsive to the society it serves" (Eaton, 2003, p. 6). To fulfill this obligation, accrediting organizations must ensure that institutions/programs abide by their social contract.

Beginning with this segment of the document, the authors delineate a series of recommendations.

1. Recommendation. That accrediting bodies undertake a strategic planning process that gives strong consideration to reaffirming the social contract as an obligation of the educational institution.

DIVERSITY AS PART OF THE SOCIAL CONTRACT

Immigration continues to add to the growing diversity of the U.S. population. Generalist physicians can now expect a high percentage of their patients to be from minority cultures (Cross et al., 1989). The differences among minority cultures significantly impact health care delivery, thus creating a critical need for diversity in the health professions. Higher education in part fulfills its societal contract by developing a diverse health professions' workforce that truly reflects our society. It best accomplishes this by having diverse faculties and admitting and maintaining diverse student bodies.

Demographic changes will become increasingly apparent among future U.S. workers. "By the year 2050, one of every two workers will be African American, Latino, Asian American, Pacific Islander, or Native American," noted the Institute of Medicine in a 2001 report (IOM, 2001, p. 1). The increasing number of minorities will continue to create social and political changes throughout society, particularly in health care, where pressures on the financing and delivery systems increase to close the gap in health status between minorities and majority populations.

Using data from the Commonwealth Fund 1994 National Comparative Survey of Minority Health Care (survey sample of 3,789 adults with minorities oversampled,) authors Saha and colleagues (2002) reported their findings in an article in *Health Affairs* entitled "Do Patients Choose Physicians of their Own Race?" The authors found that a significant correlation existed between African-American and Latino patients' ability to choose their physicians and to see physicians of their own race. Approximately a quarter of those African Americans and Latinos surveyed were patients of racially concordant physicians (explicitly considered physician race or ethnicity when selecting their physicians). Among Latinos, 42 percent factored language into their choice of a physician.

In a May 2003 article in *Academic Medicine,* Bollinger states, "Because we know that minority physicians are more likely to practice in areas that contain high concentrations of minorities, diversity among practicing physicians and medical administrators increases the availability of health care within underrepresented minority communities" (Bollinger, 2003, p. 435). The late Dr. Herbert Nickens postulated that minority physicians are more "culturally sensitive to their populations and organize the delivery system in ways more congruent with the needs of a minority population." (Nickens, 1992, p. 2395).

Several medical schools in the United States have achieved diversity in their student bodies through a focused mission or by means of special programs. For example, the University of New Mexico Health Sciences Center has as an institutional mission to provide a diverse workforce and has in place methods by which to assess longitudinal outcome data to determine whether the school is meeting this goal. A 10-year retrospective study demonstrates that the school has been highly successful from its initial identification of a cohort of minority students that ultimately engages in practice in the rural and underserved areas of the state. This mission is supported throughout all levels of the institution (University of New Mexico, unpublished data, 2003). Another school, the University of Illinois at Chicago College of Medicine, graduates one of the largest cohorts of minority students in the country. The college has developed programs to encourage applications from qualified individuals from medically underserved areas of Illinois. The college maintains a professional staff to provide guidance and counseling to motivated students from minority ethnic groups and those resident candidates whose backgrounds indicate potential for practice in underserved areas of the state (AAMC, 2001–2002). The Drew/University of California at Los Angeles (UCLA) medical program offers 24 of the 145 UCLA entering places to students interested in addressing the concerns of an underserved population. Students spend the first 2 years at UCLA and their second 2 years at the Martin Luther King, Jr./Charles R. Drew Medical Center in south central Los Angeles.

Nearly 50 years ago, in *Brown v. Board of Education,* the Supreme Court observed that education is "the very foundation of good citizenship" (*Brown v. Board of Education,* 1954). The court's affirmative decision on the constitutionality that diversity is convincing reinforcement that "Effective participation by members of all racial and ethnic groups in the civic life of our nation is essential if the dream of one Nation, indivisible, is to be realized." (Supreme Court of the United States, 2003, *Grutter et al. v. Bollinger et al.,* 539 U.S. p. 19).

Diversity in Admissions

The Impact of the Supreme Court Decision

The major impact of the Supreme Court decision rendered on June 23, 2003, as it pertains to accreditation, centers squarely on the admissions process and an institution's ability to produce a diverse health care workforce. The University of Michigan cases, *Grutter et al. v. Bollinger et al.* and *Gratz et al. v. Bollinger et al.,* were the most significant tests of affirmative action to reach the courts in generations in that they challenged the university's "ability to compose a student body that enables it to achieve its educational mission and fulfill its obligations to the larger society" (*The Compelling Need,* 1999, p. 7). Two different admissions policies were at issue.

The *Grutter et al. v. Bollinger et al.* case challenged the university's law school admissions policy giving African American, Latino, and Native American applicants a loosely defined special consideration that helped ensure a "critical mass" of such applicants in each new class. A statement released by the Associated Press on June 23, 2003, questioned "whether this policy unconstitutionally discriminated against white students" (AP, 2003). The Supreme Court ruling in this case preserves the concept of affirmative action for minorities who otherwise might be underrepresented on top campuses, while clearly denoting that racial preferences must be used sparingly. The Court majority appeared to advise that if universities were willing to invest the resources to follow the Michigan Law School model and to "painstakingly evaluate each applicant as an 'individual' and not as a mere jumble of statistics, then they too would most likely find themselves on the right side of the law in trying to assemble a diverse class" (Steinberg, 2003, p. A25).

With this decision, the justices effectively overruled major portions of the 1996 U.S. Court of Appeals ruling for the Fifth Circuit in *Hopwood v. Texas* and will allow colleges and universities in the states of Texas, Louisiana, and Mississippi to use race-conscious admissions policies designed to advance diversity. State laws in California, Washington, and Florida still prohibit universities from employing such admissions policies. However, private universities can use properly designed race-conscious policies consistent with their obligations under Title VI of the Civil Rights Act of 1964 and other federal laws (Joint Statement, 2003). AAMC President Dr. Cohen commented that the recent Supreme Court decision gave medical schools (and presumably all health professions' schools) the power to fulfill one of our most solemn obligations: the development of a health professions workforce that truly mirrors our society (Cohen, 2003).

The second case, *Gratz et al. v. Bollinger et al.*, challenged the University of Michigan's undergraduate admissions policy attempting to create a critical mass of African American, Latino, and Native American enrollments by giving these applicants an automatic 20-point bonus on the school's 150-point "selection index." The justices ruled against this policy, holding that it was not tailored narrowly enough to advance an interest in diversity because it lacked flexibility and provided insufficient individualized consideration to applicants (*The Compelling Need*, 1999). The Supreme Court's decision momentarily calms the affirmative action/diversity waters for private and other selective undergraduate and graduate institutions with the resources to comply within the parameters of the decision. Although race cannot be the exclusive or predominant factor in an admissions decision, institutions have some deference in defining the qualifications and composition of their student bodies. A race-conscious admissions policy must consider at least some nonracial factors to ensure that "all

IN THE NATION'S COMPELLING INTEREST

factors that may contribute to the student body diversity are meaningfully considered" (Joint Statement, 2003).

In light of this decision, and given the economic realities of higher education, some large-enrollment and less prosperous colleges and universities may decide to abandon race as an admissions characteristic altogether. Should large institutions choose this route, challenges will accrue to health professions schools hoping to find a cadre of diverse students seeking admission, let alone expecting to graduate a group of students who leave their college years enriched by diversity experiences.

> **2. Recommendation. Given the Supreme Court ruling on June 23, 2003, medical schools should team up with other health professions to discern how to effectively work within the law to find ways in which to increase diversity in the admissions process.**

> **3. Recommendation. Accrediting bodies should carefully review existing standards and develop more specific references to racial and ethnic diversity both in the student admissions processes and in faculty recruitment.**

Achieving Diverse Enrollments

Alan B. Krueger, Benheim Professor of Economics and Public Affairs at Princeton University and a co-editor of *The Journal of the European Economic Association*, recently observed, "A quarter century from now, the Supreme Court will have a tougher call as to whether diversity is still a compelling state" (Krueger, 2003, p. C2). The legacy of discrimination is a powerful retardant to progress in attaining a diverse health-care workforce. However, the Supreme Court has masterfully crafted a constitutional rationale and set an optimistic agenda that is realistic in terms of diversity in higher education, particularly in leadership producing graduate professional programs. Because it addresses and resolves discrimination at its core, diversity, if established as an accreditation requirement, will hasten the elimination of race consciousness in college and university admissions.

Core Competencies as Part of the Social Contract

In fulfilling the social contract, institutions/programs have an obligation to ensure that health profession and medical school graduates demonstrate achievement through outcome measures as specified in the accreditation standards. In addition, they must meet graduation requirements, pass appropriate licensure exams, pass appropriate certification exams, and satisfy other criteria that measure competency as deemed appropriate by the institution/program. The question arises as to whether these requirements have succeeded in producing graduates with the full range of qualifications. As tools of the "social contract," diversity and the core competencies presage a better likelihood that health care professionals have the capability and sensitivity necessary to treat all patients with the respect and understanding they deserve.

Leaders in health education, accrediting bodies, and federal agencies have debated the subject of competencies for many years, focusing on defining those they consider essential, attempting to determine indicators of achievement, and devising measurable outcomes. In recent years the Accreditation Council for Graduate Medical Education (ACGME) has worked with the American Board of Medical Specialties (ABMS) to delineate core competencies that must be attained by those in residency training and practice (ACGME, 2001). We believe that full implementation of such requirements will eventually alter the culture across all areas of medicine. It certainly appears likely that accreditation, particularly with inclusion and emphasis on diversity and cultural competence, also will be able to effect significant change. Modeling aspects of the approaches taken by ACGME and ABMS would provide a major step toward attaining the goal of producing a diverse workforce capable of proffering quality care to a diverse society.

In June 2002, the IOM held a Health Professions Education Summit that brought together 150 expert participants to generate a report on whether "doctors, nurses and other health-care professionals are being adequately prepared to provide the highest quality and safest medical care possible" (IOM, 2003a, p. 7). Their report stressed the importance of integrating a core set of competencies across professions, recommending that all programs that educate and train health professionals adopt these five core competencies: "the abilities to deliver patient-centered care, work as a member of an interdisciplinary team, engage in evidence-based practice, apply quality improvement approaches, and use information technology. The report calls on accreditation, licensing, and certification organizations to make certain that students and working professionals develop and maintain proficiency in these core areas." (IOM, 2003b).

Cultural Competency as Part of the Social Contract

Cultural competency has been described as "a set of academic and personal skills that allow us to increase . . . understanding and appreciation of cultural differences among groups" (Archbold, 1996, pp. A1, A5). In light of this, cultural competency realistically falls under the objective of the IOM recommended core competency, the "ability to deliver patient-centered care."

In her recent article, "Insurgent Multiculturalism: Rethinking How and

Why We Teach Culture in Medical Education," Wear states, "Very few academic medical educators would deny the need for students to understand and respect differences among people based on gender, race, ethnicity, social class, physical or intellectual abilities, sexual identity or religious beliefs. Yet racial disparities in health have been documented throughout history . . . " (Wear, 2003, p. 550). Cultural competency requires that health practitioners not only recognize and treat patients' illnesses, but that they understand the illnesses within the context of each patient's social and cultural backgrounds.

> **4. Recommendation. That high-profile organizations such as the IOM, Department of Health and Human Services, CHEA, ASPA, LCME, and ACGME, along with key foundations and health professions' organizations, convene for the purpose of (1) agreeing upon a core set of competencies that includes diversity and cultural competency, and (2) developing a clear and uniform definition of the core competencies.**

> **5. Recommendation. That accrediting organizations translate the core competencies into standards. Individual accrediting bodies (nursing, medicine, etc.) would need to work out the details of standards that focus on best practices for their disciplines.**

Although many institutions currently grapple with finding methods of teaching and assessing cultural competency in students, few have considered doing the same for their faculty. Obviously having a culturally competent faculty and admitting students with the potential for fully developing cultural competency skills would greatly aid schools/programs in their effort to graduate caring, compassionate students with respect for people of all types.

> **6. Recommendation. Accrediting organizations should require universities and their health-care programs to revise their mission statements to include more specific references to racial and ethnic diversity, cultural competency, and culturally appropriate care for diverse populations. Such standards could further suggest including faculty developmental processes to enhance the teaching of cultural competency.**

Student treatment has become an important and well-understood part of the educational environment in all health professions schools. Many institutions/programs have standards relating to student treatment, with outcome measures provided through student questionnaires. One of these, the 2002 AAMC Graduation Questionnaire, asked students in the 126 U.S. medical schools to rate two important issues: (1) cultural differences and health-related behaviors/customs (71.5 percent indicated their education in this area was "appropriate," while 23.5 percent rated it "inadequate"); and

(2) culturally appropriate care for diverse populations (71.2 percent rated their education in this area "appropriate," and 24.2 percent denoted it as "inadequate") (AAMC, 2002). With one-quarter of approximately 17,000 medical students considering their educational experiences in these cultural issues inadequate, it becomes apparent that greater emphasis needs to be placed on teaching and assessing cultural competency.

If our nation were homogeneous, we would have universal cultural values, belief systems, and language, with health-care providers who share the same set of values, beliefs, and rituals as their patients. Obviously this is not the case, and because educational diversity requires that caregivers provide quality care to a diverse population, they must be taught cultural competency through a developmental process. As Wear notes, "cultural competency, agreed upon as a core value and ostensibly modeled in clinical settings, has taken hold in curriculum decision making at all levels, from medical school to residency to continuing medical education." In considering new curriculum models for cultural competency, Wear admonishes schools to broaden their approach: "Medical education rarely looks outside its own literature to examine how culture is conceived and taught in other domains" (Wear, 2003, p. 550).

A recent article by Halpern, Lee, Boulter, and Phillips synthesized nine major reports on physician competencies and concluded that "medical education and training programs have been slow to introduce curriculum content that reflects the important changes in practice organizations and health care delivery" (Halpern et al., 2001, p. 606). The authors recognized challenges in implementing curriculum reform and stated that competencies need to be "organized and sequenced for stage of training and specialty, and barriers to change require strategic and operational planning." We believe that accreditation could serve as a major force in meeting these challenges.

7. Recommendation. Leaders from different health disciplines should meet biennially to promote ways to integrate the core competencies into health professions education.

8. Recommendation. Accrediting bodies should develop standards mandating that institutions/programs incorporate cultural competency into the curriculum. Because some of the other health professions' standards already emphasize the importance of teaching cultural competency (reviewed later in this paper), collaboration on best practices could be especially helpful in devising effective standards. Such standards should require that schools/programs incorporate curricular elements that involve continuous, first-hand experiences with diverse patients. The school/program would need to include how it intends to assess whether the teaching and experiences offered did in fact increase cultural competency.

9. Recommendation. That accrediting bodies devise new standards that address ways in which institutions/programs can better judge student readiness in areas of professionalism, communication, and interpersonal skills. Accrediting bodies should work closely with licensing agencies that test for core competencies in graduates of health professions programs in the process of change, such that as new core competencies are developed, these might be included in assessments for licensure. Testing that has consequences always serves as a powerful incentive, particularly when the reward centers on achieving licensure, certification, or recertification.

10. Recommendation. Once new standards have been established, accrediting bodies could offer national workshops or seminars to schools/programs that would review the intent and meaning of the new standards. In addition, the accrediting bodies could create a website that lists key resources and best practices and offers opportunities to site visit programs that showcase best practices. To keep the public aware of efforts being made, the website could contain results of yearly research in education that offers the latest in assessment or development of new information on health and illness in various ethnic and minority groups.

Accreditation requires that institutions demonstrate through outcome measures that what schools teach is being successfully incorporated and practiced by their graduates. As accrediting bodies include cultural competency and other areas of competencies (e.g., professionalism, communication, interpersonal skills) in their established standards, institutions/programs will need to develop new tools to assess these more abstract qualities. The development of these new tools could best be accomplished through a collective effort across the health professions. A coalition of organizations such as the National Board of Medical Examiners, the Federation of State Medical Boards, and specialty certifying boards would aid significantly in achieving this goal.

THREE HEALTH PROFESSIONS' ACCREDITING BODIES' STANDARDS RELATING TO DIVERSITY

The standards of health professions' accrediting organizations differ in regard to core competencies. However, most have developed a limited number of standards requiring that students achieve a degree of competence in matters of diversity and that programs establish diversity in admissions. A few have created standards in an attempt to establish diversity among faculty. (Analysis of LCME standards for medicine is in a later section of this paper, along with recommendations for change.) When reading the standards (where they exist) of the three major health professions to be reviewed, it becomes clear that they do place a high value on diversity while varying in strength of statement.

Dentistry

The American Dental Association's Commission on Dental Accreditation Programs is the specialized accrediting agency recognized by ED to accredit programs that provide basic preparation for licensure or certification in dentistry and related disciplines (ADA, 2002). The Accreditation Standards for Dental Education Programs document states: "Institutional definitions and operations . . . ensure patients' preferences and that their social, economic and emotional circumstances are sensitively considered." (DEP standards, 1998, p. 6). In keeping with this commitment, DEP has established standards for dental education programs that directly pertain to achieving diversity in admissions: "Admissions policies and procedures *must* be designed to include recruitment and admission of a diverse student population." Another standard states, "Graduates must be competent in managing a diverse patient population and have the interpersonal and communication skills to function successfully in a multicultural environment." It should be noted that all of the dental accreditation standards contain the word "must," thus disallowing circumstantial means of noncompliance. These authors have no evidence as to how effective the dental profession has been in providing programmatic support to meet the standards, nor what assessment tools enable the profession to effectively measure the outcomes sought through the standards. It would be helpful to learn from the dental profession whether the word "must" has been effective in its recruitment and retention of a diverse student body.

Psychology

Accrediting bodies for this field govern education for advanced-level psychology students attaining training primarily in the understanding and intricacies of health and human development. The Committee on Accreditation for Professional Programs in Psychology includes in its scope of accreditation (APA, 2002): (1) the doctoral graduate training program; (2) the internship carried out during the doctoral training; and (3) postdoctoral residencies in professional psychology. The following selections from psychology accreditation standards give evidence to the commitment of establishing diversity and retaining culturally competent faculty and students.

• Standard five under this domain reads: "The program engages in actions that indicate respect for and understanding of cultural and individual diversity . . . with regard to personal and demographic characteristics, not limited to: age, color, disabilities, ethnicity, gender, language, national origin, race, religion, sexual orientation and socioeconomic status." Standard five continues: "Respect for and understanding of culture and individual diversity is reflected in the program's policies for the recruitment, retention, and development of faculty and students, and in its curriculum and field placements" (p. 8).

• Standard three under Domain B, *Program Philosophy, Objectives and Curriculum Plan,* states, "In achieving its objectives, the program has and implements a clear and coherent curriculum plan that provides the means whereby all students can acquire and demonstrate substantial understanding of and competence in the following areas . . . (d) Issues of cultural and individual diversity that are relevant to all of the above" (p. 9).

• Standard one under Domain D, *Cultural and Individual Differences and Diversity,* references the need for "programs to make systematic, coherent, and long-term efforts to attract and retain faculty from differing ethnic, racial and personal backgrounds into the program" (p. 12).

• Standard two under Domain D states that a program "has and implements a thoughtful and coherent plan to provide students with relevant knowledge and experience about the role of cultural and individual diversity in psychological phenomena as they relate to the science and practice of professional psychology" (p. 12).

Nursing

ED recognizes two accreditation bodies for the nursing profession. The older of the two, the National League for Nursing Accrediting Commission (NLNAC), has responsibility for the specialized accreditation of all types of nursing education programs, both postsecondary and higher degree, that offer a certificate, diploma, or a recognized professional degree. NLNAC has as one of its goals that of promulgating a common core of standards and criteria for the accreditation of nursing programs (NLNAC, 2002). Although NLNAC currently has no standards directed toward achieving diversity, in 2002 the organization voiced support of the Pew Health Commission Competencies for 2005 (1991 report) and the *21 Competencies for the Twenty-First Century* (1998 report). The *1991 Pew Report—Healthy America: Practitioners for 2005, Agenda for Action,* calls for "a change in strategies wherein both the state and federal government assume a responsible role in health care and education. The Report recommends that the federal government encourage accreditation bodies to work closely with schools as they develop their responses to a changing environment" (Shugars et al., 1991, p. 24). In the report *21 Competencies for the Twenty-First Century*, only one of the core competencies relates to diversity: Competency 12 advocates the need to provide culturally sensitive care to a diverse society by: "creating a diverse learning environment by recruiting a culturally and racially diverse faculty and student body" (O'Neil and the Pew Health Commission, 1998, pp. 36–37). NLNAC's support of these 21 competencies acknowledges their value by asking nursing programs to interpret skills and competencies in the content, context, function, and structure of their programs.

ED also recognizes the Commission on Collegiate Nursing Education (CCNE). This specialized/professional accrediting organization is designed to evaluate and make judgments about the quality of baccalaureate and U.S. graduate programs in nursing (CCNE, 1998). Conceived by the American Association of Colleges of Nursing in 1996, CCNE began accrediting operations in 1998. A board of commissioners governs the body and serves as the final authority on all policy and accreditation matters. CCNE currently has no standards regarding diversity in admissions.

Another agency that has been working toward creating diversity in the nursing profession is the National Advisory Council on Nurse Education and Practice (NACNEP). Authorized under Title VIII of the Public Health Service Act, NACNEP provides advice and recommendations to the Secretary and Congress concerning the range of issues relating to the nurse workforce, education, and practice improvement. In its 1996 report to the Secretary of Health and Human Services and Congress on the Nursing Workforce, NACNEP identified as a critical goal that of increasing the racial/ethnic diversity of the registered nurse workforce to meet the nursing needs of the population. In 2000, the National Agenda for the Nursing Workforce met and subsequently issued a report to the Secretary of Health and Human Services (NACNEP, 2000, p. xi) that contains this statement, "The health of the nation depends on an adequate supply of nurses and a nursing workforce that reflects the racial and ethnic diversity of the population." The report continues with the admonition that "Without significant interventions the nursing workforce will continue to be out of balance with the health care demands imposed by the changing population demographics." The report recommends specific goals and actions that can serve as a national action agenda to be undertaken to address these issues.

As seen from this brief review, these three health professions have two common goals: to graduate students who possess cultural competencies and to achieve diversity through admissions. Accrediting bodies for dentistry, medicine (described in the next section), and psychology have relatively consonant standards relating to the acquisition of core competencies pertaining to diversity. As for nursing, NLNAC has adopted the Pew 21 Core Competencies with an admonition to nursing programs to incorporate these competencies into their educational programs. Existing standards, however, lack uniformity of language and greater explication on ways by which to assess outcomes.

THE LCME'S COMMITMENT TO ACHIEVING DIVERSITY IN ADMISSIONS

The LCME regularly holds retreats to examine the accreditation process and to review the role and range of its activities. At a retreat held several years ago, the question was raised as to what role the LCME should take in effecting social change. At that time the group concluded that because issues such as racial and ethnic diversity were societal, and that the role of an accrediting body was to set educational standards, the LCME's scope of effort did not include attempting to address societal issues. Since that time, AAMC President Dr. Cohen has voiced his opinion: "A diverse healthcare workforce will help expand health care access for the underserved, foster research in neglected areas of societal need, and enrich the pool of managers and policymakers to meet the needs of a diversity society." (Cohen et al., 2002, p. 91).

Within the scope of this commitment, the LCME has established standards geared toward increasing racial and ethnic diversity in the student body and on medical school faculty. Currently 5 of the 126 standards listed in the LCME standards document, *Functions and Structure of a Medical School*, pertain directly to diversity. Over the past several years, the LCME has sought to tighten the language and provide annotation of the standards in order to effectively communicate its full intent (LCME, 2002).

Analysis and Recommendations Regarding the Five LCME Accreditation Standards on Diversity

Five LCME standards pertain specifically to diversity. A brief discussion of each follows, along with recommendations. The authors have taken into consideration whether site team visitors can easily analyze those standards requiring specific outcomes and means of assessment.

1. ED–21: "The faculty and students *must* demonstrate an understanding of the manner in which people of diverse cultures and belief systems perceive health and illness and respond to various symptoms, diseases and treatments."

Although this standard has as its goal a very well intentioned outcome, its double-pronged approach, directed toward both faculty and students, renders it virtually ineffective. Most schools have few, if any, provisions on how to effectively abide by the standard relevant for both. The ability to measure outcomes for this standard remains marginal; even the best informed LCME site visitors have no way to assess whether both faculty *and* students have met the cultural competency (understanding) as set forth. In all likelihood, the visiting team's focus would center on assessing the types of cultural competency curricular programs available for students and the content of faculty development programs being offered to address this issue.

11. Recommendation. Considering the intent and scope of this standard, we recommend crafting standards directed toward achieving the two separate outcomes currently stated in ED–21 and developing measurable outcomes to assess cultural competency (understanding) in the separate standards.

Having been a site team visitor to several institutions, this author (Wagoner) suggests that once the LCME has strengthened existing standards and instituted new ones, the organization provide a more comprehensive training program for site visitors on how to properly interpret standards.

2. ED–22: "Medical students *must* learn to recognize and appropriately address gender and cultural biases in themselves and others, and in the process of health care delivery."

This critically important standard essentially speaks to the matter of trust, a subject much discussed in health professions' literature. Trust in the doctor-patient relationship can only be established when physicians overcome preconceived biases and acquire insight and understanding into another person's values, beliefs, and needs. In the article, "Trust, Patient Well-Being and Affirmative Action in Medical School," DeVille highlights the importance of trust, calling it "central to the individual physician's ability to practice good medicine." He notes that minorities' historical and current experience with the medical profession and health delivery system frequently breeds suspicion rather than faith. He concludes: "Society and the medical profession have a compelling interest and duty to produce physicians who inspire trust" (DeVille, 1999, p. 247). Although schools can be cited for noncompliance of this standard, this author (Wagoner) knows of no institution that has been cited for failure to achieve the outcome specified by ED–22 or for lacking a mechanism by which to assist individual students in overcoming biases.

12. Recommendation. Standard ED–22 hinges on the development of measurable core competencies. Once accrediting bodies have developed the core competencies, they should place a high priority on determining how the competencies are being achieved. An array of assessment instruments could furnish this information.

3. MS–8: "Each medical school *should* have policies and practices ensuring the gender, racial, cultural and economic diversity of its students."

This broad-based standard acknowledges the LCME's commitment to the stated goal of diversity in students entering medicine, although the standard is weakened by use of the word "should" rather than "must." The intention of this standard mirrors that of dentistry in its focus on the recruitment and retention of diverse students. At present, site visit teams can assess the school's admissions selection process and the extent to which diversity exists by evaluating medical school data. Therefore, unlike the previous two standards, this one has outcomes that can be measured by specific instruments. However, as written, the standard fails to acknowledge the importance of diversity in the context of a quality education or in the quality of health-care access or delivery for an ever-increasing diverse population.

13. Recommendation: Reframe the standard to emphasize the importance of having a diverse, culturally competent workforce in order to provide the highest quality health care. Ensure that the standard's wording is changed from "should" to "must" in all current and newly created standards.

The subtext of this standard states: "The extent of diversity needed will depend on the school's missions, goals, and educational objectives, expectations of the community in which it operates, and its implied or explicit social contract at the local, state and national levels." This subtext gives institutions tremendous latitude to gear their policies and practices toward their current missions, goals, educational objectives, and social contract, which may be woefully inadequate to create a diverse student body or to train medical students to be racially, culturally, and gender sensitive. Unless an institution's leadership has a strong commitment to the goal of diversity, achieving this standard in its full measure will be a matter of circumstance rather than advocacy.

4. MS–31: "In the admissions process and throughout medical school, there *should* be no discrimination on the basis of gender, sexual orientation, age, race, creed or national origin."

14. Recommendation. That the word "should" be replaced by the word "must."

This standard encompasses verbiage found in most medical school admissions handbooks that puts them in compliance with the Equal Employment Opportunity Commission laws disallowing discrimination in the admissions process on the listed bases. Although well intentioned, the standard provides no means of determining whether schools/programs are conforming in the admissions process, particularly in how they handle/consider/recruit individual candidates. Assessment by LCME site visitors at this microlevel would be well beyond the purview of their responsibility. In essence, they have to trust the school's word that it is in compliance.

15. Recommendation. In order to provide measurable outcomes, this standard needs to require (1) that each school/program publish yearly statistics regarding its class diversity, and (2) that each institution/ program have its mission statement readily available for inspection by students so that those seeking an institution that values diversity could more effectively target their applications. This sort of public accountability also would enable patients to recognize programs that have a commitment to creating a diverse workforce.

5. FA–1: "The recruitment and development of a medical school's faculty *should* take into account its mission, the diversity of its student body and the population it serves."

For the past three decades, the number of women on medical school faculties has increased. The 2001 AAMC Faculty Roster source shows that women constitute 32.6 percent of U.S. faculty (AAMC, 2001). However, the same has not been true for minorities, whose number does not come close to reflecting the patient population or, in many instances, the student population at any particular medical school. In the IOM Symposium on Diversity in the Health Professions entitled *The Right Thing to Do, The Smart Thing To Do,* in his chapter on "How Do We Retain Minority Health Professions Students?" Dr. Michael Rainey stated, "There is a severe shortage of underrepresented minority (URM) faculty teaching core courses. Although African Americans, Native Americans, Mexican Americans, and Mainland Puerto Ricans make up almost 25% of the U.S. population, they account for less than 8% of all practicing physicians. Only 3% of medical school faculty members belong to one of these minority groups." In 1989, URM faculty represented only 2.9 percent of clinical faculty in U.S. medical schools (Rainey, 2001).

THE ROLE OF OTHER ORGANIZATIONS IN AIDING ACCREDITATION

We believe that select governmental organizations, private foundations, accrediting organizations, and national health professions share a common interest in supporting diversity and developing a set of core competencies applicable to all health professions. We offer the following suggestions for cooperative undertakings:

- Offer grant incentives to support change:
  — to health professions' schools to build bridges between their institutions/programs and public undergraduate institutions and select private schools. This liaison would help ensure a future pipeline of diverse students prepared to meet the health care challenges of the 21st century;
  — and to health professions' schools to increase faculty/student diversity.
- Facilitate multidisciplinary partnering of health professions' schools committed to promoting diversity and cultural competency through the development of educational modules (clinical case studies) for institutions/ programs for online testing and self-learning. Other modules could be devised to establish programs that aid in the development of cultural competency skills. This might include references to articles and other literature that offer insight into how effective programs at other institutions (across disciplines) accomplish their educational objectives.
- Take explicit actions to identify diversity-related issues within the education and work settings and develop strategies to address them. "A laissez-faire approach will not confront the unconscious practice biases that exist" (Schmieding, 1991, p. 70). Reporting the results of such efforts will prove critical to the success of diversity.
- Honor institutions by giving yearly monetary awards to encourage and acknowledge those that have demonstrated excellence in developing outstanding educational modules. In order to foster collaboration across the health professions, emphasis should be on interdisciplinary educational modules that promote team approaches to care, quality improvement, and the use of educational technology. Other modules could include those that address challenges of health care access, health-care delivery, cultural competency, patient education, and any other modules that better the quality of health care and increase patient safety. It will be imperative to continuously monitor any efforts undertaken by any or all of these organizations to identify, support, and pursue diversity within the health professions student body, workforce, faculty, and staff. To demonstrate public accountability, the agencies and organizations should publish their benchmark progress toward policy goals and articulated action items.

CONCLUSION

The importance of accreditation in fulfilling the health professions' social contract cannot be understated. As stewards of the public's trust and guardians of the social contract, accrediting organizations have an obligation to use their authority to help increase competency and racial and ethnic diversity in the health professions. They can accomplish this by ensuring that all institutions and programs identify these as necessary objectives. At present, accreditation standards vary widely in their mandates and may not achieve the objectives to the extent required to promote diversity or to educate competent health-care professionals. Accomplishing this lofty goal will require the creation of a comprehensive, symbiotic, and open relationship among health-care leadership organizations, accrediting organizations, and the health professions. Together these groups can collaborate on all relevant issues regarding the attainment of diversity; the design, measurement, and assessment of core competencies; and the methods by which to encourage the development of educational materials. Accrediting bodies are exceptionally positioned to spearhead this cooperative effort.

REFERENCES

AAMC (Association of American Medical Colleges). 2001. *Women Faculty by Department.* AAMC Faculty Roster System. [Online]. Available: http://www.aamc.org/members/wim/statistics/stats01/01table4.pdf [accessed August 22, 2003].

AAMC. 2001–2002. *Information About U.S. Medical Schools Accredited by the LCME. Medical School Admission Requirements.* Part 2. Washington, DC: AAMC. Pp. 16 and 61.

AAMC. 2002. *LCME Graduation Questionnaire.* Washington, DC: AAMC.

ACGME (Accreditation Council for Graduate Medical Education). 2001. *ACGME Outcome Project.* [Online]. Available: http://www.acgme.org/outcome/comp/compFull.asp [accessed May 31, 2002].

ADA (American Dental Association). 2002. *Accreditation Standards for Dental Education Programs.* Chicago: Commission on Dental Accreditation.

AP (Associated Press). 2003, June 23. Court upholds Michigan affirmative action: Supreme Court upholds affirmative action in University of Michigan Law School's admissions.

APA (American Psychological Association). 2002. Committee on Accreditation for Professional Programs in Psychology. *Guidelines and Principles for Accreditation of Programs in Professional Psychology, Education Directorate.* [Online]. Available: http://www.apa.org/ed/G7P2.pdf [accessed August 4, 2003].

Archbold M. 1996. Medicine spoken here. King County Journal Newspapers. *South County Journal,* pp. A1 and A5, November 16, 1996.

Bollinger LC. 2003. The need for diversity in higher education. *Academic Medicine* 78(5): 431–436.

Borsellino M. 2003. Wanted: Social accountability. *Medical Post* 39(3):1–4.

CCNE (Commission on Collegiate Nursing Education). 1998. *Standards for Accreditation of Baccalaureate and Graduate Nursing Education Programs.* [Online]. Available: http://www.aacn.ncche.edu/accreditation/standrds.htm [accessed October 28, 2002].

Cohen J. 2003. *Supreme Court Ruling Supports Greater Diversity in Medicine.* AAMC Newsroom. [Online]. Available: http://www.aamc.org/newsroom/pressrel/2003/030623.htm [accessed June 24, 2003].

Cohen J, Gabriel BA, Terrell, C. 2002. The case for diversity in the health care workforce. *Health Affairs* 21(5):90–102.

Colloton J. 1989. Academic medicine's changing covenant with society. *Academic Medicine* 64(2):55–60.

The Compelling Need for Diversity in Higher Education. 1999. Expert reports prepared for *Gratz et al. v. Bollinger et al.* No. 97-75231 (E.D. Mich.) and *Grutter et al. v. Bollinger et al.* No. 97-75928 (E.D. Mich.). [Online]. Available: http://www.umich.edu/~urel/admissions/legal/expert [accessed August 7, 2003].

Cross TL, Bazron BJ, Dennis KW, Isaacs MR. 1989. *Towards a Culturally Competent System of Care: Volume I.* Washington, DC: CASSP Technical Assistance Center, Georgetown University Child Development Center. [Online]. Available: http://www.amsa.org/programs/gpit/cultural.cfm [accessed July 8, 2003].

DEP (Dental Education Programs standards). 1998. *Commission on Dental Accreditation, Accreditation Standards for Dental Education Program.* Chicago: American Dental Association. Pp. 9–20.

DeVille K. 1999. Trust, patient well-being and affirmative action in medical school admissions. *Mount Sinai Journal of Medicine* 66(4):247–256.

Eaton J. 2003. *Letter from the President, The Value of Accreditation: Four Pivotal Roles.* Council for Higher Education Accreditation. [Online]. Available: http://www.chea.org/Research/Value%20%20of%20Accrd%20lt%205-03%20combo.pdf [accessed August 3, 2003].

Flexner A. 1910. *Medical Education in the United States and Canada.* Bulletin #4. New York: Carnegie Foundation for the Advancement of Teaching.

Halpern R, Lee MY, Boulter PR, Phillips RR. 2001. A synthesis of nine major reports on physicians' competencies for the emerging practice environment. *Academic Medicine* 76(6):606–615.

IOM (Institute of Medicine). 2001. Enhancing diversity in the health professions. In: Smedley BD, Stith AY, Colburn L, Evans CH. *The Right Thing to Do, The Smart Thing to Do.* Washington, DC: National Academy Press.

IOM. 2003a. *Health Professions Education: A Bridge to Quality.* Washington, DC: The National Academies Press. Executive Summary, pp. 1–18.

IOM. 2003b. Press Release, April 8, 2003. Health professionals' education must be overhauled to ensure safety, quality of care. [Online]. Available: http://www4.nationalacademies.org/news.nsf/isbn/0309087236?OpenDocument [accessed August 1, 2003].

Joint Statement of Constitutional Law Scholars (regarding *Grutter et al. v. Bollinger, et al.*, 123 S. Ct. 2344). 2003. *Reaffirming Diversity: A Legal Analysis of the University of Michigan Affirmative Action Cases.* Cambridge, MA: The Civil Rights Project at Harvard University.

Krueger AB. 2003, July 24. Why affirmative action matters. *The New York Times*, p. C2.

LCME (Liaison Committee on Medical Education). 2002. Overview of the Accreditation of the LCME. *Functions and Structure of a Medical School and Guide to Institutional Self-Study.* [Online]. Available: http://www.aamc.org/publications/functionsandstructure.htm [accessed May 7, 2003].

LCME. 2003. *Guide to the Institutional Self-Study for Programs of Medical Education Leading to the M.D. Degree.* Chicago and Washington, DC: LCME.

NACNEP (National Advisory Council on Nurse Education and Practice). 2000. *National Agenda for Nursing Workforce Racial/Ethnic Diversity.* [Online]. Available: http://bhpr.hrsa.gov/nursing/nacnep/diversity.htm [accessed August 4, 2003].

Nickens, H. 1992. The rationale for minority-targeted programs in the 1990's. *Journal of the American Medical Association* 267(17):2390–2395.

NLNAC (National League for Nursing Accrediting Commission). 1999. *1999 Standards and Criteria and Interpretive Guidelines.* [Online]. Available: http://www.nlnac.org/Manual%20&%20Ig/01_accreditation_manual.htm [accessed July 20, 2003].

NLNAC (National League for Nursing Accrediting Commission) 2002. *Interpretative Guidelines by Program Type: 2002 Standards and Criteria.* [Online]. Available: http://www.nlnac.org/Manual%20&20IG/01_am_-_stds_&_criteria.htm [accessed October 30, 2002].

O'Neil EH, Pew Health Professions Commission. 1998. *Recreating Health Professional Practice for a New Century. The Fourth Report.* San Francisco: Pew Health Professions Commission.

Parboosing J. 2003. Medical schools' social contract: More than just education and research. Association of Canadian Medical Colleges' Working Group on Social Accountability. *Canadian Medical Assocation Journal,* 68(7):852–853.

Rainey M. 2001. How do we retain minority health professions students? In: *The Right Thing to Do, The Smart Thing to Do: Enhancing Diversity in Health Professions.* Smedley BD, Stith AY, Colburn L, Evans CH, eds. Washington, DC: National Academy Press. Pp. 328–360.

Saha S, Taggart SH, Komarony M, Bindman AB. 2002. Do patients choose physicians of their own race? *Health Affairs* 19(4):76–83.

Schmieding NJ. 1991. A novel approach to recruitment, retention, and advancement of minority nurses in a health care organization. *Nursing Administration Quarterly* 15(4): 69–76.

Schroeder S, Zones JS, Showstack JA. 1989. Academic medicine as a public trust. *Journal of the American Medical Association* 262:803–812.

Shugars DA, O'Neil EH, Bader JD, eds. 1991. *Healthy America: Practitioners for 2005. An Agenda for Action of U.S. Health Professional Schools.* San Francisco: The Pew Health Professions Commission.

Steinberg J. 2003, June 24. An admissions guide. *The New York Times,* p. A25.

U.S. Department of State. 2003. *Short Term Study, Accreditation.* [Online]. Available: http://www.educcationusa.state.gov/admissions/study/accreditation.htp [accessed July 14, 2003].

Wear D. 2003. Insurgent multiculturalism: Rethinking how and why we teach culture in medical education. *Academic Medicine* 78(6):549–554.

APPENDIX TO PAPER CONTRIBUTION C

The U.S. Department of Education oversees the LCME. Public Law 96–88 of October 1979 authorizing the organization of the ED defined its mission. The following areas are considered ED's purview:

• Strengthen the federal commitment to ensuring access to equal educational opportunity for every individual.

• Supplement and complement the efforts of states, the local school systems, other instrumentalities of the states, the private sector, public and private nonprofit educational research institutions, community-based organizations, parents, and students to improve the quality of education.

• Encourage the increased involvement of the public, parents, and students in federal education programs.

• Promote improvements in the quality and usefulness of education through federally supported research, evaluation, and sharing of information.

• Improve the coordination of federal education programs.

• Improve the management of federal education activities.

• Increase the accountability of federal education programs to the president, Congress, and the public.

Paper Contribution D

Diversity Considerations in Health Professions Education

Jeffrey F. Milem, Eric L. Dey, and Casey B. White,

"Effective participation by members of all racial and ethnic groups in the civic life of our Nation is essential if the dream of one Nation, indivisible, is to be realized."
— Justice O'Connor in Grutter v. Bollinger

INTRODUCTION

The recent decisions by the U.S. Supreme Court in two cases that challenged the use of affirmative action in undergraduate admissions and in law school admissions at the University of Michigan helped to provide some clarity to an ongoing debate regarding the educational value of diversity, and specifically, racial and ethnic diversity, on our nation's college campuses. In the opinion that upheld the constitutionality of the admissions process used for selecting law school students at Michigan, Justice O'Connor wrote that a majority of the court agreed that diversity served a compelling interest for institutions of higher education as well as for our society. The University of Michigan successfully demonstrated to the Court that diversity was essential in helping it to achieve its education mission because more diverse colleges and universities provide opportunities for teaching and learning that are not available in institutions that are less diverse. The university was able to make this case, in large part, because of the array of empirical evidence that it and other organizations provided that established how diversity enhanced the learning outcomes for students at Michigan and at colleges and universities across the country.

The primary goal of this paper is to examine the ways in which existing evidence about diversity in higher education and its effects on students, institutions, and society can be used to inform and improve the quality of education received by students in health professions. Published reviews of the literature on undergraduate college students clearly demonstrate that various aspects of racial and ethnic diversity within higher education help promote benefits of assorted kinds (Milem, 2003; Hurtado et al., 2003; Milem and Hakuta, 2000; Gurin, 1999, Appendix A). These reviews indicate that diversity-related benefits are far ranging, spanning from benefits to individual students and the institutions in which they enroll, to private enterprise, the economy, and the broader society.

The benefits that accrue to individuals through enhancements to their educational experiences and educational outcomes (including process outcomes that help influence subsequent outcomes of these students; see Milem, 2003; Astin, 1991) are perhaps the most commonly recognized; diversity has been shown to enhance the ability of colleges and universities to achieve their missions—particularly as they relate to the missions of teaching, research, and service. Economic and private-sector benefits are reflected in the ways in which diversity enhances the economy and the functioning of organizations and businesses in the private sector. Societal benefits differ in that they transcend the boundaries of individual organizations and are related to the achievement of democratic ideals, the development of an educated and involved citizenry, and the ways in which underserved groups (e.g., low-income, elderly, those who lack insufficient health care) are able to receive the services they require. Recent original research efforts reinforce this viewpoint in higher education generally (Bowen and Bok, 1998), and specifically in medical education (Whitla et al., 2003).

It is important to note that research on the benefits of diversity indicates that these benefits *do not automatically* accrue to students who attend institutions that are, in terms of student or faculty composition, racially and ethnically diverse. Rather, if the benefits of diversity in higher education are to be realized, close attention must be paid to the institutional context in which that diversity is enacted. In other words, it is not enough to simply bring together a diverse group of students. Although this is an important first step in creating opportunities for students to learn from diversity, it cannot be the only step that is taken. Diverse learning environments provide unique challenges and opportunities that must be considered if we are to maximize the learning opportunities that they present.

If we are to change educational environments in ways that allow us to maximize the opportunities and minimize the challenges that are presented by diversity, we must first understand the conditions under which students are able to learn from diversity. In the pages that follow, we summarize the literature that does this. To begin, we review the literature drawn from studies of higher education generally, followed by a focused consideration of issues related specifically to health professions education (with an emphasis on medical education). To begin our discussion of higher education generally, we summarize and extend the key components of a framework for understanding campus diversity issues first developed by Hurtado and colleagues (1998, 1999). This provides a useful frame for understanding the different dimensions of campus diversity and their importance. Having provided some conceptual definitions of diversity, we turn to research linking diversity and learning, emphasizing in turn cognitive and emotional development issues, contextual issues and learning environments, and pedagogy.

The focused discussion of health professions issues follows a similar logic, beginning with a consideration of the importance of diversity in these fields and unique characteristics of these fields of study (including goals, standards, and curricular structure). The status of current curricular approaches that support diversity-related education is discussed as are problems and issues with current approaches. An extension of cognitive and emotional development concerns related to health professions education is presented, followed by a discussion of how educational settings and learning environments can influence learning related to diversity issues, as well as pedagogy that can promote transformative learning. These two strands of work—higher education generally, and health professions specifically—are brought together in a set of recommendations intended to guide the transformation of education in the health professions so that students in these fields realize the educational benefits of diversity, and so that all members of our society will be better served by the professionals who provide them with health care.

DEFINING DIVERSITY

In considering how we maximize the benefits of diverse learning environments, it is important to define precisely what we mean by *diversity*. Although other dimensions exist, for the purpose of this paper we will focus on diversity with respect to race and ethnicity. Recent work by Hurtado and colleagues (1998, 1999) provides a useful framework for conceptualizing and understanding the impact of various dimensions of the campus racial climate and documents the importance of an institution's context in shaping student outcomes. This framework was first introduced in a study of the climate for Latino students (Hurtado, 1994) and further developed in syntheses of research done for policy makers and practitioners (Hurtado et al., 1998, 1999).

The campus climate described by Hurtado and colleagues differs from earlier research that defined the climate as reflecting common participant attitudes, perceptions, or observations about the environment (Peterson and Spencer, 1990). These common attitudes and perceptions are identified as malleable and distinguishable from the stable norms and beliefs that may constitute an organizational culture. Although this work has been important in distinguishing the climate from the culture of an organization, it is most important in establishing that the climate is malleable and that the current patterns of beliefs and behaviors are amenable to planned efforts to change or improve the climate. The framework discussed by Hurtado et al. (1998, 1999) builds on this earlier work by expanding our thinking about climate by asserting that the psychological climate (perceptions and attitudes) is linked to a range of social phenomenon that have to do with structure, history, and actual interactions across diverse communities within the environment. Central to their conceptualization of a campus climate for diversity is the notion that students are educated in distinct racial contexts. Both external and internal (institutional) forces shape these contexts in higher education.

The external components of climate represent the impact of *governmental policy, programs, and initiatives* as well as the impact of *sociohistorical forces* on campus racial climate. The authors indicate that governmental contextual factors that influence the climate for diversity on college campuses include financial aid policies and programs, state and federal policy regarding affirmative action, court decisions related to the desegregation of higher education, and the manner in which states provide for institutional differentiation within their state system of higher education. Hurtado et al. (1998, 1999) describe sociohistoric forces that influence the climate for diversity on campus as events or issues in the larger society that are connected to the ways in which people view racial diversity in society. One recent example of this is the impact that the ongoing debate over affirmative action in college admissions had on the climate for diversity at colleges and universities across the country. Although these forces are usually initiated outside of the context of the institution, they frequently serve as a stimulus for discussion or other activity within the campus context. Because "[n]o policy can be isolated from the social arena in which it is enacted" (Tierney, 1997, p. 177), it is important to note that these two forces mutually influence each other.

The *institutional context* contains multiple dimensions that are a function of educational programs and practices. These include an institution's *historical legacy of inclusion or exclusion* of various racial/ethnic groups; its *compositional diversity*[1] in terms of the numerical and proportional

---

[1]Much of the relevant research describes this dimension of climate as structural diversity. However, we prefer the term compositional diversity as it more accurately reflects how this concept has been operationalized in diversity research, without being confused with other aspects of campus structure—such as the curriculum, decision-making practices, reward structures, hiring practices, admissions practices, tenure decisions, and other factors that function as part of the day-to-day "business" on our campuses. Although the term "compositional" is divergent from existing research, we employ it here in hopes of being more direct in describing the concept we are discussing.

representation of various racial/ethnic groups; the *psychological climate*, which includes perceptions and attitudes between and among groups; as well as a *behavioral climate* dimension that is characterized by the nature of intergroup relations on campus. Hurtado et al. (1998, 1999) conceptualize the institutional climate as a product of these dimensions. These dimensions are not discrete; rather, they are connected with each other. For example, a historical vestige of segregation has an impact on an institution's ability to improve its racial/ethnic student enrollments, and the underrepresentation of specific groups contributes to stereotypical attitudes among individuals within the learning and work environment that affect the psychological and behavioral climate. While some institutions take a "multilayered" approach toward assessing diversity on their campuses and are developing programs to address the climate on campus, most institutions fail to recognize the importance of the dynamics of these interrelated elements of the climate.

Historical Legacy of Inclusion or Exclusion

Hurtado et al. (1998, 1999) argue that the historical vestiges of segregated schools and colleges continue to affect the climate for racial/ethnic diversity on college campuses. Evidence can be seen in resistance to desegregation in communities and specific campus settings, maintenance of old campus policies at predominantly white institutions (PWIs) that best serve a homogeneous population, and attitudes and behaviors that prevent interaction across race and ethnicity. Duster (1993) argued that many campuses sustain benefits for particular student groups that go largely unrecognized because these institutions are embedded in a culture of a historically segregated environment. While some campuses have a history of admitting and graduating students of color since their founding (i.e., historically black colleges and universities), most PWIs have a history of limited access and exclusion (Thelin, 1985). These institutions have a longer history of segregation and exclusion than they do of inclusion. An institution's historical legacy of exclusion has a significant impact on the prevailing climate that influences current policies and practices at the institution (Hurtado, 1992; Hurtado et al., 1998, 1999).

Institutions that are clear about their history of exclusion and the detrimental impact that this history has had may be able to gain broader support for their efforts to become more diverse through the use of affirmative action and other programs and services designed to improve the climate for diversity. Furthermore, institutions that acknowledge a history of exclusion may be able to demonstrate to people of color that the institution is willing to acknowledge its past transgressions and is working to rid itself of its exclusionary past.

Compositional Diversity

Increasing the compositional diversity of an institution is an important initial step toward improving the climate (Hurtado et al., 1998, 1999). The distribution of students in a particular environment shapes the dynamics of social interaction in that environment (Kanter, 1977). For example, Chang (1999) has shown that the likelihood that students will engage with students who are different from them increases as the compositional diversity of the campus increases. Conversely, campuses with high proportions of white students provide limited opportunities for interaction across race/ethnicity and limit student learning experiences with socially, culturally diverse groups (Hurtado et al., 1994).

Moreover, in environments that lack diverse populations, underrepresented groups are frequently viewed as tokens. Tokenism contributes to the heightened visibility of the underrepresented group, overstatement of group differences, and the alteration of images to fit existing stereotypes (Kanter, 1977). In addition, the fact that racial and ethnic students remain minorities in majority white environments contributes to social stigma that can adversely affect their achievement (e.g., see Steele, 1992, 1997, 1998; Steele and Aronson, 1995) and can produce minority status stressors (Prillerman et al., 1989; Smedley et al., 1993). Finally, an institution's stance on increasing the representation of diverse racial/ethnic groups communicates to external and internal constituencies the importance of maintaining a multicultural environment (Hurtado et al., 1998, 1999).

Institutional leaders should not expect that they will substantially improve the campus racial climate merely by increasing the compositional diversity of their institution. As stated earlier, problems may arise if efforts are not made to address and improve other dimensions of the campus climate. However, if increased compositional diversity is accompanied by institutional efforts to become more "student centered" in approaches to teaching and learning (Hurtado, 1992; Hurtado et al., 1998, 1999), and if regular and ongoing opportunities for students to come together to communicate and interact cross-racially are provided (Chang, 1999), increased compositional diversity is likely to be beneficial. Increasing compositional diversity is an important *first step* in improving the campus climate.

The Psychological Climate

The psychological dimension of the campus climate includes individuals' views of group relations and institutional responses to diversity, perceptions of discrimination or racial conflict, and attitudes held toward individuals from different racial/ethnic backgrounds. Increasingly, studies have shown that racially and ethnically diverse administrators, students, and faculty are likely to view the campus climate differently. Thus, an individual's position and power within the organization as well as her/his view as "insider" or "outsider" are likely to contribute to different views or standpoints (Collins, 1986). Hurtado et al. (1998, 1999) summarized this phenomenon by asserting that who you are and where you are positioned in an institution affects the way in which you experience and view the institution. These differences in perception of the college experience are significant because perception is both a product of the environment and a potential determinant of future interactions and outcomes (Astin, 1968; Berger and Milem, 1999; Milem and Berger, 1997; Tierney, 1987).

Research on the impact of peer groups and other reference groups is helpful in understanding another important aspect of the psychological dimension of climate on campus. Peer groups exert influence over the attitudes and the behavior of students through the norms that they communicate to their members. While faculty play an important role in the educational development of students, most researchers believe that student peer groups are principally responsible for much of the socialization that transpires (Astin, 1993; Chickering, 1969; Dey, 1996, 1997; Feldman and Newcomb, 1969; Milem, 1998). This is not meant to diminish the role that faculty play; rather, it suggests that the normative influence of faculty is likely to be amplified or attenuated by the interactions students have with their peers. Recent research on diverse friendship groups suggests that such dynamics are especially strong in areas where students are in the process of transforming their attitudes related to issues of race and ethnicity as well as those of their peers (Antonio, 2001).

The Behavioral Climate

The behavioral dimension of the institutional climate consists of general social interaction, interaction between and among individuals from different racial/ethnic backgrounds, as well as the nature of intergroup relations on campus. The prevailing view, particularly in reports forwarded by the popular media, is that campus race relations are poor and that segregation has increased on college campuses among minority groups. However, several research studies present a different picture of students' actual interactions and relations on campus. For example, while in one study, white students interpreted ethnic group clustering as racial segregation, students of color described this behavior as their attempt to find sources of cultural support within an unsupportive environment (Loo and Rolison, 1986). Another study that examined the nature of cross-racial interaction among college students found that Mexican American, Asian American, and African American students reported widespread and frequent interaction across race/ethnicity in various informal situations (i.e., dining, roommates, dating, socializing), while white students were least likely to report engaging in these activities across race (Hurtado et al., 1994). Moreover, it is clear that the absence of interracial contact influences students' views toward others, their support for important campus initiatives, and key educational outcomes (Hurtado et al., 1998, 1999).

However, students who have the opportunity to engage diverse peers in regular and ongoing structured interaction are more likely to show greater growth on a number of critical educational outcomes. The findings from research on the impact of campus initiatives that bring students from diverse groups together to engage in structured intergroup dialogues indicate that students who participate in these activities are more likely to report growth in their affinity for others. In addition, they are more likely to report enhanced enjoyment in learning about their own background as well as the backgrounds of diverse others. Moreover, these students are likely to report more positive views of conflict and to hold the perception that diversity does not need to be divisive in our society. Gurin (1999) argues that these are essential skills required of all citizens in an increasingly diverse democracy.

An important aspect of the behavioral climate involves the extent to which students have the opportunity to engage diverse others as well as diverse information and diverse ideas in their classes. These opportunities are enhanced in classrooms where faculty members use active teaching methods. In these classrooms, students are able to interact with peers from diverse backgrounds through class discussions, collaborative learning methods, and group projects. These activities contribute to a campus climate that is more supportive of diversity and leads to positive outcomes for the students involved (see, for example, Astin, 1993; Gurin, 1999; Hurtado et al., 1998, 1999; Milem, 2003; Milem and Hakuta, 2000; Smith & Associates, 1997). Clearly, there are some disciplines in which it is much easier for students to engage diverse information through course content (e.g., fields such as education, English, humanities, history, political science, psychology, sociology). However, when faculty are conscientious about incorporating active pedagogical methods into the courses they teach, students have frequent opportunities to learn from diverse peers—even in fields that do not appear to readily lend themselves to the incorporation of diverse content and subject matter (e.g., the physical sciences). As we will discuss later in this manuscript, the use of active learning or student-centered pedagogical methods in classes enhances a variety of important learning outcomes for students, including mastery of content in particular disciplines. However, the opportunities that students have to learn from diverse peers in classes that use these active learning methods, even in classes where the content does not deal explicitly with diversity issues, can help students to build bridges across communities of difference.

The Consequences of Diversity Climate

Within the context of an institution's diversity climate, the effects of diversity play themselves out along a variety of dimensions. The works of Gurin (1999), Chang (1999), Milem (2003), and Milem and Hakuta (2000) argue that, in addition to compositional diversity, there are two additional types of diversity that can have an impact on important educational outcomes. Diversity of interactions is a second type shown to be influential in creating educational benefits and is represented by students' exchanges with racially and ethnically diverse people *and* diverse ideas, information, and experiences. People are influenced by their interactions with diverse ideas and information as well as with diverse people. The final type of diversity is characterized by different *diversity-related initiatives* (i.e., core diversity course requirements, ethnic studies course/programs, diversity enhancement workshops, intergroup dialogue programs, and others) that occur on college and university campuses. While shifts or changes in the compositional diversity of campuses often provide stimulus for the creation and implementation of diversity-related initiatives (Chang, 1999), increasingly more colleges and universities are implementing these initiatives even though their campuses are quite racially and ethnically homogeneous.

These types of diversity are not discrete. We are most frequently exposed to diverse information and ideas through the interactions that we have with diverse people. Moreover, while diversity-related initiatives benefit students who are exposed to them—even on campuses that are almost exclusively white—their impact on students is much more powerful on campuses that have greater compositional diversity (Chang, 1999, 2002). Although each type of diversity has the potential to confer significant positive effects on educational outcomes, the impact of each type of diversity is enhanced by the presence of the others (Chang, 1999, 2002; Gurin, 1999; Gurin et al., 2002; Hurtado et al., 1998, 1999; Hurtado et al., 2003; Milem, 2003; Milem and Hakuta, 2000). Conversely, the impact of each type of diversity is diminished in environments where the other types are absent.

Chang's work (1999, 2002) is very helpful in illustrating the three types of diversity we have discussed and the impact they have on students. Chang (1999) found that maximizing cross-racial interaction and encouraging ongoing discussions about race were educational practices that produced positive educational outcomes for students. The findings from Chang's study revealed that socializing across race and discussing racial/ethnic issues had a positive effect on the likelihood that students would stay enrolled in college, be more satisfied with their college experience, and report higher levels of intellectual and social self-concept (Chang, 1999). However, Chang found that when the effects of higher levels of compositional diversity were considered without involvement in activities that provided students with opportunities to interact in meaningful ways cross-racially, students of color were likely to report less overall satisfaction with their college experience (Chang, 1999). In other words, increasing *only* the compositional diversity of an institution without considering the influence that these changes will have on other dimensions of the campus racial climate is likely to produce problems for students at these institutions. This finding is consistent with scholarship on race relations, which indicates that as organizations become more racially diverse, the likelihood of conflict increases (Blalock, 1967).

Chang's work also shows that students who attended more compositionally diverse institutions had more frequent opportunities to engage students from different racial/ethnic backgrounds. In other words, as compositional diversity increases, so does the likelihood that students will engage with students who are different from them. This work establishes that compositional diversity (represented by the enrollment of students of color at an institution) is an essential ingredient in providing opportunities for this interaction to occur.

LINKING DIVERSITY AND LEARNING

It is important to have a framework that helps us to understand the ways in which diversity can be connected to student learning. The most current and relevant framework for understanding the link between diversity and learning can be found in the material developed and tested as part of the Michigan legal cases (Gurin, 1999; Gurin et al., 2002, 2003) and is drawn largely from social psychological theories and research.

As part of the Michigan legal cases, Gurin (1999) argued persuasively that higher education institutions are uniquely positioned to enhance the cognitive and psychosocial development of students. Building on previous research and conceptual frameworks, she argued that students are at a critical stage in their human growth and development in which diversity, broadly defined, can facilitate greater awareness of the learning process, better critical thinking skills, and better preparation for the complex challenges they face as involved citizens in a democratic, multiracial society.

Conceptions of Development

Erikson's work (1946, 1956, cited in Gurin, 1999) regarding psychosocial development indicated that individuals' social and personal identity is formed during late adolescence and early adulthood—the time when many students attend college and graduate/professional school. Institutions of higher education can facilitate the development of individual identity. For example, among the conditions in college that facilitate the development of identity is the opportunity to be exposed to people, experiences, and ideas that differ from one's past milieu (Gurin, 1999). Moreover, as mentioned earlier, the learning environment in higher education is likely to accentuate the normative influence of peer groups. Diversity and complexity in the college environment "encourage intellectual experimentation and recognition of varied future possibilities" (Gurin, 1999, p. 103). These conditions are critical to the successful development of identity.

Gurin (1999) used the work of Piaget (1971, 1975/1985) as a conceptual and theoretical rationale for how diversity facilitates students' cognitive development. Piaget argued that cognitive growth is facilitated by disequilibrium, or periods of incongruity and dissonance. For adolescents to develop the ability to understand and appreciate the perspectives and feelings of others, they must interact with diverse individuals in roughly equal status situations. These conditions foster a process of "perspective taking" and allow students to progress in intellectual and moral development. For "perspective taking" to occur, both diversity and equality must be present in the learning environment (Gurin, 1999).

While Piaget's work was done primarily with children and adolescents, the applicability of this work to the development processes of college-age students was well documented in the work of William Perry. Perry's (1970) work with college students laid a foundation for understanding development that occurs in the college environment. At Harvard, over a 15-year period in the 1950s and 1960s, Perry and his colleagues conducted a series of interviews with a population of men at the end of each year of college. From these interviews Perry and his team constructed a schema of cognitive and personal development involving a progression from viewing knowledge as right or wrong (dualism), to beginning to understand a dimension of uncertainty related to knowledge (multiplicity), to accepting knowledge as contingent and contextual (relativism; i.e., not only are there alternate views, but some may be better than others). In the final position, students make a commitment to living in a world with many answers, some good and some bad, and they reinforce this commitment by constructing their own values and opinions.

Perry's model used an explicitly Piagetian perspective in tracing the development of students' thinking about the nature of knowledge, truth, values, and the meaning of life and responsibilities (King, 1978). Specifically, Perry's theory examined students' intellect (how they understand the world and the nature of knowledge) and their identity (how they find meaning for their place in the world) (King, 1978). Key to the successful progression of students through the developmental stages in this theory is the ability to recognize the existence of multiple viewpoints and "'the indeterminacies' of 'Truth'" (Pascarella and Terenzini, 1991, p. 29). The process of developing these commitments is dynamic and changeable and is prompted by the exposure that students have to new experiences, new ideas, and new people. Perry (1981) argued that this developmental process extends over the entire lifespan.

Belenky and colleagues (1986) extended Perry's model to include women. Through their study of women of different ages, cultures, and educational levels, Belenkyand colleagues created a model comprising five distinct epistemological positions, with transitions between them. "Silence" was described as an overwhelming sense of isolation and fear. Silent women, of whom none had a college education, had little sense of self and perceived their identity strictly through others' opinions of them. "Received knowers" (whose epistemology was very similar to men who were at the "dualism" stage in Perry's model) perceived those in authority as having the one and only truth. "Subjective knowers" found a voice and a sense of self, and although they still believed there was an absolute right and an absolute wrong, they also believed they had authority and could make their own decisions about who was right or wrong. "Procedural knowers" focused on processes to get to the truth, such as thinking, reflecting, and analyzing. Finally, "constructed knowers" made the self an object of study and sense making; they integrated their self, their mind, and their voice in meaning making and understood knowledge to be mutable and fluid.

In his exploration of "the mental demands of modern life," Kegan (1994) included men and women in a study that explored coping and development in the different contexts of everyday life, including adolescence, parenting, work, and learning. He and his team charted five "orders of consciousness" through which individuals progress in the context of how they think, feel, and relate to themselves and others.

In the first order—running from infancy to about age 7 or 8—children make meaning (i.e., create knowledge) based on their perceptions. If their perception of an object changes, the object itself changes. The second order extends from around age 8 until adolescence and comprises the ability to construct "durable categories," within which physical objects and other people possess characteristics separate from self. In the second order, children, seeing themselves as distinct, begin to develop a self-concept. The transition from the second to the third order begins during adolescence, and the third order is often achieved upon entry to college. In the third order, boundaries are extended beyond the self, and as the context of the self changes, so does the concept. Another way to say this is that individuals undergo a process during which they simultaneously learn to be autonomous and interdependent. Individuals in the third order are able to extend their thinking beyond their own world and to think more abstractly. A growing understanding of self and the ability or even necessity to live life full-time in one's own context (rather than part-time in contexts created by others) leads to a need for more independent thinking. The struggle to separate the self from what others expect occurs here.

Self-authorship is achieved in the fourth order. Individuals become the creators of their own lives, with their own sets of values and convictions to guide them. They are able to self-reflect, self-assess, and self-direct. Based on his research, Kegan theorizes that one-half to two-thirds of adults never reach the fourth level of consciousness, implying that this level is not commonly achieved in the traditional undergraduate college years, though it may occur during postgraduate studies.

Contextual Issues and Learning Environments

Within the span of human development stages and transformations, there are certain contexts and environments that are particularly suited to promoting student change with respect to diversity issues as conceptualized here. When a curriculum deals explicitly with social and cultural diversity, and when a learning environment encourages students to interact frequently with others who differ from themselves in significant ways, the *content* of what students learn will naturally be affected. Less obvious, however, is the notion that features of the learning environment affect students' *mode of thought*, and that diversity is a feature that produces more active thinking and can inspire intellectual engagement and motivation. Both of these aspects of learning situations are important features of how diversity connects to learning.

Many terms in the social and cognitive psychology literature have been used to describe two basically different modes of thinking that can be thought of as being on a continuum of automaticity, from completely automatic thinking without any conscious control to more intentional and controllable mental processes (Manstead and Hewstone, 1995; Bargh, 1994). Research in social psychology in the past 20 years has shown that active engagement in learning cannot be assumed, confirming that much apparent thinking and thoughtful action are actually automatic, or what Langer (1978) calls "mindless." To some extent, mindlessness is the result of previous learning routinized such that an individual can simply rely on automatically activated scripts or schemas, as opposed to active thinking.

Automatic thinking is pervasive in most aspects of everyday life, and in some instances it is a necessary strategy for coping with multiple stimuli in a complex environment. Bargh has shown that automatic thinking is often evident not only in perceptual processes and in the execution of skills such as driving and typing, but also in evaluation, emotional reactions, determination of goals, and social behavior itself (Bargh, 1994; Gurin et al., 2002). One of our important tasks as educators is to interrupt these kinds of automatic processes so that we can facilitate active thinking in our students.

Certain conditions encourage mindful, conscious modes of thought. Novel situations for which people have no script or with which they have had no experience do not allow them to rely on their routinized or automated scripts. Situations that promote active thinking can also be ones that are not entirely novel but not entirely familiar either; situations like these demand more than their scripts and experiences will allow people to grasp (Langer, 1978). Such situations, in which people have to think about what is going on and struggle to make sense of the situation, have been called complex social structures (Coser, 1975). These situations tend to be composed of many rather than a few individuals, people who are transitory rather than stable participants in the situation, and people who hold multiple, even contradictory, perspectives and expectations of each other, thus creating some instability, unpredictability, and discrepancy. In contrast, a simple social structure is one where a small number of familiar people interact with common perspectives over a long period of time. Coser's work has shown that people develop both a greater sense of individuality and a fuller understanding of the social world when they are faced with complex rather than simple social structures.

The features of an environment that promote mental activity are compatible with cognitive-developmental theories. In general, those theories suggest that cognitive growth is fostered by *novelty, instability, discontinuity,* and *discrepancy.* To grow cognitively, we need to be in situations that lead to a state of uncertainty, and even possibly anxiety (Piaget, 1971, 1975/1985; Ruble, 1994a; Acredolo and O'Connor, 1991; Berlyne, 1970; Doise and Palmonaari, 1984). Diverse learning environments help to create these kinds of conditions and thereby stimulate active, conscious, nonautomatic thinking that stimulates cognitive development and identity.

The literature on transformative learning also provides another point of entry into understanding how students are affected by diversity experiences. Mezirow (2000a, pp. 7–8) describes transformative learning as a process that transforms "taken-for-granted frames of reference (meaning perspectives, habits of mind, mind-sets) to make them more inclusive, discriminating, open, emotionally capable of change, and reflective." On a cognitive level, this perspective aligns well with Langer's notions of mindful learning and links with aspects of identity development related to emotional maturity.

In contrast to informative learning that is focused largely on increasing what students know—a content orientation—transformative learning has as its goal a change in *how* students know (Kegan, 1994), facilitating the generation, among other things, of new perspective-taking skills that facilitate subsequent encounters with learning opportunities. Constructive discourse is key to helping students benefit from the experiences of others, and as a result attaining the goal of transformative insight (Mezirow, 2000a).

Many undergraduate efforts focused on diversity-related learning employ techniques that emphasize focused discourse surrounding issues of difference (Zuñiga and Nagda, 1993; Zuñiga et al., 2002).

Individuals transform their perspectives, or frames of reference, by becoming critically reflective of assumptions of themselves and others and aware of their context (Mezirow, 2000b). Similar context issues exist in all fields of study and provide both opportunities and challenges for those seeking to maximize the effectiveness of diversity as an educational tool. Of particular interest for health professions education is the potential for transformative learning to shape an individual's orientation toward lifelong learning. Kegan (1994) argues that an individual's transformative learning history is an important consideration in creating settings intended to create bridges to transformation, while also creating a path toward continuing transformation over the life course.

Creating the conditions for students to perceive differences both within groups and between groups is a primary reason that educators need to be concerned with ensuring that there are sufficient numbers of students of various groups in relevant educational environments. The most extreme kinds of racial imbalance from an educational perspective occur when a minority student or faculty member is alone as a solo or a token. Kanter's (1977) pathfinding research underlies our understanding of token status in organizations, concluding that being a token in an environment was associated with three negative phenomena (i.e., heightened visibility, difference accentuation, and role encapsulation). Later research supports these conclusions (Yoder, 1994; Spangler et al., 1978), showing that solos (the only one) and tokens (a tiny minority) have negative experiences when they interact with majority group members.

Pedagogy

Other conditions that can influence student learning are those created by faculty members and how they choose to structure their educational interactions in classrooms and other learning settings. The benefits of student-centered teaching practices are detailed in a comprehensive report by Chickering and Gamson (1987), who identified educational conditions that result in powerful and enduring undergraduate educational experiences and combat common criticisms of higher education (e.g., apathetic students, illiterate graduates, incompetent teaching, and impersonal campuses). The authors advocate that education should encourage cooperation and collaboration, rather than competitive or isolated learning situations. They believe that working with others and sharing ideas increases involvement and deepens understanding. This is supported by Johnson and Johnson's (1989) comprehensive review of cooperative learning methods at the college level. The review concluded that cooperative learning groups increase productivity, develop commitment and positive relationships among group members, increase social support, and enhance self-esteem. In addition, research on peer-teaching indicates that both peer-teachers and learners benefit from the cooperative relationships generated and gain a better understanding of the subject matter (Goldschmid and Goldschmid, 1976; Whitman, 1988). McKeachie and colleagues (1986) found that cooperative teaching methods such as group projects and student-led discussions were more likely than instructor-dominated methods (e.g., lecturing) to improve the problem-solving, motivation, and leadership skills of students.

In addition, research by Astin (1984) and Pace (1984) on student learning and development emphasizes the importance of a student's active involvement in the educational process. Their research suggests that the greater the student's involvement in academic work or college experience, the greater the level of knowledge acquired. Pascarella and Terenzini (1991) suggest that the most influential educational component of student involvement is the instructional approach used. In a review of the literature, they found that alternative teaching methods, such as active learning, peer teaching, and cooperative structures, have substantial advantages over traditional teaching formats in eliciting active participation. In addition, Pascarella and Terenzini (1991) indicate that content learning and cognitive development is greater in classrooms where students are engaged by the instructional and learning processes. Furthermore, they assert that academic involvement—which is more likely to occur in cooperative situations—also increases psychosocial dimensions such as nonauthoritarianism, tolerance, independence, intellectual disposition, and reflective judgment.

Taken together, these perspectives (and supporting research evidence) underscore a number of general conditions through which campus diversity—if managed through effective, thoughtful processes—can positively affect student learning outcomes. One example of such an effort can be found in the University of Michigan's Program on Intergroup Relations (IGR), which explicitly articulates these conditions and provides students with differing—and potentially conflicting—social identities opportunities to come together to understand and learn from their differences. Through courses and other learning opportunities, IGR helps students learn to talk across race and ethnicity (and across other differences as well) in a public way, learning to address group differences in a balanced and positive fashion. The conditions that facilitate this process include the presence of diverse peers, discontinuity from previous social background, equality among peers, discussion under rules of civil discourse, and normalization and negotiation of conflict (Zuñiga and Nagda, 1993; Zuñiga et al., 2002; Gurin et al., 2002).

A study based on data drawn from this program reveal that it is not simply diversity-related content that is influential in promoting student learning, but also the active learning techniques that are embedded in the program (Lopez et al., 1998). In contrast, postprogram actions were influenced not by content, but by the active learning aspects of the courses within the program. Providing students with content through lectures and readings *alone* does not generate this kind of learning.

While programs modeled after the IGR program at Michigan have begun to appear on other college campuses (e.g., Arizona State University, University of Denver, University of Maryland, University of Massachusetts at Amherst), they remain more the exception than the rule in higher education.

The Impact of Diverse Faculty on Teaching and Learning

Our discussion about the benefits of diversity up until now has focused almost exclusively on the ways in which having a diverse student body can provide important educational and societal benefits. However, it is also important to consider the impact that a diverse faculty has on institutions of higher education. In a recent study that examined the contributions made by diverse faculty to the research, teaching, and service missions of the university, Milem (1999) found that women faculty and faculty of color contributed to the diverse missions of the university in important and unique ways. Specifically, the study analyzed the relationship between the race/ethnicity and gender of faculty members and a variety of variables related to the three central missions (teaching, research, and service) of higher education institutions.

Milem found that race and gender served as significant positive predictors of the use of active teaching methods in the classroom—methods that have been shown to enhance the learning of students in the classes in which they are used. Moreover, the use of active pedagogy provides students with opportunities to interact with peers from different backgrounds through class discussions, collaborative learning methods, and group projects. These activities contribute to a campus climate that is more supportive of diversity and lead to positive outcomes for the students involved (see, e.g., Astin, 1993; Gurin, 1999; Hurtado et al., 1998, 1999; Milem, 2003; Milem and Hakuta, 2000; Smith & Associates, 1997).

Milem (1999) also found that diverse faculty members provided students with more opportunities to encounter readings and research that address the experiences of women and members of different racial/ethnic groups. Interacting with diverse course content provides students with opportunities to understand the experiences of individuals and groups who differ from them in various ways. Moreover, by engaging diversity through readings and class materials, students of color are given opportunities to see themselves and aspects of their experiences in the curriculum. Takaki (1993) has argued that the significance of providing these opportunities to students should not be underestimated. "What happens . . . when someone with the authority of a teacher describes our society, and you are not in it? Such an experience can be disorienting—a moment of psychic disequilibrium, as if you looked into a mirror and saw nothing" (Takaki, 1993, p. 16).

Regarding the research mission of the university, Milem (1999) argued that faculty of color and women faculty expand the boundaries of current knowledge through the questions they explore in the research they do. They are much more likely to engage in research that extends our knowledge of issues pertaining to race/ethnicity and women/gender in society. Finally, Milem found that faculty of color and women were more likely to engage in service-related activities than their other colleagues.

To summarize, Milem (1999) argued that students who attend institutions with higher proportions of women faculty and faculty of color are more likely to be exposed to faculty who are student centered in their orientation to teaching and learning. They also are more likely to experience a curriculum that is more inclusive in its representation of the experiences and contributions of women and people of color in our society. Finally, students who attend institutions with more women and faculty of color are more likely to interact with faculty who are engaged in research on issues of race and gender. On the basis of these analyses, Milem (1999) argued that women and faculty of color play a distinctive and fundamental role in the teaching and learning process through the unique contributions that they make to the three missions of higher education (research, teaching, and service).

Summary

In summary, the higher education literature identifies a number of important issues that link diversity to student learning, including factors related to individual development and the environments within which students are educated. The literature suggests that individual development is enhanced when individuals encounter novel ideas and new social situations, forcing them to abandon automated scripts and think in mindful ways. Given the continuing pattern of segregation in American society, the first time that many individuals encounter racial and ethnic diversity is at college, creating a rich and complex social situation that can be effectively used to promote student learning and development. As the diversity of American society progressively increases, so does the opportunity to make educational use of diversity as does the importance of doing so.

Maintaining or increasing compositional diversity is an important first step for campuses to take in this area, but it is not sufficient to simply diversify an educational program. Intentional actions that create meaningful interactions between individuals and ideas through the formal curriculum and its implementation, as well as through peer-to-peer interactions in informal settings, help create conditions that enhance student learning. Crafted and managed carefully, such experiences can help transform the ways people learn not only about issues of racial, power, and social justice, but how they approach the learning task itself.

INSTITUTIONALIZING DIVERSITY

If the value-added educational benefits associated with diversity are to be realized, then institutions of higher education and their faculties must be actively involved in a process of institutional change and transformation (Chang, 2002; Smith, 1995; Smith & Associates, 1997). Earlier research that examined the impact of increased compositional diversity on college campuses indicated that as the representation of students of color increased on campus, institutions felt greater pressure to change. Evidence of these early pressures to change can be seen in the development of ethnic studies programs, creation of diverse student organizations, implementation of specific academic support programs, and presentation of various diversity enhancement programs (Treviño, 1992; Muñoz, 1989; Peterson et al., 1978).

Garcia and Smith (1996) argue that the pressure that institutions face to change themselves as they become more diverse goes to the heart of the educational enterprise in terms of what is to be taught, who is to teach it, and how it is to be taught. Those who view diversity as a stimulus for institutional change and transformation believe that institutions of higher education should be held accountable to basic democratic ideals that require that they be more equitable and inclusive. Diversity initiatives are transformational in nature because they challenge traditional assumptions about learning as well as other forms of privilege that are associated with learning (Chang, 2002).

Chang (2002) provides a helpful way with which to consider how educators and leaders at individual institutions view diversity. Specifically, he asserts that two primary forms of discourse dominate our thinking about diversity in higher education. He labels these as a discourse of preservation and a discourse of transformation. Somewhat paradoxically, a discourse of preservation has as its key (if not exclusive) focus, increasing the compositional diversity of campuses. Chang (2002) argues that a discourse of preservation is limiting because it overlooks the full historical development of diversity-related efforts on college campuses, focuses on admissions as the primary goal, ignores transformative aims, and thereby underestimates the impact of diversity on student learning.

Chang argues that we should engage in a discourse of transformation when it comes to campus diversity, which is based not only on compositional changes, but also deeper kinds of institutional changes. However, this is very difficult because the transformative aims of diversity often clash with deep-seated institutional assumptions and values. The educational benefits of diversity emanate from institutional changes that challenge prevailing educational sensibilities and that enhance educational participation. Clearly, if the educational benefits that diverse educational environments offer are to be realized, we must be acutely aware of the context in which this diversity is enacted. When the discourse about campus diversity is transformative, important questions should shape the discussions:

- Who deserves an opportunity to learn?
- How is the potential for learning evaluated?
- What is learned?
- Who decides what is important to learn?
- Who oversees learning?
- What conditions advance learning for all students?

Although the discourses described by Chang are important to begin the process of transforming institutions, diversity must eventually become institutionalized as an integral and seamless part of the organizational fabric of our colleges and universities. However, evidence from scholarship that examines organizational behavior in higher education suggests that this is a task that is not easy. A number of organizational forces at work in institutions of higher education make it difficult to institutionalize diversity. In the section that follows, we describe some of the forces that can impede progress in institutionalizing diversity in institutions of higher education.

In a report that summarized the impact of affirmative action in employment, Reskin (1998) indicated that much of the race and sex discrimination that exist in the workplace are a function of the business practices of firms in which such discrimination takes place. To illustrate this concept, Reskin offered two examples of factors that contribute to employment discrimination. The first occurs when employers rely heavily on informal networks to recruit their employees. The second occurs when firms require job credentials that are not necessary to do a job effectively. Reskin (1998, p. 35) suggested that "structural discrimination persists because, once in place, discriminatory practices in bureaucratic organizations are hard to change."

Reskin argued that bureaucratic organizations develop an inertia that tends to preserve these practices unless the organization is faced with genuine pressures to change itself. These observations about the role of organizational inertia in the business sector suggest that similar forces exist in colleges and universities. This is very likely when we consider that colleges and universities, like many private businesses and firms, tend to be highly bureaucratic organizations. Moreover, organizations that provide health care also tend to be highly bureaucratic. Hence, it is important to examine the organizational behaviors that are likely to impede efforts to incorporate diversity as a central part of our institutional missions.

While the American higher education system is large, diverse, complex, and decentralized, it is also extremely homogeneous (Astin, 1985). This homogeneity can be seen in comparable approaches to undergraduate curriculum, great conformity in the training and preparation of faculty, and very similar administrative structures. This tendency toward conformity is complicated by the fact that most educators and educational administrators view the higher education system from an institutional perspective as opposed to a systems perspective. This tendency toward overreliance on an institutional perspective tends to lead to the implementation of policies and practices that weaken the system as a whole (Astin, 1985).

A related perspective on these processes can be found in the concept of institutional isomorphism, an idea first introduced by Riesman (1956). This concept also has been described as "institutional homogenization" or "institutional imitation" (Jencks and Riesman, 1968; Pace, 1974; DiMaggio and Powell, 1983; Astin, 1985; Levinson, 1989; Hackett, 1990; Scott, 1995). "There is no doubt that colleges and universities in this country model themselves upon each other. . . . All one has to do is read catalogues to realize the extent of this isomorphism," Riesman (1956, p. 25) wrote. Riesman depicted the higher education system as an "academic procession," which he described as a snake-like entity in which the most prestigious institutions in the hierarchy are at the head of the snake, followed by the middle group, with the least prestigious schools forming the tail of the snake. The most elite institutions carefully watch each other as they jockey for position in the hierarchy. In the meantime, schools in the middle are busy trying to catch up with the head of the snake by imitating the high-prestige institutions. As a result, schools in the middle of the procession begin to look more like the top institutions while the institutions in the tail pursue the middle-range schools. As a consequence of this type of organizational behavior, institutional forms become less distinctive, relatively little real change occurs in the hierarchy, and the system of higher education struggles to move forward. It is important to note the similarity in outcomes of isomorphic behavior to Reskin's (1998) discussion of the consequences of organizational inertia. Namely, institutions of higher education are likely to resist efforts at change unless they are forced to do so. Jencks and Riesman (1968) suggested that strong economic and professional pres-

sures drive isomorphism in higher education and concluded that homogenization occurs faster than differentiation.

One consequence of this type of organizational behavior can be seen in
its effect on admissions policies and procedures. When students are viewed
as resources, there is immense pressure to rely on narrow definitions of
individual merit and to make institutional admissions policies more selective. Under these circumstances, decisions to seek applicants with higher
standardized test scores are not made for any compelling pedagogical or
educational reasons; rather, based on this traditional view of merit, institutional leaders believe that higher standardized test scores bolster an
institution's reputation. Faculty and administrators come to view selective
admissions policies as being essential to the maintenance of academic excellence or standards. As a result, institutional excellence is defined by the
"quality" of the people who are admitted and not by the nature of the
educational experiences that students have while attending the institution
(Astin, 1985). Despite the tendency for many educational leaders and policy
makers to think otherwise, this extremely narrow definition of excellence
does not serve colleges and universities, their constituencies, or our society
well.

HEALTH PROFESSIONS EDUCATION

It is important to note that much of the research documenting the
benefits of diversity and addressing the campus climate for diversity has
been conducted using data collected from undergraduate students. Although
this might suggest a limited utility of the perspectives generated from the
general higher education literature for health care education, we suggest
that this literature provides a good platform for addressing the common as
well as the unique aspects associated with training in health care professions.

Some of the health professions disciplines are centered in baccalaureate
programs (e.g., nursing, some allied health fields), while others are post-
graduate in nature (e.g., medicine, dentistry). Thus, while many students in
health professions education are subject to the same or similar cognitive
and developmental issues as students enrolled in other postsecondary settings, many may have achieved a more advanced stage.

Structurally, because much of health professions education occurs
within the larger organizational setting known as higher education, it is
subject to institutional forces similar to those found in undergraduate and
graduate/professional settings. What is unique in most health professions
educational programs is the body of learning that occurs outside the traditional educational settings (i.e., lecture halls, classrooms, and laboratories),
and within the settings where health care is actually delivered. Although

this two-part educational model is essential to health professions education, the format and venue for the clinical components of the programs can limit the intended influences and outcomes of the programs.

Finally, but perhaps more importantly, goals that guide health professions education include educating students to interact with and care for patients. The higher education literature discusses the need to ensure "equal status" among students from different cultures in order to achieve and enhance learning outcomes. Health professions educators need to take this one step further by helping students understand the importance of equal status in the context of interactions between health-care providers and patients, where differences in professional status as well as culture greatly influence the quality of health care provided.

Structure of Medical Education

History and Traditional Pedagogy

In 1910 Abraham Flexner—a high school principal with funding from the Carnegie Foundation—published a report on the state of medical education in the United States and Canada (Flexner, 1910). In the report, which was actually an exposé on the disorganized state of medical education, Flexner outlined specific problems and recommendations for improvement. The medical schools that survived after his report were the ones that complied with its recommendations; this resulted in medical training that was very similar in format across many of the schools, and that remained largely intact for nearly 75 years.

In general, the first 2 years of medical education were composed of lectures offered by scientists in specific biomedical science disciplines (e.g., biochemistry, physiology, pharmacology, microbiology) and accompanying laboratory exercises, some with human cadavers and animals. There was also preclinical skills instruction, mostly consisting of students practicing basic physical examination techniques on each other and occasionally using mannequins under a physician's guidance.

In the third year, instruction shifted from classroom lectures and lab exercises to an apprenticeship format. Students, known as "clinical clerks," followed physicians and residents around the hospital wards. Patients were available day and night for the students to interview, examine, and present during medical teaching rounds. Physicians who were providing patient care and teaching residents instructed medical students as they rotated through clerkships in the basic medical disciplines (e.g., internal medicine, surgery, obstetrics/gynecology, pediatrics, psychiatry).

While over the years there was a significant decrease in laboratory exercises—especially animal-based physiology and pharmacology labs for first- and second-year students—this format for learning how to practice medicine remained largely unchanged until the mid-1980s. At that time, the Association of American Medical Colleges (AAMC, 1984), with support from the Liaison Committee on Medical Education (the accrediting agency for U.S. medical schools), encouraged medical schools to reform their curricula to integrate more active methodologies as a way of ensuring lifelong learning skills in physicians. By the early 1990s, many medical schools had responded to this call by reviewing and revising their educational programs. Most of the major revisions have been limited to the first 2 years of the curriculum and consist of additional small-group discussions and an earlier introduction to caring for patients. Some schools, however, took a more dramatic step and adopted the problem-based learning (PBL) format that had been in place in a few medical schools for 20 to 30 years, because of a belief that it promised more effective outcomes by placing learning in the problem-solving context in which medicine would be practiced.

More recently, medical schools have been working to respond to health-care concerns that result from an increasingly diverse patient population in the United States. These concerns have been translated into educational standards and goals by oversight agencies, including state licensing boards and AAMC. As a result, medical schools have begun to design, implement, and evaluate learning modules that address issues and topics such as communication skills, cultural competence, spirituality and health beliefs, palliative care, and approaches that integrate non-Western therapies with more traditional Western therapies.

Problem-Based Learning

To address the matter of integrating more active learning into programs that relied so heavily on lectures, medical educators looked to a few medical schools that had adopted PBL, a student-centered methodology in which small groups of students led by tutors learn through clinical problem solving. PBL programs, pure or blended with more traditional approaches, have been adopted in the first 2 (preclinical) years of medical education. However, few medical schools have implemented significant changes in the clinical clerkships that were created shortly after the Flexner report.

The PBL approach in undergraduate medical education had been established by Case Western Reserve Medical School in the 1950s and McMaster University (in Canada) in the 1960s. At McMaster, Barrows saw PBL as a way for medical students to integrate knowledge across subject boundaries and at the same time develop problem-solving skills (Maudsley, 1999). PBL assessment was innovative as well, involving tutors and peers as well as students assessing themselves. Barrows (2000) described "pure" or "authentic" PBL as "modeled on the skills and activities that will be expected of students when they are practicing their profession. It avoids requiring any learning behaviors that are not of value to the students' future role as physicians" (e.g., rote memorization and answering multiple-choice questions).

Years later, medical educators who are critical of PBL have highlighted the inconsistency in approaches taken to PBL across medical schools, PBL's questionable effectiveness, and the paucity of longer-term sustainability of benefits. Maudsley (1999) reported that various claims had been made for PBL about gains in knowledge, understanding, and thinking, but the label PBL had been used to describe "heterogeneous" approaches to educational activities, and few medical schools have even agreed on the basic characteristics of the method.

Colliver (2000) conducted a comprehensive meta-analysis of research related to the PBL method, comparing the performance of students in PBL programs with performance of students in the more traditional programs. He found no or small effect sizes in the comparisons and concluded that while PBL programs might provide a more challenging, motivating, and enjoyable approach to medical education, the "educational superiority" of PBL relative to the more traditional approach taken in medical education had not been clearly established.

Medical Education Goals and Objectives

A common overarching goal of medical education is to educate physicians who are prepared to practice medicine. In addition to this and to their own more specific goals for medical student education related to achieving cultural competency, U.S. medical schools are guided by educational objectives and standards established by two prominent national organizations.

AAMC, as part of its "Medical School Objectives Project" (AAMC, 1998), has described attributes that graduating medical students should possess. High on this list of important attributes are knowledge of the biomedical sciences and an understanding of the power of the scientific method, as well as the ability to obtain medical histories and perform physical examinations. Other qualities identified by AAMC as being important are the ability to communicate effectively, both orally and in writing, with patients, patients' families, colleagues, and others; knowledge of the nonbiological determinants of poor health and of the economic, psychological, and cultural factors that contribute to the development and/or continuation of maladies; and a commitment to provide care to patients who are unable to pay and to advocate for access to health care for members of medically underserved populations.

Educational Standards and Accreditation

In addition to the guidance provided by AAMC, each medical school in the United States undergoes an accreditation process every 7 years that is conducted by the Liaison Committee for Medical Education (LCME). In contrast to educational programs that are evaluated by other accrediting agencies that rely largely on self-assessment activities, medical schools are assessed by a group of external experts using a specific set of educational standards, which are outlined in a publication titled *Functions and Structure of a Medical School* (LCME, 2002). Schools are advised about what they need to do to meet these explicit accreditation standards. These include providing students with content in their curricula and other discipline-based learning opportunities for broader, proficiency-based content, such as preparing students for their role in addressing the medical consequences of common societal problems; ensuring that graduating students have an understanding of the manner in which people of diverse cultures and belief systems perceive health and illness and respond to various symptoms, diseases, and treatments; and developing in students the ability to recognize and appropriately address gender and cultural biases in themselves and others.

External Assessments of Learning

An external measure of the knowledge and skills students acquire during medical school is the United States Medical Licensure Examination (USMLE), administered by the National Board of Medical Educators. Two steps of this three-step process toward licensure specifically assess medical student learning (the first two steps usually occur during medical school; the third step usually occurs during residency). Step 2 now has two parts (effective 2004), the second of which is a specific test of clinical skills, including communication skills (called the Step 2 CSE, or clinical skills examination).

Step 1 assesses whether students understand and can apply important concepts of the sciences basic to the practice of medicine, with special emphasis on principles and mechanisms underlying health, disease, and modes of therapy. Step 1 ensures mastery of the sciences that provide a foundation for the safe and competent practice of medicine in the present as well as the scientific principles required for maintenance of competence through lifelong learning. Step 2 assesses whether students can apply medical knowledge, skills, and understanding of clinical science essential for the provision of patient care under supervision with an emphasis on health promotion and disease prevention. Step 2 ensures that proper attention is devoted to principles of clinical science and basic patient-centered skills that provide the foundation for the safe and competent practice of medicine.

Current Diversity-Related Pedagogy in Medical Education

Knowledge and Skills

In response to societal concerns and educational goals and standards set by state licensing boards and the medical school accrediting agency, there has been an increase in the number of courses and experiences designed by medical schools to teach medical students to be clinically competent in providing health care to a socially diverse society.

The *cultural competency approach* (Wear, 2003) described by several medical schools highlights the language and customs of particular minority groups, especially their beliefs related to health. Nuñez (2000) asserts that this method is designed to help students increase their understanding of cultural differences and similarities within, among, and between different groups. While students learn characteristics that differ from their own, this is usually done using broad groupings of people (e.g., Latino), rather than using characteristics related to Latino subgroups (i.e., Mexican American, Puerto Rican American, Cuban American) or other dimensions of difference (urban versus rural, lower versus higher socioeconomic status) that exist within these broad categories. Critics of this methodology note that it characterizes culture as a static, "distinctive set of beliefs, values, morals, customs, and institutions which people inherit," rather than "a process in which views and practices are dynamically affected by social transformations, social conflicts, power relationships, and migrations" (Guarnaccia and Rodriguez, 1996). One obvious negative effect of this approach is its tendency to perpetuate rigid stereotypes about members of particular groups and their needs, beliefs, and behaviors (Taylor, 2003).

A second approach, the *communication skills approach*, helps students to elicit important and relevant information from the patient through use of the patient's own words. An added benefit of this approach is that students who use this method are able to communicate better with all patients, regardless of ethnicity or belief systems. This approach considers individual patients and their experiences rather than adhering to a rigid checklist of ethnic traits (Chin and Humikowski, 2002). Kleinman and colleagues' model (1978) is one example of how health-care providers can use this approach to solicit input from patients in explaining their complaint or illness in their own words, thereby providing information to the provider about the patient's cultural, social, economic, and environmental context (Table PCD-1). The model, which can work effectively in the educational and practice settings, helps health-care providers develop a more thorough

TABLE PCD-1 Questions to Be Posed in Kleinman's Explanatory Model

- What do you call the problem?
- What do you think has caused the problem?
- Why do you think it started when it did?
- What do you think the sickness does to you? How does it work?
- How severe is the sickness? Will it have a short or long course?
- What kind of treatment do you think you need? What are the most important results you hope to receive from this treatment?
- What are the chief problems the sickness has caused?
- What do you fear most about the sickness?

SOURCE: Kleinman et al., 1978.

understanding of how the individual patient is experiencing his or her illness.

A third approach to incorporating diversity-related content and pedagogy in medical education combines the previous two and recognizes "the dynamic and ever-changing nature of cultures that occur within cultural groups" using longitudinal paradigm of "key themes and components of culture in health care" (Tervalon, 2003, p. 573). Proponents of this approach assert that students should learn about core cultural issues rather than lists of traits or characteristics, and that it is important to explore with each patient her/his particular cultural belief systems. This combined *knowledge/skills method* is supported by medical educators who concur with Chin and Humikowski's (2002) assertion that "although individualization of care is most important . . . it would be foolhardy not to take into account common beliefs and cultural issues in a community."

Learning Formats

The findings from recent survey data (Flores et al., 2000) indicate that only 8 percent of U.S. medical schools reported having a separate course to address cultural issues; 87 percent reported that learning was embedded in other courses (in 1 to 3 lecture hours); and 16 percent reported offering a separate elective (the percentages exceed 100 percent because some schools offer more than one format). Case-based (59 percent) and didactic (57 percent) designs were the primary teaching methods, which is consistent with the focus in medical education on acquiring accurate knowledge (transmitted through didactic lectures) and developing appropriate behaviors and skills (practiced using cases).

While most medical schools provided opportunities to learn about diversity-related issues in the first (84 percent) and second years (72 percent), surprisingly, only 6 percent of medical schools provided opportunities for any formal learning about these issues in the third year (which is usually characterized by intensive clinical training). This finding suggests that the assumption is that the learning about diversity that occurs in the first 2 (preclinical) years of medical school will be transferred to the clinical setting in the third year. However, this approach provides inconsistent reinforcement of what students learn, which is essential to the long-term maintenance and continued improvement of knowledge and skills.

Although this survey did not address how and when learning is assessed by the medical schools that responded, assessment can play an important role in student learning. Through the use of assessment activities that require students to interact with a simulated patient (such as Objective Structured Clinical Examinations, or OSCEs), faculty observe and provide feedback to each student, or the simulated patient can be trained to do the same (Betancourt, 2003). If the OSCE is administered at the end of the third-year clerkships, as many are, this can be used to help reinforce what students learned in their first 2 years as well as during their clinical skills practice in the third year.

Attitudes

Embedded in the approaches that we have described so far are various efforts to address students' attitudes about diverse cultures. These approaches assume that health-care providers need to be aware of their own biases, prejudices, and stereotypes about culture and the influence these have in health-care encounters with patients if they are to provide culturally competent health care. Some proposed methods designed to do this include the use of learning situations where students describe their own cultural identities (Carillo et al., 1999) and activities that help students identify the sources of bias, prejudice, and discrimination in their own personal experiences (Welch, 1998). Humility, empathy, curiosity, respect, and sensitivity are important attributes in the delivery of effective, culturally competent care. Learning methods that help to develop these attributes include reflective journal entries (Crandall et al., 2003), small-group discussions (Tang et al., in press), student role-playing specific cases with feedback from faculty, exercises with simulated patients (Betancourt, 2003), and guest speakers and tutorials (Beagan, 2003). However, efforts to shape or change student attitudes can be exceptionally difficult. This point is illustrated in the experience of one author who observed a tendency for students and faculty "to focus on content rather than self-awareness" (Beagan, 2003, p. 613), and another who argued that "efforts to change attitudes are labor-intensive, difficult, and complex to evaluate" (Betancourt, 2003, p. 562).

Negative Reinforcements to Learning

Despite numerous attempts to develop and implement diversity-related curricula, medical educators have documented an educational paradox: This paradox highlights the conflict that exists between the explicit curriculum as articulated and enacted in medical classrooms and the implicit or hidden curriculum that is part of the underlying culture of medicine (Hafferty and Franks, 1994). They observe that "only a fraction of medical culture is to be found or can be conveyed within those curriculum-based hours formally allocated to medical students' instruction"(1994, p. 864). Most of what medical students internalize in terms of the values, attitudes, and beliefs comes from the hidden curriculum, and these messages frequently stand in opposition to the formal curriculum (Hafferty, 1998).

M.J.D. Good (1995) argued that the "hidden culture" of medicine can undermine formal learning. One of the processes by which medical students demonstrate their medical competence is through crafting clinical narratives that transform the language used by patients into the language used by physicians. Good reported that this process leaves no room for students to elicit cultural information from their patients. B. Good (1994) found that the clinical narratives were a systematic process of disregarding the patient's story. Hafferty (1998) wrote that in exercises where medical students were encouraged "to create medically meaningful arguments and plots with therapeutic consequences for patients," the psychosocial dimensions of patients' illnesses were regarded as "inadmissible evidence" during medical rounds. Thus, medical competence is regarded by many medical professionals—and so also by medical students—as the *real* competence (Taylor, 2003). Hence, as taught and demonstrated, this leaves no room for patients to tell their story, which would allow them to provide important information to the health-care provider about their social/cultural context.

Educators express caution with another kind of hidden curriculum (which may be more accurately described as the "unintended curriculum") that can undermine the primary curriculum by sending unintended messages to students through their content or format. In an analysis of patient cases integrated throughout first- and second-year courses at the University of Minnesota (these cases were not part of a cultural diversity course or sequence), Turbes et al. (2002) explored whether the cases supported or undermined explicit messages to the students about diverse patient populations. The authors reported that there was an underrepresentation of women in the cases (which was likely to minimize the importance of discussions about women's health issues), little mention of racial or ethnic identifiers in the cases (which, the authors explained, occurred within a cultural environment in which whiteness is often assumed), and almost no mention of sexual orientation (which leads to an assumption of heterosexuality).

TABLE PCD-2 Examples of Advice Given to Health-Care Providers That Can Reinforce Stereotypes

* Sexual problems and venereal diseases can be difficult topics for Arab American patients to discuss (Purnell and Paulanka, 1998).
* An Albanian patient may expect the need for medication in order to become healthy (University of Washington Medical Center, 1999).
* Avoid using phrases such as "you people" or "culturally deprived," which may be considered culturally insensitive (University of Michigan Health System, 2003).

Hafferty and Frank (1994) described a hidden and unintentional curriculum in classrooms or clinical settings where faculty unwittingly present case reports to illustrate concepts that may convey images perpetuating a variety of stereotypes. Stories and jokes shared by students and faculty are often part of the shared culture of medicine and can be an enormously influential component of medical education. As students move from the classrooms to the stressful, arduous clinical training environment, they may cope with their stress by dehumanizing patients, transforming them into objects of work and sources of antagonism and assigning disparaging labels such as "hits" and "gomers" to their patients.

Finally, there are times when advice given to health-care personnel, although accompanied by documentation, can unwittingly reinforce stereotypes or aim so low as to elicit a negative response from the recipients (examples of a few of these are listed in Table PCD-2). This advice, which is generally available to all faculty, staff, practitioners, and their students in academic medical settings, can undermine educational goals rather than foster efforts to appreciate and understand the diverse cultures and complex health care needs represented in the patient population.

The pedagogy that is currently in place in many U.S. medical schools to ensure that graduating medical students are culturally competent tends to focus on the acquisition of accurate knowledge, respectful attitudes, and appropriate behaviors for interacting with patients. Although some medical schools report approaches that are designed to help students reflect on how their biases and prejudices may influence the quality of care they provide to patients, (e.g., Tervalon, 2003; Crandall et al., 2003), by and large, the approach taken at most medical schools to teaching cultural competence is consigned to courses in cultural sensitivity or provider-patient communication (Chin and Humikowski, 2002).

Current Status of Medical Education

If internal and external goals and standards requiring graduating medical students to be culturally competent in caring for patients are to be achieved, medical educators must grapple with a number of difficult challenges. Current medical pedagogy tends to underestimate or even ignore the power of the hidden and informal curricula, where "students learn about the core values of medicine and medical work" (Hafferty and Frank, 1994), which can be in sharp contrast to the core values underlying the formal educational goals of the curriculum. There can also be a "disconnect" between early clinical skills training where students learn about the importance of cultural competence and later clinical training where they learn that patients' social and cultural contexts are irrelevant to competent medical practice (Good, 1994; Good, 1995).

While increasing numbers of women are now entering medical school—nearly half of the entering class in 2002 consisted of women, an increase from 42 percent in 1992 (AAMC, 2003), the majority of physicians are white men who were raised and educated in racially homogeneous environments where nonwhite cultures were not present or represented (Project 3000 by 2000, 1994). Whites continue to be the predominant racial group in entering medical school classes, representing nearly two-thirds of medical school matriculants in 2002 (AAMC, 2003). Given this underrepresentation of people of color in medical school and the use of existing diversity-related teaching methods in medical education that focus on knowledge and skills that enable students to communicate with cultures other than their own, students are likely to adopt a perspective called "othering" (Beagan, 2003), in which students lump individuals from diverse cultures and subcultures together, viewing them through a lens in which difference is tantamount to disadvantage. This view prevents students from recognizing the privileges and advantages that are inherent in being a member of the dominant culture, which is key to recognizing and understanding the perspectives of individuals from nondominant cultures (Beagan, 2003).

Finally, high standards have been set regarding the need to include diversity-related learning opportunities for students in medical education that require medical educators to do more than assist in the acquisition of knowledge, skills, and behaviors. The goals and standards for medical education that have been adopted insist that these experiences enable medical professions to demonstrate scrupulous ethical principles and the capacity to recognize and accept their own limitations (AAMC, 1998), an understanding of the manner in which people of diverse cultures and belief systems perceive health and illness, and the ability to recognize and address gender and cultural biases in themselves and others (LCME, 2002). Achieving these goals requires that medical educators develop in their students attributes such as critical self-awareness and self-assessment, abstract thinking, understanding the perspectives of others, and the ability to understand and value diverse perspectives.

Student Development

There is a substantial body of evidence already described in this paper on models of moral, emotional, and cognitive development from childhood through college and adulthood. Beginning with Piaget's observations of children and continuing through the twentieth century to Kegan's orders of consciousness (how we make meaning or create knowledge), educators have been interested in the intersections between and the mutual influences of developmental stage and learning.

Kegan's model is particularly compelling for health professions educators because of its focus on self-authorship in the fourth order he describes and the strong connections between the qualities and characteristics demonstrated by self-authors and the expectations of those striving to deliver effective, competent, and compassionate health care. As Kegan wrote (1994, p. 169), "Self-evaluating and self-correcting demands an internal standard; it requires a theory or a philosophy of what makes something valuable, a meta-leap beyond the third order." Self-authorship in practice includes the ability to function independently, construct one's own vision, make informed decisions, act appropriately, and take responsibility for one's actions (Baxter Magolda, 1999), all of which are characteristics that society expects of its health-care providers. AAMC, LCME, and many medical schools have institutionalized these expectations by articulating goals for self-assessment as a vital component for self-directed (and self-correcting) lifelong learning.

There is also an important interpersonal dimension woven centrally into Kegan's concept of self-authorship. Bruffee's (1993, p. 2) medical example nicely describes the importance of interweaving the two dimensions (cognitive and interpersonal): "There is a perception by many in the medical profession itself that although traditional medical education stuffs young physicians full of facts, it leaves their diagnostic judgment rudimentary and does not develop their ability to interact socially, with either colleagues or patients, over complex, demanding, perhaps life-and-death issues." Given the importance of communication skills in effectively working across cultural and other differences, it is important to ensure that both of these dimensions are clearly evident in intention and practice.

Of particular interest to medical educators is Kegan's belief that one-half to two-thirds of the adult population never reach the level at which self-authorship is possible. He does, however, provide insight into an approach to learning that can help students become self-authors. Kegan noted that educators can create learning opportunities and set expectations to help students become self-directed learners, understanding that in doing so, many of them will need to change the ways in which they understand themselves and everything in their world. He describes students who have

achieved self-authorship as "self-directed learners" who are able to "examine themselves, their culture, and their milieu in order to understand how to
separate what they feel from what they should feel, what they value from
what they should value, and what they want from what they should want.
They develop critical thinking, individual initiative, and a sense of themselves as co-creators of the culture that shapes them" (Kegan, 1994, p.
274). Kegan cautioned that using training as a method for teaching individuals to respect diversity would run the risk of reducing respect to a skill.
Paradoxically, this could send the message that respecting diversity (i.e.,
mastering the skill) means to "keep our negative attributions and characterizations to ourselves, rather than to learn that our negative attributions and
characterizations are in themselves a failure to respect diversity" (Kegan,
1994, p. 196).

Transformative Learning

Through a process called "transformative learning" (Mezirow, 2000a),
individuals can transform their perspectives, or frames of reference, by
becoming critically reflective of assumptions of themselves and others and
aware of their context. Transformative learning theory and principles are
particularly compelling when they are viewed in light of recent reports by
Tatum (2003), Maher and Tetreault (2003), and Vacarr (2003). These
authors encourage and describe transformative frameworks for learning
about diversity that are problem based and focused on social issues, including race and racism, prejudice, dominant cultures and voices, and
positionality. As noted by Tatum (2003, p. 156), who developed strategies
for promoting racial identity development and improving interracial dialogue in the classroom, "It is certainly common to witness beginning transformations in classes with race-related content." Such principles are not
inconsistent with Baxter Magolda's research and resulting principles that
underlie pedagogical efforts to help students achieve self-authorship. She
wrote, "Promoting self-authorship is a matter of helping students transform their assumptions about knowledge and about themselves" (Baxter
Magolda, 1994, p. 97).

Current medical education literature is not void of thought-provoking
suggestions for medical curricula that combine active learning formats with
deeper and broader levels of self-reflection and understanding so vital to
true cultural competence. Wear (2003) describes an approach to educating
medical students based on Giroux's antiracist pedagogy—a pedagogy that
extends beyond the limitations of "communicative competence" and the
"celebration of tolerance." This approach calls for students to analyze
unequal distributions of power that advantage dominant groups, and the
relevant policies, attitudes, and rituals (i.e., culture) within these groups,

including their own medical school and health care environment. West (1989) wrote about how central such an approach is to recognizing the culture of those who are oppressed, rather than focusing on what makes them different, which runs the risk of marginalizing them even further. Ayers (1998) calls this "teaching for social justice" and argues that it serves as the very foundation of cultural competency efforts. Such experiences are designed to help students understand themselves as individuals who are "positioned" (or situated) in specific social and economic contexts that influence every interaction they have with patients, by providing them with "opportunities to look at their biases, challenge their assumptions, know people beyond labels, and confront the effects of power and privilege" (Wear, 2003). As noted earlier, by creating experiences that allow students to engage peers from different backgrounds in ongoing, structured interactions, students show greater achievement of critical educational outcomes (Gurin, 1999; Gurin et al., 2003). Likewise, faculty can provide opportunities for these interactions by adopting active-learning and student-centered formats (e.g., learning groups, peer teaching, group projects) that provide the students from different cultures with important opportunities to build bridges across their differences.

Medical educators have been working for more than a decade to integrate more active learning into their curricula, so some of this information is not new to them. The long philosophical leap they are asked to make here is to consider reexamining the principles underlying current medical school pedagogy that are focused on helping students to master the knowledge, skills, and attitudes that will in theory make them culturally competent. The higher education and psychology literatures on development, social justice pedagogy, active and interactive educational formats, and transformative learning provide convincing frameworks for development and learning that are better matches with attributes for delivering culturally competent health care that all interested parties—particularly some members of society—believe medical school graduates and physicians should possess. Medical educators can synthesize these literatures to develop an ideology that will guide them in constructing experiences that address the particular challenges they face in ensuring that medical students can effectively achieve cultural competency.

Medical Student Composition

As mentioned earlier in this paper, in the University of Michigan's affirmative action deposition to the U.S. Supreme Court, Gurin (1999) used Piaget's work (1971, 1975/1985) to support the contention that diversity in the student body facilitates students' cognitive and identity development. Specifically, when students interact with diverse individuals—in "safe" environments where all have an equal opportunity to participate and be heard—the process of perspective taking, which stimulates development, is fostered. However, there is a strong correlation between the ethnic/racial composition of the student body and the educational benefits to be gained from such diversity-related initiatives. For example, Chang (1999) provided evidence about the diminished benefits of diversity-related pedagogy and approaches when they are adopted with little or no change in student body composition. Currently, the number and percentage of medical school matriculants in the United States remains predominantly white, with little change in underrepresented minorities over the past 10 years. Given this, efforts to engage medical students from diverse backgrounds in educational initiatives to achieve goals for cultural competence will have diminished impact if student diversity is not increased.

Although our manuscript does not focus on admissions practices in medical school or health professions programs, deans and admissions directors should consider the connections that we have shown exist between a diverse student body and educational initiatives that help students achieve cultural competence as they reflect on the criteria they use for admissions to their programs. This is an important consideration to make in pondering ways to achieve greater diversity in these programs.

Bowen and Bok (1998) wrote about society's increasing dependence on the character of the individuals who serve society in professional roles. Levin (1996) said, "Academic excellence must remain the most important single criterion for admission . . . but we should continue to look for something more—for those elusive qualities of character that give young men and women the potential to have an impact on the world, to make contributions to the larger society through their scholarly, artistic, and professional achievements, and to work and to encourage others to work for the betterment of the human condition."

Recent reports detailing health-care disparities (e.g., Institute of Medicine, 2003) underscore the need to address more directly "the betterment of the human condition" by ensuring access to health care to certain populations in the United States. By achieving greater nonwhite diversity among their students, medical schools can play a key role in the longer-term solutions to these disparities. Studies conducted by Komaromy and colleagues (1996, reported in Bowen and Bok, 1998) and Keith and colleagues (1985, reported in Bowen and Bok, 1998) provide important evidence that black and Hispanic physicians are much more likely to treat patients in minority communities that include poor people and that minority physicians are twice as likely to treat patients in locations where there are health-care shortages (as identified by the federal government). Medical schools may want to consider documented outcomes like this or evidence about the predictive value of admissions criteria as they contemplate increasing diversity in the medical student population.

For example, a recent analysis of predictors of medical school performance (White et al., unpublished) showed that for underrepresented minority students at one medical school, academic performance (i.e., the undergraduate grade point average) is a better predictor of academic performance in medical school (measured at three time points, progressively) than standardized test scores (i.e., the Medical College Admissions Test, or MCAT), which reliably predicted only scores on future standardized tests (i.e., USMLE Step 1 examination).

Extending the Transformation into the Clinical Years

We ask medical educators to consider how studies reported in the higher education and psychology literatures (and to a lesser degree in the medical education literature), many of which are presented here, can be used to develop approaches that ensure medical student achievement of cultural competence. The methods and pedagogies discussed in this paper can potentially help medical students transform their perspectives about diversity and at the same time progress toward achievement of self-authorship, which provides a foundation for understanding the perspectives of those from other cultures and backgrounds.

However, in considering a comprehensive educational approach within the medical education context, the "negative reinforcement" issues also must be addressed. When students begin clinical training, they leave behind the sheltered environment of the classrooms and clinical skills laboratories, and the day-to-day influence of the faculty members who have taught them in the first 2 years. As they enter the clinics, hospitals, and operating rooms, the "hidden curriculum" (Hafferty, 1998) and "hidden culture" (Taylor, 2003) largely dictate the cultural norms students will need to survive or even thrive. As noted by Hafferty (1998), the values underlying these informal curricula might be in direct conflict with the values underlying the goals of the formal curriculum. The challenge for medical educators is how to extend learning into a very influential milieu over which they have limited control and which in fact may serve to undermine or undo learning that has occurred.

In this paper we have encouraged medical educators to contemplate connections between attributes associated with specific developmental levels and those associated with educational standards and goals for cultural competence. As noted, language in the standards describing desired attributes of physicians closely mirrors language that Perry (1970), Kegan (1994) and others use to describe a high (or in some cases the highest) level of cognitive and interpersonal development—one in which individuals become the creators of their own lives, with their own sets of values and convictions to guide them, along with the abilities to self-reflect, self-assess, and self-direct. It might be reasonable to anticipate that students who have achieved self-authorship prior to being sent into the realm of the informal curriculum have in essence been "armed" with the capability to create and rely on their own value structures, thus possibly diminishing (at least in the short term, until they gain more professional autonomy) the undermining influence of the informal curriculum. Comprehensive assessments already in place in most medical schools can be used to monitor the longitudinal effectiveness of newly adopted pedagogies and approaches by measuring mastery of specific learning outcomes into and after one or both of the intensive clinical years.

It is also not impossible to imagine a health-care world where educational values correlate more closely with conflicting cultural values. Standards developed by the Joint Commission on Accreditation of Healthcare Organizations (2003) include quality of patient care, which many institutions are assessing through surveys of patient satisfaction. This process provides a direct evaluation link between health-care organizations and the individuals they serve and underlies efforts that can be made to modify and influence behavior of those who are providing health care. Whether such efforts can influence the "moral underbelly" (Hafferty, 1998) of health care organizations remains to be seen, but with regard to influence over student values related to cultural competence, they are a move in the right direction.

CONCLUDING THOUGHTS

In this paper we have presented an evidence-based argument to support the importance and benefits of diversity in higher and health professions education. To understand specifically what we mean by "diversity in higher education," we began with a description of the factors within college/university campus climates that impact educational diversity: historical legacy (resistance to desegregation and unrecognized, embedded advantages for dominant cultures), psychological climate (perceptions of discrimination and attitudes toward individuals from different cultures), behavioral climate (social and educational interactions among students and faculty), and compositional diversity (racial/ethnic composition of the student body).

In a discussion about linking diversity with learning, we presented information about college student cognitive and emotional development; approaches to learning that are active and student-centered and provide the discontinuity and discrepancy that stimulate development within a cognitive framework; and specific learning methodologies that encourage cooperation, deepen understanding, and enhance self-esteem.

Finally, we presented information on the increased benefits of combining student composition with educational initiatives, impediments to institutionalizing diversity-based programs, and principles that might guide thinking and action related to integrating diversity-based initiatives into college and university life.

We then linked this body of evidence to health professions education, in a specific medical education context, where the argument supporting the educational value of diversity is even more compelling given the goals and standards related to the competent care of patients in an increasingly diverse U.S. population.

Specifically, we presented a brief history and described the structure of medical education programs, and described external goals and standards that guide medical educators in developing specific institutional goals and learning outcomes. We explained current educational initiatives in the medical education literature designed to achieve cultural competence and suggested a potential "disconnect" between current approaches and educational goals and standards.

We linked student development to potentially effective pedagogies, building on the higher education research on transformative learning and adding information about social justice educational principles and pedagogies from the higher education and medical education literatures. Although not a primary concern of this paper because of the evidence that cautions educators about important connections between the racial and ethnic composition of student bodies and diversity-based initiatives to achieve educational outcomes, we briefly discussed the current composition of students in U.S. medical schools.

Finally, we recognized that changes in curriculum and composition alone will not address the negative reinforcements that can undermine educational goals and standards. We asked readers of this paper to think about how pedagogy and experience to help medical students achieve self-authorship not only yields benefits related to learning and autonomy, but might also serve to at least diminish the influence of negative reinforcements that can weaken efforts to achieve clinical competence.

To achieve these benefits and maximize the opportunities for teaching and learning that diverse learning environments provide, it is important to give careful consideration to the context in which the diversity is enacted. Merely bringing diverse people together in an institution or an educational program does not ensure that the benefits of diversity will be achieved. Although it is an important *first* step, it cannot be the *only* step that this taken. In reviewing the relevant literatures, we have attempted to identify some general principles that can guide efforts to enhance the goals of diversity in health professions education.

REFERENCES

AAMC (Association of American Medical Colleges). 1984. *Physicians for the Twenty-First Century: The GPEP Report.* Washington, DC: AAMC.

AAMC. 1998. *Report I: Learning Objectives for Medical Student Education: Guidelines for Medical Schools.* Medical School Objectives Project. Washington, DC: AAMC.

AAMC. 2003. *FACTS—Applicants, Matriculants, and Graduates.* [Online]. Available: http://www.aamc.org/data/facts [accessed September 5, 2003].

Acredolo C, O'Connor J. 1991. On the difficulty of detecting cognitive uncertainty. *Human Development* 34:204–223.

Antonio AL. 2001. Diversity and the influence of friendship groups in college. *Review of Higher Education* 25(1):63–89.

Association of American Colleges. 1990. *Liberal Learning and the Arts and Sciences Major.* Vol. 2. Reports from the Field. Washington, DC: AAC.

Astin AW. 1968. *The College Environment.* Washington, DC: American Council on Education.

Astin AW. 1984. Student involvement: A developmental theory for higher education. *Journal of College Student Personnel* 25:297–308

Astin AW. 1985. *Achieving Educational Excellence.* San Francisco: Jossey-Bass.

Astin AW. 1991. *Assessment for Excellence: The Philosophy and Practice of Assessment and Evaluation in Higher Education.* New York: Macmillan.

Astin AW. 1993. *What Matters in College? Four Critical Years Revisited.* San Francisco: Jossey-Bass.

Ayers W. 1998. Popular education—teaching for social justice. In: Ayers W, Hunt JA, Quinn T, eds. *Teaching for Social Justice.* New York: New Press and Teachers College Press. Pp. xvii–xxvi.

Bargh JA. 1984. Automatic and conscious processing of social information. In: Wyer RS Jr., Srull TK, eds. *Handbook of Social Cognition.* Vol. 3. Hillsdale, NJ: Erlbaum.

Bargh JA. 1994. The four horsemen of automaticity: awareness, intention, efficiency, and control in social cognition. In: Wyer RS Jr., Srull TK, eds. *Handbook of Social Cognition. Vol. 1: Basic Processes* (2nd ed.). Hillsdale, NJ: Erlbaum.

Barrows HS. 2000. Authentic problem-based learning. In: Distlehorst LH, Dunnington GL, Folse JR, eds. *Teaching and Learning in Medical and Surgical Education: Lessons Learned for the 21st Century.* Mahwah, NJ: Erlbaum Associates.

Baxter Magolda MB. 1999. *Creating Contexts for Learning and Self-Authorship: Constructive-Developmental Pedagogy.* Nashville, TN: Vanderbilt University Press.

Beagan BL. 2003. Teaching social and cultural awareness to medical students: "It's all very nice to talk about it in theory, but ultimately it makes no difference." *Academic Medicine* 78(6):605–614.

Belenky MF, Clinchy BM, Goldberger N, Tarule J. 1986. *Women's Ways of Knowing: The Development of Self, Voice and Mind.* New York: Basic Books, Inc.

Berger JB, Milem JF. 1999. The role of student involvement and perceptions of integration in a causal model of student persistence. *Research in Higher Education* 40(6):641–664.

Berlyne DE. 1970. Children's reasoning and thinking. In: Mussen PH, ed. *Carmichael's Manual of Child Psychology.* Vol. 1. New York: Wiley. Pp. 939–981.

Betancourt JR. 2003. Cross-cultural medical education: Conceptual approaches and frameworks for evaluation. *Academic Medicine* 78(6):560–569.

Blalock JM. 1967. *Toward a Theory of Minority-Group Relations.* New York: Wiley.

Bowen WG, Bok D. 1998. *The Shape of the River: Long-Term Consequences of Considering Race in College and University Admissions.* Princeton, NJ: Princeton University Press.

Bruffee KA. 1993. *Collaborative Learning: Higher Education, Independence, and the Authority of Knowledge*. Baltimore: Johns Hopkins University Press.

Carillo JE, Green AR, Betancourt JR. 1999. Cross-cultural primary care: A patient-based approach. *Annals of Internal Medicine* 10:829–834.

Chang MJ. 1999. Does racial diversity matter? The educational impact of a racially diverse undergraduate population. *Journal of College Student Development* 40(4):377–395.

Chang MJ. 2002. Preservation or transformation: Where's the real educational discourse on diversity? *Review of Higher Education* 25(2):125–140.

Chickering AW. 1969. *Education and Identity*. San Francisco: Jossey-Bass.

Chickering AW, Gamson Z. 1987. Seven principles of good practice in undergraduate education. *AAHE Bulletin* 39:3–7.

Chin MH, Humikowski CA. 2002. When is risk stratification by race or ethnicity justified in medical care? *Academic Medicine* 77(3):202–208.

Collins PH. 1986. Learning from the outsider within: The sociological significance of black feminist thought. *Social Problems* 33(3):514–532.

Colliver JA. 2000. Effectiveness of problem-based learning curricula: Research and theory. *Academic Medicine* 75(3):259–266.

Coser R. 1975. The complexity of roles as a seedbed of individual autonomy. In: Coser LA, ed. *The Idea of Social Structure: Papers in Honor of Robert Merton*. New York: Harcourt Brace Jovanovich.

Crandall SJ, George G, Marion GS, Davis S. 2003. Applying theory to the design of competency training for medical students: A case study. *Academic Medicine* 78(6):588–594.

Dey EL. 1996. Undergraduate political attitudes: An examination of peer, faculty, and social influences. *Research in Higher Education* 37(5):535–554.

Dey EL. 1997. Undergraduate political attitudes: Peer influence in changing social contexts. *Journal of Higher Education* 68(4):398–413.

DiMaggio P, Powell W. 1983. The iron cage revisited: Institutional isomorphism and collective rationality in organizational fields. *American Sociological Review* 48:147–160.

Doise W, Palmonaari A, eds. 1984. *Social Interaction in Individual Development*. New York: Cambridge University Press.

Duster T. 1993. The diversity of California at Berkeley: An emerging reformulation of competence: in an increasingly multicultural world. In: Thompson BW, Tyagi S, eds. *Beyond a Dream Deferred: Multicultural Education and the Politics of Excellence*. Minneapolis: University of Minnesota Press.

Erikson E. 1946. Ego development and historical change. *Psychoanalytic Study of the Child* 2:359–396.

Erikson E. 1956. The problem of ego identity. *Journal of American Psychoanalytic Association* 4:56–121.

Feldman KA, Newcomb TM. 1969. *The Impact of College on Students*. San Francisco: Jossey-Bass.

Flexner A. 1910. *Medical Education in the United States and Canada: A Report to the Carnegie Foundation for the Advancement of Teaching*. New York: Carnegie Foundation.

Flores G, Gee D, Kastner B. 2000. The teaching of cultural issues in U.S. and Canadian medical schools. *Academic Medicine* 75(5):451–455.

Garcia M, Smith DG. 1996. Reflecting inclusiveness in the college curriculum. In: Garcia M, ed. *Affirmative Action's Testament of Hope: Strategies for a New Era in Higher Education*. Albany: State University of New York Press.

Goldschmid B, Goldschmid M. 1976. Peer teaching in higher education: A review. *Higher Education* 5:9–33.

Good B. 1994. *Medicine, Rationality and Experience: An Anthropological Perspective.* Cambridge, England: Cambridge University Press.

Good MJD. 1995. *American Medicine: The Quest for Competence.* Berkeley: University of California Press.

Guarnaccia PJ, Rodriguez O. 1996. Concepts of culture and their role in the development of culturally-competent mental health services. *Hispanic Journal of Behavioral Sciences* 18: 419–443.

Gurin P. 1999. Expert Report, *The Compelling Need for Diversity in Higher Education,* prepared for *Gratz et al. v. Bollinger et al.* No. 97-75231 (E.D. Mich.) and *Grutter et al. v. Bollinger et al.* No. 97-75928 (E.D. Mich.).

Gurin P, Dey EL, Hurtado S, Gurin G. 2002. Diversity and higher education: Theory and impact on educational outcomes. *Harvard Educational Review* 72(3):330–366.

Gurin PY, Dey EL, Gurin G, Hurtado, S. 2003. How does racial/ethnic diversity promote education? *Western Journal of Black Studies* 27(1):20–29.

Hackett EJ. 1990. Science as vocation in the 1990s: The changing organizational culture of academic science. *Journal of Higher Education* 61(3):241–279.

Hafferty FW. 1998. Beyond curriculum reform: Confronting medicine's hidden curriculum. *Academic Medicine* 73(4):403–407.

Hafferty FW, Franks R. 1994. The hidden curriculum, ethics teaching, and the structure of medical education. *Academic Medicine* 69(11):861–871.

Hurtado S. 1992. The campus racial climate: Contexts of conflict. *Journal of Higher Education* 63(5):539–569.

Hurtado S. 1994. The institutional climate for talented Latino students. *Research in Higher Education* 35(1):21–41.

Hurtado S, Dey EL, Trevino JG. 1994, April. *Exclusion or Self-Segregation? Interaction Across Racial/Ethnic Groups on Campus.* Paper presented at the Annual Meeting of the American Educational Research Association, New Orleans.

Hurtado S, Milem JF, Clayton-Pedersen AR, Allen WR. 1998. Enhancing campus climates for racial/ethnic diversity through educational policy and practice [20th Anniversary Edition]. *The Review of Higher Education* 21(3):279–302.

Hurtado S, Milem JF, Clayton-Pederson AR, Allen WR. 1999. *Enacting diverse learning environments: Improving the climate for racial/ethnic diversity in higher education.* San Francisco: Jossey-Bass.

Hurtado S, Dey,EL, Gurin PY, Gurin G. 2003. The college environment, diversity, and student learning. In: Smart, J., ed. *Higher Education: Handbook of Theory and Research.* Amsterdam: Kluwer Academic Press. Pp. 143–189.

Institute of Medicine. 2003. *Unequal Treatment: Confronting Racial and Ethnic Disparities in Health Care.* Washington, DC: The National Academies Press.

Jencks C, Riesman D. 1968. *The Academic Revolution.* Garden City, NY: Doubleday.

Johnson DW, Johnson RT. 1989. *Cooperation and Competition: Theory and Research.* Edina, MN: Interaction Book Company.

Joint Commission on Accreditation of Healthcare Organizations. 2003. *Standards.* [Online]. Available: http://www.jcaho.org/accredited+organizations/hopsitals/standards/standards.html [accessed September 5, 2003].

Kanter RM. 1977. Some effects of proportions on group life: Skewed sex ratios and responses to token women. *American Journal of Sociology* 82:965–990.

Kegan R. 1994. *In Over Our Heads: The Mental Demands of Modern Life.* Cambridge, MA: Harvard University Press.

King P. 1978. William Perry's theory of intellectual and ethical development. In: Knefelkamp L, Widick C, Parker C, eds. *Applying New Developmental Findings (New Directions for Student Services No. 4).* San Francisco: Jossey-Bass.

Kleinman A, Eisenberg L, Good B. 1978. Culture, illness, and care: Clinical lessons from anthropologic and cross-cultural research. *Annals of Internal Medicine* 88:251–258.

Langer EJ. 1978. Rethinking the role of thought in social interaction. In: Harvey J, Ickes W, Kiss R, eds. *New Directions in Attribution Research*. Hillsdale, NJ: Erlbaum.

LCME (Liaison Committee on Medical Education). 2002. *Functions and Structure of a Medical School*. Washington, DC: Liaison Committee on Medical Education.

Levin RC. 1998, October 26. *Preparing for Yale's Fourth Century*. Essay prepared for the Association of Yale Alumni Assembly, New Haven, CT.

Levinson RM. 1989. The faculty and institutional isomorphism. *Academe* 75(1):23–27.

Loo CM, Rolison G. 1986. Alienation of ethnic minority students at a predominately white university. *Journal of Higher Education* 57(1):58–77.

Lopez GE, Gurin P, Nagda BA. 1998. Education and understanding structural causes for group inequalities. *Journal of Political Psychology* 19(2):305–329.

MacPhee D, Kreutzer JC, Fritz JJ. 1994. Infusing a diversity perspective into human development courses. *Child Development* 65(2):699–715.

Maher FA, Tetreault MKT. 2003. Learning in the dark: How assumptions of whiteness shape classroom knowledge. In: Howell A, Tuitt F, eds. *Race and Higher Education*. Harvard Educational Review, No. 36.

Manstead ASR, Hewstone M, eds. 1995. *The Blackwell Encyclopedia of Social Psychology*. Cambridge: Basil Blackwell.

Maudsley G. 1999. Do we all mean the same thing by "problem-based learning"? A review of the concepts and a formulation of ground rules. *Academic Medicine* 74(2):178–185.

McKeachie WJ, Pintrich PR, Lin YG, Smith DAE. 1986. *Teaching and Learning in the College Classroom: A Review of the Research Literature*. Ann Arbor, MI: National Center for Research and Improvement on Postsecondary Teaching and Learning.

Mezirow J. 2000a. Learning to think like an adult: Core concepts of transformation theory. In: Mezirow J & Associates, eds. *Learning as Transformation: Critical Perspectives on a Theory in Progress*. San Francisco: Jossey-Bass.

Mezirow J. 2000b. How critical reflection triggers transformative learning. In: J Mezirow & Associates, eds. *Fostering Critical Reflection in Adulthood: A Guide to Transformative and Emancipatory Learning*. San Francisco: Jossey Bass.

Milem JF. 1998. Attitude change in college students: Examining the effects of college peer groups and faculty reference groups. *Journal of Higher Education* 69(2):117–140.

Milem JF. 1999, January. *The Importance of Faculty Diversity to Student Learning and to the Mission of Higher Education*. Paper presented at A Symposium and Working Research Meeting on Diversity and Affirmative Action, sponsored by the American Council on Education, Washington, DC.

Milem JF. 2003. The educational benefits of diversity: Evidence from multiple sectors. In: Chang M, Witt D, Jones J, Hakuta K, eds. *Compelling Interest: Examining the Evidence on Racial Dynamics in Higher Education*. Palo Alto, CA: Stanford University Press.

Milem JF, Berger JB. 1997. A modified model of college student persistence: The relationship between Astin's theory of involvement and Tinto's theory of student departure. *Journal of College Student Development* 38(4):387–400.

Milem JF, Hakuta K. 2000. The benefits of racial and ethnic diversity in higher education. Featured report. In: Wilds D, author. *Minorities in Higher Education: Seventeenth Annual Status Report*. Washington, DC: American Council on Education. Pp. 39–67.

Muñoz C. 1989. *Youth, Identity, and Power in the Chicano Movement*. New York: Vesco.

Nuñez AE. 2000. Transforming cultural competence into cross-cultural efficacy in women's health education. *Academic Medicine* 75(11):1071–1080.

Pace CR. 1974. *The Demise of Diversity? A Comparative Profile of Eight Types of Institutions*. Berkeley, CA: Carnegie Commission on Higher Education.

Pace CR. 1984. *Measuring the Quality of College Student Experiences.* Los Angeles: Higher Education Research Institute, UCLA.

Pascarella ET, Terenzini PT. 1991. *How College Affects Students.* San Francisco: Jossey-Bass.

Perry WG. 1970. *Forms of Intellectual and Ethical Development in the College Years: A Scheme.* New York: Holt, Rinehart and Winston.

Perry WG. 1981. Cognitive and ethical growth. In: A Chickering, & Associates, eds. *The Modern American College: Responding to the New Realities of Diverse Students and a Changing Society.* San Francisco: Jossey-Bass.

Peterson MW, Spencer MG. 1990. Understanding academic culture and climate. In: Tierney WG, ed. *Assessing Academic Climates and Cultures. New Directions for Institutional Research* (No. 68). San Francisco: Jossey-Bass.

Peterson MW, Blackburn RT, Gamson ZF, Arce CH, Davenport RW, Mingle JR. 1978. *Black Students on White Campuses: The Impacts of Increased Black Enrollment.* Ann Arbor, MI: Institute for Social Research.

Piaget J. 1971. The theory of stages in cognitive development. In: Green DR, Ford MP, Flamer GB, eds. *Measurement and Piaget.* New York: McGraw-Hill. Pp. 1–11.

Piaget J. 1975/1985. *The Equilibrium of Cognitive Structures: The Central Problem of Intellectual Development.* Chicago: University of Chicago Press.

Prillerman SL, Myers HF, Smedley BD. 1989. Stress, well-being, and academic achievement in college. In: Berry GL, Asamen JK, eds. *Black Students: Psychosocial Issues and Academic Achievement.* Newbury Park, CA: Sage.

Project 3000 by 2000. 1994. Racial and ethnic diversity in U.S. medical schools. *New England Journal of Medicine* 331:472–476.

Purnell LD, Paulanka BJ. 1998. *Transcultural Health Care: A Culturally Competent Approach.* Philadelphia: F.A. Davis.

Reskin BF. 1998. *The Realities of Affirmative Action in Employment.* Washington, DC: American Sociological Association.

Riesman D. 1956. *The Academic Procession. Constraint and Variety in American Higher Education.* Lincoln: University of Nebraska Press.

Ruble D. 1994a. A phase model of transitions: Cognitive and motivational consequences. *Advances in Experimental Social Psychology* 26:163–214.

Ruble D. 1994b. Developmental changes in achievement evaluation: Motivational implications of self-other differences. *Child Development* 65:1095–1110.

Scott WR. 1995. *Institutions and Organizations.* Thousand Oaks, CA: Sage.

Smedley BD, Myers HF, Harrell SP. 1993. Minority-status stresses and the college adjustment of ethnic minority freshmen. *Journal of Higher Education* 64(4):434–452.

Smith DG. 1995. *The Drama of Diversity and Democracy.* Washington, DC: Association of American Colleges and Universities.

Smith DG, & Associates. 1997. *Diversity Works: The Emerging Picture of How Students Benefit.* Washington, DC: Association of American Colleges and Universities.

Spangler E, Gordon MA, Pipkin RM. 1978. Token women: An empirical test of Kanter's hypothesis. *American Journal of Sociology* 84:160–170.

Steele CM. 1992. Race and the schooling of black Americans. *The Atlantic Monthly* (April):68–78.

Steele CM. 1997. A threat in the air: How stereotypes shape intellectual identity and performance. *American Psychologist* 52(6):613–629.

Steele CM. 1998. Stereotyping and its threat are real. *American Psychologist* 53:680–681.

Steele CM, Aronson J. 1995. Stereotype threat and the intellectual test performance of African Americans. *Journal of Personality and Social Psychology* 69:797–811.

Takaki R. 1993. *A Different Mirror: A History of Multicultural America.* Boston: Little, Brown.

Tang TS, Hernandez EJ, Adams BS. In press. Learning by teaching: A peer-teaching model for diversity training in medical school. *Teaching and Learning in Medicine.*

Tatum BD. 2003. Talking about race, learning about racism: The application of racial identity development theory in the classroom. In: Howell A, Tuitt F, eds. *Race and Higher Education.* Cambridge, MA: Harvard Publication Group.

Taylor JS. 2003. Confronting "culture" in medicine's "culture of no culture." *Academic Medicine* 78(6):555–559.

Tervalon M. 2003. Components of culture in health for medical students' education. *Academic Medicine* 78(6):570–576.

Thelin J. 1985. Beyond the background music: Historical research on admissions and access in higher education. In: Smart JC, ed. *Higher Education Handbook of Theory and Research.* Vol. 1. New York: Agathon.

Tierney WG. 1987. Facts and constructs: Defining reality in higher education organizations. *Review of Higher Education* 11(1):61–73.

Tierney WG. 1997. The parameters of affirmative action: Equity and excellence in the academy. *Review of Educational Research* 67(2):165–196.

Treviño JG. 1992. *Participating in Ethnic/Racial Student Organizations.* Unpublished Ph.D. dissertation, University of California, Los Angeles.

Turbes S, Krebs E, Axtell S. 2002. The hidden curriculum in multicultural medical education: The role of case examples. *Academic Medicine* 77(3):209–216.

University of Michigan Health System. 2003. *Tools and Resources: Approaches for Cross-Cultural Relationships.* [Online]. Available: http://www.med.umich.edu/multicultural/ccp/approaches.htm [accessed September 5, 2003].

University of Washington Medical Center. 1999. *Culture Clues: Communicating With Your Albanian Patient.* Seattle: University of Washington Medical Center Staff Development Group, Patient and Family Education Committee.

Vacarr B. 2003. Moving beyond political correctness: Practicing mindfulness in the diverse classroom. In: Howell A, Tuitt F, eds. *Race and Higher Education.* Harvard Educational Review, No. 36.

Wear D. 2003. Insurgent multiculturalism: Rethinking how and why we teach culture in medical education. *Academic Medicine* 78(6):549–554.

Welch M. 1998. *Enhancing Awareness and Improving Cultural Competence in Health Care: A Partnership Guide for Teaching Diversity and Cross-Cultural Concepts in Health Professional Training.* San Francisco: University of California.

West C. 1989. Black culture and postmodernism. In: Kruger B, Mariani P, eds. *Remaking History.* Port Townsend, WA: Bay Press.

White CB, Dey EL, Fantone JC. Unpublished. *Predictors of Clinical Performance in Medical School.* Unpublished manuscript. University of Michigan at Ann Arbor.

Whitla DK, Orfield G, Silen W, Teperow C, Howard C, Reede J. 2003. The educational benefits of diversity in medical school: A survey of students. *Academic Medicine* 78(5): 460–466.

Whitman, NA. 1988. *Peer Teaching: To Teach Is to Learn Twice* (ASHE-ERIC Higher Education Report No. 4). Washington, DC: ERIC Clearinghouse on Higher Education, George Washington University and Association for the Study of Higher Education.

Yoder JD. 1994. Looking beyond numbers: The effects of gender status, job prestige, and occupational gender-typing on tokenism processes. *Social Psychology Quarterly* 57:150–159.

Zúñiga X, Nagda BA. 1993. Dialogue groups: An innovative approach to multicultural learning. In: Schoem D, Frankel L, Zúñiga X, Lewis E, eds. *Multicultural Teaching in the University.* Westport, CT: Praeger. Pp. 233–248.

Zúñiga X, Nagda BA, Sevig TD. 2002. Intergroup dialogues: An educational model for cultivating student engagement across differences. *Equity and Excellence in Education* 35(1):7–17.

Index

A

Office of Program Consultation and
  Accreditation, 135
recruitment and retention initiatives,
  249-251
Suinn Minority Achievement Awards,
  163, 250
Area Health Education Centers, 110, 276-
  277, 285, 295, 297, 300
Arizona State University, 361
Arkansas, financial aid programs, 294, 295
Armed Forces Health Professions
  Scholarship Program, 289
Asian Americans/Pacific Islanders
  access to care, 26
  cross-racial interactions, 351-352
  debt impacts, 102
  faculty, 41-42, 48, 50
  financial status of families, 89-90
  in health professions workforce, 42-43,
    46, 48, 274-275
  initiative, 282
  satisfaction with care, 32
  school enrollment and graduation
    trends, 40, 51, 72-73, 74, 253
  standardized test performance, 63, 64,
    65-66, 70
  U.S. population, 23
Association of Academic Health Centers,
  309
Association of American Medical Colleges
  (AAMC), 3 n.1, 7, 27-28, 38, 78-79,
  236, 238, 243, 244, 245, 261, 273
  n.1, 275, 304, 309, 321, 323, 324,
  327, 330-331, 336, 368, 369
Association of Canadian Medical Colleges,
  321, 324
Association of Hispanic-Serving Health
  Professions Schools, 282
Association of Specialized and Professional
  Accreditors, 130, 320
Atkinson, Richard C., 233, 256
Atlanta University Center, 163

B

Bakke, Allan, 239
Beason, Charlotte, 131
Binet, Alfred, 56
Bob Jones University, 181, 197
Brigham, Carl, 57
Bush, George H.W., 182

C

California
  admissions policies, 71, 84, 241, 256-
    257, 261, 327
  community benefit standard applied to
    nonprofit health care organizations,
    183, 185, 187, 188, 189, 193
  diversity in health professions, 30, 31,
    244
  financial aid programs, 294, 296
  minority access to care, 26, 30, 234
  minority population, 23, 235
  Office of Statewide Health Planning and
    Development, 113, 187
  Proposition 209 (Civil Rights Initiative),
    4, 24, 240, 256-257
California Endowment, 11, 112-113, 252,
  283, 309
California HealthCare Foundation, 309
California Wellness Foundation, 11, 112,
  113-114
Canadian Medical Association, Council on
  Medical Education, 321
Carnegie Foundation, 321
Case Western Reserve Medical School, 368
Catholic Health Association of the United
  States, 190
Cecil G. Sheps Center for Health Services
  Research, 286
Center for California Health Workforce
  Studies, 283
Center for Medicare and Medicaid Services,
  114, 291, 298, 302, 305, 307-308,
  311
Centers for Disease Control and Prevention,
  305
Centers of Excellence (COP) program, 108-
  109, 110, 276-277, 284, 300
Centers of Research Excellence in Science
  and Technology, 282-283, 293
Children's Hospitals Graduate Medical
  Education Program, 278-279, 286-
  287
Civil Rights Act of 1964, 327
Civil Rights movement, 243
Clark-Atlanta University, 163
Clinical research
  benefits of diversity, 237
  minority enrollment in, 35-36
Clinical Training grants, 280-281

E

data and research needs, 18, 205-206
defined, 25
education of stakeholders, 18, 206-208
leadership needs, 256-257
rationale for examining, 23-24, 26-27
recommendations, 18, 20, 210, 256-257
state referenda, 4, 24
supportive mechanisms, 205-210
Institutional climate for diversity
and academic performance, 68-70, 147, 161, 170
accreditation and, 330-331, 370
admissions policies and, 83, 145, 146, 160-161, 169-171, 173-174, 249, 251, 256-257, 326, 345, 348
affiliations with community health care facilities, 14, 15, 163, 170-171, 173-174, 175
attitudes and, 145, 146, 148, 157, 350, 354, 373
behavioral, 13, 146, 172, 349, 351-352
campus-related initiatives, 13, 145, 148, 171-172
and clinical practice, 381-382
compositional diversity and, 143, 146-147, 148, 348-349, 350, 353-354, 363, 379-380, 381-382
cross-cultural curriculum, 34-35, 165-169, 174
cross-racial interactions, 13, 351-352, 353
cultural audit of, 153, 154
curricular and cocurricular activities, 34-35, 155-156, 165-169, 174
defining, 13, 144-147, 171, 347-354
and democracy outcomes, 147, 148, 172
in dentistry, 169-171
design principles for improving, 13-14, 152-156, 172-173
external influences, 145-146, 348
faculty recruitment, hiring, and retention strategies and, 14, 15, 143, 145, 157-160, 161, 171, 173, 174, 361-362
financial aid policies and, 102, 146, 161, 164, 171, 348
holistic approach to change, 13-14, 144, 152, 172-173, 346-347
leadership and, 144, 152, 153, 156-157, 204, 350
and learning outcomes, 6, 34-35, 147-152, 158, 172, 262-263, 354-363, 368-369, 370-371, 374-375, 378-379

long-term perspective, 144
mediation mechanisms, 15, 165, 175
in medical education, 366-382
mission statement and, 14, 159, 173, 174, 346
monitoring and evaluation of intervention strategies, 13-14, 144, 152, 153, 167, 171, 175, 370-371
organizational impediments, 364-366
orientation for students, 14, 164, 174
pedagogy and, 143, 145, 155, 158, 164, 171, 352, 359-361, 367-368, 371-376
peer group influences, 351, 352, 355, 360, 363
psychological, 13, 145, 146, 172, 348, 349, 350-351
recommendations, 2, 15, 19, 174-175
resource allocation and, 144, 152
segregation and, 13, 145, 146, 151-152, 155, 156, 172, 237-242, 348-349, 351
sensitivity training of staff, 14-15, 156
student development, 155-156, 377-379
student recruitment, 14, 83, 143, 145, 160-161, 162-163, 169-171, 173-174, 249, 262
student retention, 14-15, 161-165, 169-171, 173-174
support services and programming, 14, 156, 164-165, 170, 174
Institutional culture, 146, 347-348
Institutional isomorphism, 365
International medical graduates, 302
Intervention strategies. *See also* Affirmative action; Institutional and policy-level strategies
academic advising, 243-244, 264
in admissions policies and practices, 2, 75-83, 254-264
community-based learning experiences, 119-120
data collection and analysis, 305-306
early matriculation programs, 262-263
financial aid, 11, 95, 119-123, 294-299, 308-310, 311
institutional climate improvements, 13-14, 144, 152-171, 175, 370-371
monitoring and evaluation of, 13-14, 144, 152, 153, 167, 171, 175, 370-371

Y

Z